Integrated Clinical and Fiscal Management in Mental Health: A Guidebook

Developments in Clinical Psychology

Series Editor

Glenn R. Caddy
Nova University

MMPI-168 Codebook, by Ken R. Vincent, Iliana Castillo, Robert I. Hauser, H. James Stuart, Javier A. Zapata, Cal K. Cohn, and Gregory O'Shanick, 1984

Integrated Clinical and Fiscal Management in Mental Health: A Guidebook, by Fred Newman and James Sorensen, 1985

In Preparation:

Advances in the Treatment of Addictive Behaviors, edited by Ted D. Nirenberg

The Behavioral Management of the Cardiac Patient, by D. G. Byrne

Clinical Applications of Hypnosis, edited by Frank A. DePiano and Herman C. Salzberg, 1986

Language and Psychopathology, by Stephen Schwartz

The Professional Practice of Psychology, edited by Georgiana Shick Tryon, 1986

Integrated Clinical and Fiscal Management in Mental Health: *A Guidebook*

Frederick L. Newman
Northwestern University

James E. Sorensen
University of Denver

ABLEX PUBLISHING CORPORATION
NORWOOD, NEW JERSEY

Printed in the United States of America.

Library of Congress Cataloging in Publication Data

Newman, Frederick L.
Integrated clinical and fiscal management in mental health.

(Developments in clinical psychology)
Includes bibliographies and index.
1. Mental health services—Management. 2. Mental health services—Finance. 3. Mental health services—Medical records. I. Sorensen, James E. II. Title.
[DNLM: 1. Financial Management. 2. Mental Health Services—organization & administration. WM 30 N5695i]
RA790.5.N484 1985 362.2′068 85–6219
ISBN 0–89391–233–6

Ablex Publishing Corporation
355 Chestnut Street
Norwood, New Jersey 07648

CONTENTS

SECTION VII MANAGEMENT SUPPORT—PART II: DATA ANALYSIS FOR MANAGEMENT USE

SECTION VIII DESIGNING AND IMPLEMENTING A MANAGEMENT INFORMATION SYSTEM (MIS)

A Historical Perspective and Acknowledgments

We are the scribes and borrowers of the insights and labors of more than 60 colleagues who have made significant contributions to the *Guidebook* during the 10 years of its development and publication. These colleagues have been described as risk-taking professionals who dared to develop techniques and procedures which had not been successfully attempted before and which fit within the framework of one guiding principle: A procedure would only be judged as acceptable if it could be empirically demonstrated to help clients to function in the community. We describe the contributions of these colleagues here in a historical manner to give the reader a flavor of how the client-oriented system of integrating clinical and fiscal management was developed with the help of these colleages.

The contributions of four colleagues were vital to the early formulation of integrating clinical and fiscal management procedures which focused on the client. Two people, Stanley Nelson (administrator of Lancaster County MH/MR D/A Programs, Pennsylvania) and David Duncan (Associate Commissioner of Pennsylvania MH programs 1972–1976), provided the direction of a client-oriented system: Dollars and services must follow the needs and service goals of the client! It was under the guidance of these two visionaries that one of the authors (FLN) began to test and develop procedures which would abide by this concept.

The concept would have remained a theory without the hard work, creativity, and support of William Underhill and Barbara Burwell. These two colleagues have worked with the technical development of the system since the beginning and have contributed to this book in more ways than we can accurately count. Bill Underhill was the first (currently with Somerset State Hospital in Pennsylvania). Bill was the inventor of the cost outcome matrix (see Chapters 21–24) around which many of the quantitative analysis procedures have been developed. The cost outcome matrix technique allowed us to describe the combined impact of clinical services on client outcome and resource consumption for clients. The second author (JES) became aware of how Underhill and Newman had "borrowed" Sorensen's cost finding procedures to develop the technique of cost outcome analysis, when Bill presented data from the Reading Hospital MH Center to a Regional NIMH meeting on evaluation research in 1973. Sorensen and Newman began discussing the possibility of a joint developmental effort at that time. But we were both aware that several key components were still missing, particularly issues surrounding treatment planning and quality assurance.

Barbara Burwell, then at the Fayette County (Pennsylvania) MH/MR Center and now at the Ravenswood CMHC in Chicago, worked with us on refining a systematic procedure for defining, documenting, and describing treatment planning and quality assurance procedures which others could understand and use in their own mental health service programs. Barbara's creative contributions became an integral part of many of the technical procedures described in this text. Most notable are the procedures for describing and documenting the clinical process (Section II) and the method for documenting the relationships and connections among clinical, fiscal, and administrative information needs (Chapter 25 on "Information System Linkages" and Chapter 29 on "Developing a Procedure Manual").

While we thought that our procedures were quite original and creative, we soon discovered we were simply filling in the pieces of an outline of a visionary who in 1968 had recognized that such a system was needed; Cecil Wurster of the NIMH Division of Biometry and Epidemiology upon learning of our efforts in 1974 began guiding its development and dissemination. First, he arranged for NIMH to publish the manual on client-oriented systems (written with Dale Carter for the Pennsylvania Office of Mental Health). Second, he arranged for both authors to teach NIMH-sponsored courses (FLN on ''Client-Oriented Systems'' and JES on ''Financial Management''). Barbara Burwell worked with FLN on his course and Glyn Hanbery worked with JES on the fiscal management course. Cecil Wurster recruited Dr. Walter Leginsky and assigned him to work with us on the coordination of these courses with NIMH and State Offices of mental health. With Walt's guidance these two courses, under various formats, eventually trained personnel from every state mental health program office and from more than 80% of the community mental health and state hospital programs in the country. The Financial Management course, with the aid of Saul Feldman and Isabell Davidoff, became a mainstay in the NIMH Staff College.

One of the techniques for dissemination was also vital to the development of the procedures present in the Guidebook. We were contracted by NIMH (Biometry and Epidemology and the Staff College) and by The Applied Statistics Training Institute of The National Center for Health Statistics to involve co-trainers in the course on ''Client-Oriented Systems'' who could then become trainers on their own. Later this became the theme of an NIMH training grant, ''Training Technical Assistance Trainers.'' Taylor Anderson, Sandra Forquer, and Patricia Moore (Medical College of Pennsylvania) worked with FLN on this project. Forquer and Anderson made two critically important contributions which have been incorporated into the *Guidebook*. First, they developed techniques for implementing treatment planning and quality assurance procedures within clinical settings. As one can readily imagine, introducing quality assurance and fiscal management procedures into clinical settings is not always well received. We were also assisted by Tuan Nguyen (San Francisco County MH Program), William Dossett (Austin, Texas), David Glen (Meadville, Pennsylvania), and Bill Underhill. The results of the seminal work they had done in Pennsylvania and Georgia have been integrated into the *Guidebook*.

A key component of an integrated clinical and fiscal management system concerns the management use (or misuse) of data. Much of our practical understanding of this issue comes from a team of people, led by Paul Sherman, who have been actively studying this issue: Dwight Walker (Smokey Mt. CMHC), Gary Olsen (Salt Lake City MH Program), and Barbara Burwell. Their current work builds upon the earlier work of our colleagues Myles Cooper, Bob Minnehan, Edna Kamis, Tuan Nguyen, Bill Underhill, and Dan Hadley.

Glyn Hanbery deserves special mention, since his steady work with JES through the years has led to his thinking and efforts being woven into the fabric of the fiscal, financial management, and information systems sections of the *Guidebook*. Moreover, his good humor and teaching style have led to the further popular appeal of the fiscal issues to clinical program managers.

Pat Moore is actually the *Guidebook*'s mother. While FLN and JES claimed to have written or adapted the material into a readable form, Pat did the composing and editing through seven major revisions. Her original artwork, text design, and formatting brought the book into an integrated whole. After FLN moved to Chicago, Nancy Zabel picked up Pat's task and brought the *Guidebook* to its successful publication.

Finally, we would like to thank our spouses (Trink and Karin) and the Newman boys (Andy and Adam) for providing the personal support we needed over the last 10 years we devoted to this project.

Preface
Creating Client-Oriented Systems: A Guidebook for Design and Management

WHAT THE GUIDEBOOK CAN DO FOR YOU

Program directors and managers find themselves faced with tightening dollars and increased regulatory control, along with continuing client/consumer demands. Managing mental-health service programs under these pressures becomes very difficult and, at times, appears to be impossible. From the clients' and clinicians' perspective, one often worries that increased emphasis on cost containment, revenues, and meeting regulatory standards will obscure the needs of the client.

In light of these pressures, the *Guidebook* is designed to help managers and directors of service programs in three major ways:

(1) In the design and management of clinical services focusing on clients, service costs, and revenues.

(2) In the design and use of techniques for documenting and evaluating clinical efforts and client outcomes for:

Quality assurance review
Third-party payor justification
Program and budget planning
Policy review
Cost effectiveness analysis

(3) In complying with governmental and professional standards and regulations without losing sight of client needs.

THE *GUIDEBOOK'S* FOCUS ON THE CLIENT

A client-oriented system integrates clinical and fiscal management for efficient and effective impact on consumers. Clients are penalized if they are treated ineffectively. The more efficiently services are provided for any one consumer, the more consumers who can be served. The more effective the service is in achieving client goals, the less likely the consumer is to become an expensive burden in the future. Today's consumer can become a productive person in the community, especially if some degree of life management exists. Service programs

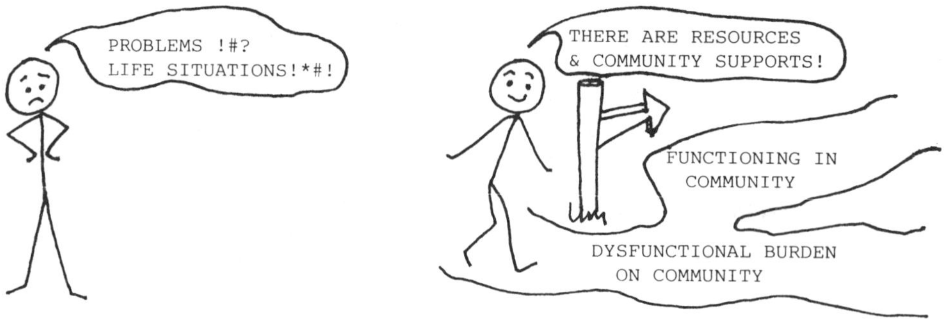
PROBLEMS !#?
LIFE SITUATIONS!*#!
THERE ARE RESOURCES
& COMMUNITY SUPPORTS!
FUNCTIONING IN
COMMUNITY
DYSFUNCTIONAL BURDEN
ON COMMUNITY

should use a minimum of resources, yet maximize the time clients spend as functioning, self respecting individuals in the community.

The *Guidebook* will show how to design an integrated clinical and fiscal management system to provide services for all needy citizens in a community. The link between clients' service needs and goals with program design and management procedures will be seen in four ways:

(1) *Clinical services are designed to achieve service goals.* Clinical procedures are developed for maximum use of available resources in achieving each client's service goals. The clinical review and supervisory procedures are tailored to specific program goals and clients' demands.
(2) *Program organizational components are designed to support service goals.* Each organizational component is developed in terms of how it supports client-related services. Lines of responsibility, authority, and coordination necessary to maintain a client-oriented program are identified.
(3) *Technical systems are designed to support the management of service goals.* The technical staff of the information systems unit, the fiscal unit, and the evaluation research unit are focused on supportive roles of the client-oriented management of clinical services.
(4) *Service costs and revenues are described in terms of client-service goals.* Service costs and revenues are related directly to client problems, goals, and outcomes. These procedures will, in turn, permit budgeting and planning services in terms of client problems and goals.

THE *GUIDEBOOK'S* FOCUS ON THE PROGRAM DIRECTOR

The program director is the keystone of a service program. Directors, however, appear to be under two opposing influences. The director must manage and lead all clinical and technical support activities to have an *economical* and effective *impact* on consumers. The director must ensure support of service goals while meeting all governmental and third-party payor regulations. The director must also balance clients' needs with available resources and revenues. The long-term survival and viability of a service program depends upon the director's ability to maintain a client-oriented program.

Others—technical staff, clinical supervisors, people in government and regulatory agencies—will benefit from the *Guidebook*. The major benefit is an understanding of how their respective roles support the client-oriented goals of a service program.

HOW OTHERS CAN BENEFIT

Technical Staff Development

The *Guidebook* provides special technical chapters for the staff of the information systems, fiscal, and evaluation research units. The technical chapters are designed to help specific technical support personnel understand their roles in supporting clinical efforts. Moreover, the technical chapters detail the procedures needed to fulfill the objectives of designing, maintaining and managing a client-oriented system.

Governmental and Regulatory Personnel

The *Guidebook* can help these persons to better understand how to develop standards and regulations. Techniques for planning and monitoring service programs in terms of client needs and outcomes will be described. The *Guidebook* can also be used by regulatory agencies as an outline and guide for local-service programs. The *Guidebook* can assist agencies in developing client-focused systems which are both manageable and accountable.

The Student in Professional-Training Programs

Students in mental health, health, and social-service fields can use the *Guidebook* to simulate the design of a service system for a course in program design and management. The *Guidebook* can also be used during the student's internship or field placement activities to identify service-system components.

CRITICAL CONCERNS ABOUT CLIENT-ORIENTED SYSTEMS

The activities of teaching and providing technical assistance on client-oriented systems have identified three major concerns many people have at the outset:

— How new or unique is a client-oriented system?
The basic concepts and procedures of a client-oriented system are not really new. The components of the system have been pieced together from elements which have been tried, tested, and proven worthwhile under a variety of circumstances. A number of the concepts will be familiar. The unique feature is the comprehensive system integrating both clinical and fiscal management techniques so that a program can focus simultaneously on client programs, goals, related service costs, clinical outcomes, and revenues.

— How flexible is the system?
Highly. No two existing client-oriented systems are structured in the same way. They are individually designed and developed. Their clinical procedures and records, their fiscal and organizational management structures, and their information systems are all uniquely tailored to the demands of clients and sociopolitical community situations.

— How expensive is the development and maintenance of the system?
Cost depends upon the current program structure. For example, if current effort and dollars are being expended on an information system, comprehensive quality assurance and utilization review, and program evaluation, then the procedures in this text will probably save effort and money. On the other hand, if none of these activities are operating, costs will increase by one to three staff people, depending upon the size of the program.

SECTION I
OVERVIEW AND SYSTEM DESIGN

Chapter 1
The Client-Oriented System

UNIQUE PROGRAMS AND UNIQUE SYSTEMS

While no two client-oriented service systems are exactly alike, an overall description of an operating client-oriented system may be helpful. Our purpose here is to illustrate:

— How client-oriented systems develop
— The client orientation of the program
— Staff involvement in system development
— The integration of clinical and fiscal data
— Sample reports and their use

Elements of the system presented represent a composite of several operating client-oriented systems. One of the greatest strengths of the client-oriented system is its versatility in a variety of organizations, including large and small hospital-based as well as free-standing centers in urban, suburban, and rural settings.

Our example represents a consensus of what has worked among those who have built client-oriented systems. As you review the example, try not to focus on its details; instead, try to grasp the conceptual framework of:

— Client orientation
— Active involvement of staff
— Staff self-management through job performance feedback to improve job performance

THE MAJOR SYSTEM COMPONENTS

The example describes how six major system components converge on the ongoing management of a mental-health program. The six major components are:

(A) *Program Design* relates program goals for consumers to services.
(B) *Clinical Process Design* describes the concerns and decisions of clients and staff during client entry, service planning and delivery, and termination from a service program.
(C) *Visible Evidence* records and supports dependable clinical communication.
(D) *Fiscal System* formulates cost-finding procedures to relate costs and clinical efforts.
(E) *Management Support* describes the supporting roles of staff in relationship to the therapeutic/service process.

(F) *Information Systems* provides the linkages among clients, staff, and managers in providing and managing service delivery.

Collectively the system produces two major products for program staff. First, staff will be able to raise questions and review data relating client characteristics, service efforts, and outcomes. Second, the system focuses on helping staff address and solve the problems which are appropriate to their role in the program.

Consider two actual incidents. In one program, the director believed the cost outcome data suggested program policies and budgets needed to be changed to achieve more favorable outcomes for black clients. When he submitted the data to the county authority for discussion and resolution, the data were somehow "leaked" to the press as an example of the director's poor management of the program. Here is how the director used the system to overcome this ordeal. As a defensive counterplay, he asked for an independent blue-ribbon, professional panel to perform a clinial and fiscal audit of the program including a review of clinical and fiscal records and client interviews. The director said, "If the audit proves me to be a poor manager, then fire me! But if the audit supports the argument that client outcomes are related to insufficient program policies and budgeting, then readjust these policies and budgets." Since the program had all six components in place and his management procedures assured their review and maintenance, the system stood up to a close audit. Three things occurred as a result of the audit. Policies were changed. So were budget allocations. And, the county authority director was fired (not the program director).

In a second case, an indecisive individual was hired as executive director of an agency using an operating client-oriented system. When the clinical director left, nine months passed before a replacement was selected; no one was assigned the clinical supervisor responsibilities of coordinating quality assurance. When poor cost outcome data started to surface, suggesting lack of clinical supervision and service coordination, the director suggested stopping reporting and analyzing the data. Nine months later he was fired.

These two examples underscore the need for all six components to be in place and periodically reviewed. Now, each component is highlighted in more detail.

PROGRAM DESIGN[1]

A program of services may define its purpose and goals in terms of impact on consumers. Two categories of consumers should be considered simultaneously: one is the dysfunctional individual, and the other is the community where these individuals reside. Once program goals are defined in terms of the potential impact on these two consumer groups, services become a means of achieving these goals.

There is a direct relationship between the behavior of individuals and the behavior of the communities where the individuals live. As an individual or group becomes less productive or independent, for whatever reason, the community acquires or exerts greater responsibility, expense, or control. For many of the programs that have developed a client-oriented system, the principal goal has been "To assist clients to attain the highest level of psychosocial functioning possible in their ordinary community setting." More specifically, a person's or group's level of functioning is defined as existing productively and independently in their ordinary community

---

[1] Adapted from Carter & Newman (1976).

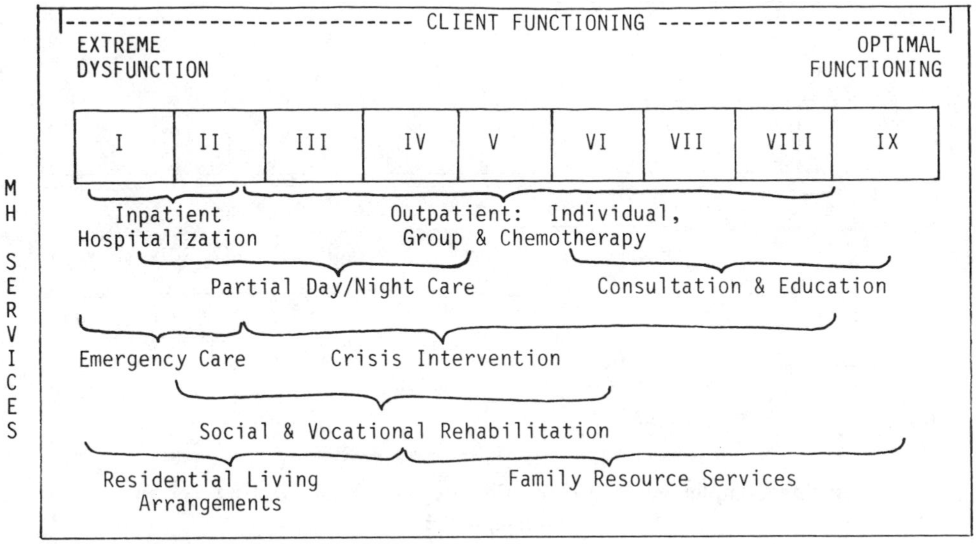

Figure 1. Designing an Array of Mental Health Services (Adapted from Nelson, Newman, & Hinkle, 1975)

setting. The goals of community service activities can be described by their impact on the level of functioning of an individual or group. Specifically:

Treatment is an activity to raise a person's or group's overall level of functioning by impacting on one or more facets of behavior or life situation.
Intervention is an activity to retard or stop a person's or group's continued movement toward lower levels of functioning.
Prevention is an activity to increase resiliency to stress, to decrease vulnerability to stress, or to decrease the potential for stress factors contributing to a person or group becoming less functional.

To describe clients' ability to function in their community, many programs use a global level of functioning scale.[2] Once a scale is adopted, programs can describe the relationships of their services to other community services by reference to the potential impact on client/consumer level of functioning. In our illustrative mental-health organization, client functioning is expected to vary over nine different levels, ranging from extreme dysfunctioning to optimal functioning. In Figure 1, each of ten separate services is mapped on the scale identifying the levels of client functioning the services address. Inpatient services, for example, are for clients in levels one or two, while outpatient services address levels three to eight. Besides describing one's own services, complementary community services can be described by the same scale. Figure 2 describes one approach to analyzing eight services related to mental-health services.

Consider the utility of Figures 1 and 2. Consultation and education staff, for example, would have a clearer view of their activities as they relate to their own services as well as those

[2] Development of a reliable and valid scale is detailed later in the text.

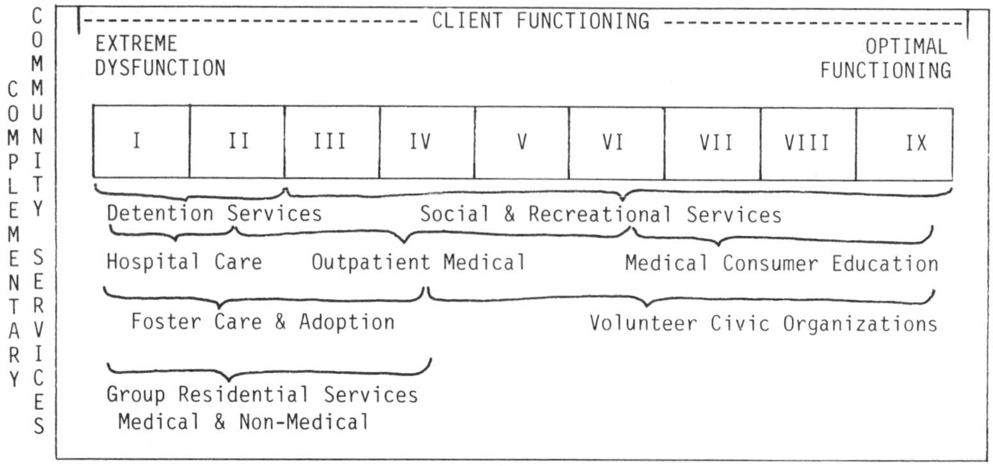

Figure 2. Analyzing Complementary Community Services (Adapted from Nelson, Newman, & Hinkle, 1975)

offered by complementary agencies. Knowledge of the levels covered by a service identifies the point at which admission and discharge should occur. Identifying the levels of functioning for admission or discharge for a service should aid in the development of criteria for admission and discharge.

Clients, however, should not be forced into service niches. Clinical staff, for example, should label client behaviors based on actual functioning behaviors of the client. There is a natural temptation to label client behavior based on the service received or planned. This issue will be discussed more completely in the units on Clinical Process Design and Management Support.

Next, we need to consider how client related data flow into and through the system.

THE CLINICAL PROCESS DESIGN AND RELATED VISIBLE EVIDENCE

How clients enter, utilize, and leave a program ought to be consistent with program goals and client goals. In a client-oriented system, the design of the clinical process is addressed by a series of questions describing the therapeutic process.

(1) *Entry*
Who is the client? Is the client at the right place?

(2) *Service-Planning*
What are the issues? What events are to happen?

(3) *Review*
Are the events occurring as planned? What changes are needed?

(4) *Termination and Followup*
Were goals met? Is followup required?

From this basic outline of clinical process, the details of the process and visible evidence in the clinical records are tailored specifically to suit local programs' unique combinations of clients and circumstances.

A more detailed outline used to develop a clinical-process design is given in Table 1. It identifies specific *concerns, who* is involved, and what *decisions* have to be made as the client moves through the therapeutic process. But even with this level of detail, a local program would still need to tailor the specific concerns and decisions to the client problems served, the socioeconomic circumstances of its service area, and its available services.

Even clinical records must be tailored to suit the unique characteristics of the clients and the services involved in the therapeutic process. The details for tailoring records to local circumstances and guidelines for developing these documents are provided in Sections II and III. The crucial feature is to develop records so they reflect the clinical process and support the communication required to fulfill therapeutic goals. Table 2 extends Table 1 by adding examples of documents providing visible evidence of the clinical process.

One common feature of all client-oriented systems is an explicit design for the clinical process with related clinical records to support the process. Once they had developed their process design and records, they found it easy to perform the minor adjustments needed to meet the standards of the National Institute of Mental Health (NIMH), the Professional Standards Review Organization (PSRO), and the Joint Commission for the Accreditation of Hospitals (JCAH). The *key* was first to develop the records to suit the process, and then to adjust to meet standards and regulations. Too often, programs create records to meet external standards and the data in the records do not always reflect the actual clinical process. The clinical data are often

Table 1. A General Outline for Designing Clinical Process, Identifying Procedures and Standards

	Characteristics at Each Stage		
Stage of Process	Concerns?	Who?	Decisions?
ENTRY Who is the client? Is the client at the right place?	Age, Family, Address? Major problems and supports?	Client/Family Receptionist Intake Worker (Crisis team on call)	Appropriate client here? Immediate action? Refer elsewhere? Regular intake?
SERVICE PLANNING What are the issues? What events are to happen?	Problems and supports? Goals? Expense? Potential income?	Client/Family Therapist/Case Manager Supervisor or Treatment Team Fiscal/Billing	Problems to be treated? Activities which may produce goals? Services providing the activities? Review strategy of what, why, who, and when?
REVIEW Are events occuring as planned? Are changes needed?	Problems and supports? Efforts, progress, and goals? Expense and income?	Client/Family Therapist/Case Manager Supervisor or Treatment Team Fiscal/Billing	Are changes in service plan needed? If so, what change? Have standards been met?
TERMINATION AND FOLLOWUP Were goals met? Is followup required?	Problems and supports? Efforts, progress, and goals? Expense and income? Client/consumer satisfaction?	Client/Family Therapist/Case Manager Supervisor or Treatment Team Fiscal/Billing	Is referral needed? Is followup needed? —Clinically? —Fiscally/bills? If so, when and how?

Table 2. Adding Visible Evidence (or Documents) to the Clinical Process

Stage of Process	Characteristics of Each Stage			Documents (Examples)
	Concerns	Who	Decisions	
ENTRY Who is the client? Is the client at the right place?				Face/History Sheet Legal/Fiscal Documents
PLANNING What are the issues? What events are to happen?				Problem/Goals List Intervention Plan Review Strategy
REVIEW Are events occurring as planned? Are changes needed?				Progress Notes Review Documents
TERMINATION Were goals met? Is follow-up required?				Discharge Summary Follow-up Documents

neither useful for the communication involved in the therapeutic process, nor for ongoing program management.

Clinical Data Dependability

The clinical and fiscal data in a client-oriented system tend to be more reliable under three conditions:

(1) *Frequent use of the data in clinical communication.* The data are an integral part of the communication among clients, direct service staff, their supervisors, and/or treatment team staff in the therapeutic process.
(2) *Use of the data in self-management.* Summaries of the data are fed back to staff at all levels to be used in their self-management in the program.
(3) *Staff development.* Training sessions are offered two to three times in a year to help staff identify factors influencing differences in clinical judgments and decisions. Staff may, for example, rate and discuss their judgments on a common set of case histories. The ratings may become the basis for estimating data reliability and validity.

When all three features are operating, several studies have shown clinical data to be reliable (Newman & Carter, 1975; Newman & Rinkus, 1978).

THE FISCAL SYSTEM

A major objective of the fiscal system is to provide estimates of the costs of each unit of service which in turn provide the basis for:

(1) *Estimating episode costs* of service effort for each client for ongoing management, e.g., utilization review and cost outcome analysis.

(2) *Setting rates and fees to be charged and billed.*
(3) *Planning resource allocation* (budgeting) to match the goals of programs and services.

Tracing costs to services can be done in many ways. Detailed examples of the various methods and their results are provided in the How-to Sections. One approach, illustrated in Figure 3, is a cost-per-hour of service in alcohol counseling services. Basically, the costs consist of:

Caseworker's salary plus fringe
Overhead including nonreimbursable activities, unaccounted-for time, paid vacation, and sick days
Support staff and administration
Other direct operating expenses of the service

Staff, administration, and the board can better see the elements of cost in providing a unit of service to alcoholism clients. Rates and charges can be evaluated. Planned versus actual use of resources can be evaluated. However, questions about how effective the service was must await data on client outcomes.

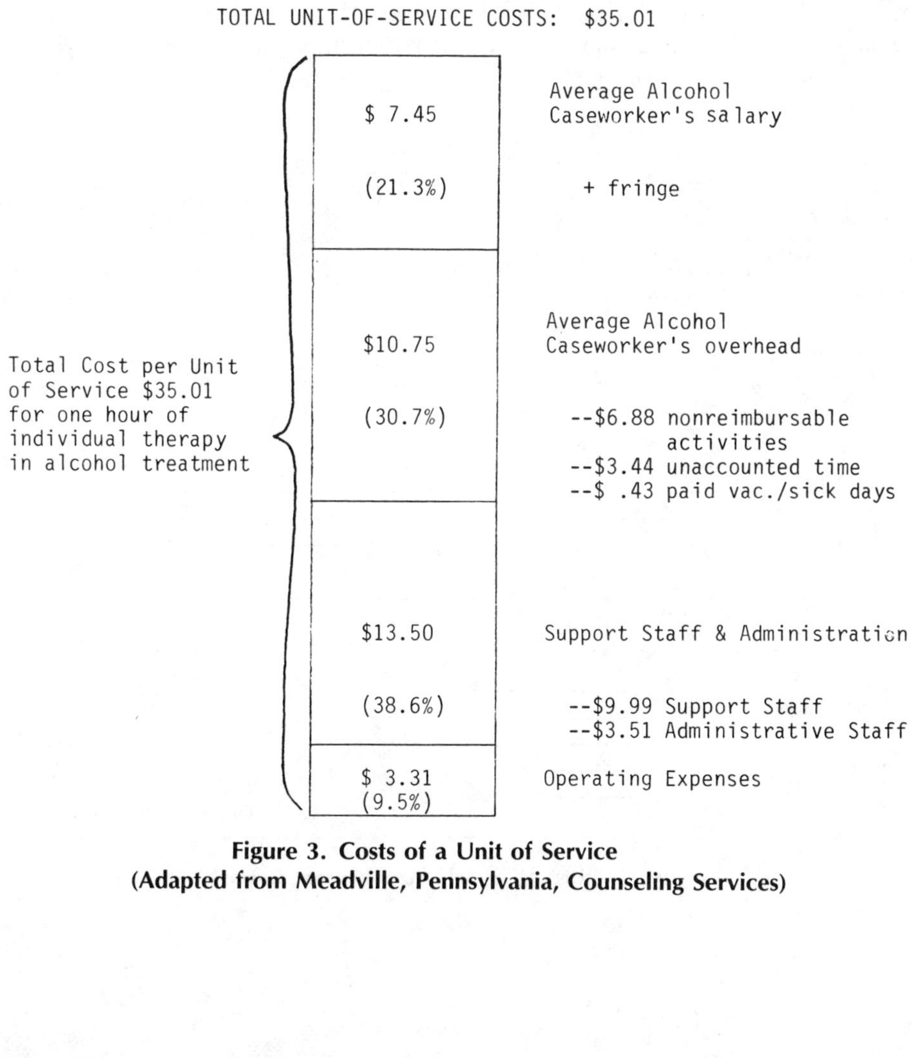

Figure 3. Costs of a Unit of Service
(Adapted from Meadville, Pennsylvania, Counseling Services)

VISIBLE EVIDENCE, INFORMATION SYSTEM, AND MANAGEMENT SUPPORT

A key feature of a client-oriented system is the smooth and reliable flow of the data needed for clinical communication, management support, and fiscal analysis. Above all, staff who supply the data must feel the data are useful in their own self-management. Reliability and submission times improve when staff feel the data will be fed back to them in a timely and useful way for their own self-management and for the ongoing management of the program. In many client-oriented systems, the principal feature linking the clinical, fiscal, and management systems is an Activity Analysis submitted by service staff. (Other flows of activity information are discussed in the units on Information Systems.)

The Activity Analysis and Self-Management

Staff can use Activity Analysis to summarize clinically relevant activities. Staff are not necessarily required to record 100% of their time. Staff cooperation and data reliability on the Activity Analysis can be achieved in two ways. First, the analysis passes through clinical records for edit checks before going to the fiscal department. Feedback to staff from clinical records and the fiscal department on what was recorded properly and the fiscal justification ("We cannot justify the billing for . . .") tends to confront staff with the responsibility for their own behavior. Second, the staff are provided monthly summaries of their activities. Figure 4 is an example of a Staff Activity Summary. Note that the staff have an opportunity to contrast their efforts with those of others in the same classification. Self-management is an underlying theme.

YOUR ACTIVITIES FOR ____________________
(Month/Year)

STAFF # ________________

Activities	Your Hours	Others in Your Classification	Total Clinic	Costs per Hour
Direct				
Indiv. Therapy	______	______	______	______
Group Therapy	______	______	______	______
↓				
Indirect-Client	______	______	______	______
Phone with Cl.	______	______	______	______
Corresp.	______	______	______	______
Recordkeeping	______	______	______	______
↓				
C & E	______	______	______	______

SUMMARY OF YOUR:	Hours	Costs		
Direct (chargeable)	______	______	Scheduled Hours	______
Client Related (nonchargeable)	______		Cancelled	______
C & E	______		Your cost per hour	______
Unaccounted Time	______			
Contracted Hours	______			

(Developed by Barbara Burwell)

Figure 4. Illustrative Self-Management Report

CLIENT TARGET GROUP

Functional Level	No Prior History		Prior History	
	Youth	Adult	Youth	Adult
1–2				
3–4				
5–6				
7–8				

(Adapted from Delaware County MH/MR)

Figure 5. Example of Individual Staff Member Monthly Caseload Report

When these reports are prepared initially, they should be kept confidential and reviewed only by the staff person and his or her immediate supervisor. Over time, each staff person will tend to work out with the supervisor a mutually satisfactory pattern of service activities. Two overriding considerations are client caseload and budget constraints. To understand the nature of an individual clinician's caseload, a monthly report can be generated for each staff person. Figure 5 provides an example of an individual staff member's monthly caseload report.

While the budget constraints are more in the realm of the supervisor, staff have input by reviewing and modifying their own activities to maximize clinical and fiscal impact. Moreover, if staff activities are documented properly, management has a stronger argument for justifying the clinical activities. A few gratifying experiences with success by management feedback to staff does wonders for staff morale and future cooperation.

With feedback and active staff involvement, staff will document 85% to 95% of their contracted time. And, if compensation for overtime is offered, then better than 100% recording is often the case.

Client Event File

Once the Staff Activity Analysis has passed through the clinical records check for accuracy and clinical justification, the data can be used for billing, statistical cost and outcome analysis, and statistical program analysis. The Client Event File (e.g., a 5″ × 8″ card in a manual system; full-page sheets in a McBee system; an event file in a computer system) has the most relevant demographic, diagnostic, and financial liability information on the top. These data are followed by a chronological listing of all relevant service information, both chargeable and nonchargeable. Minimal service information recorded on the ledger card in a manual system is illustrated in Figure 6.

The first five column entries come directly from the Staff Activity Analysis. Entries in the "Cost" column could be of two types: costs by type of service and time, or costs by staff category (Psychiatrist, Psychologist, Social Worker, etc.) and time. Costs are entered for each chargeable service event. The "Charge" information also comes from a table listing the charges permitted each service activity for each category of client financial liablity.

Practical uses of the Client Event File are plentiful. Major questions can be addressed (even if the system is manual):

CLIENT ID
DEMOGRAPHIC DATA
FINANCIAL LIABILITY

DIAGNOSTIC & SERVICE GOALS, e.g.
Sustenance or Growth Plans

Date	Level of Functioning	Service Rendered	By Whom	Time	Cost	Charge	Pay ments	Balances: Charges-Payments	Balances: Costs-Charges
2/9/79	4	313	440	1:30	$ 90	$ 60	$ 60	$0.00	-30.00
⋮	⋮	⋮	⋮	⋮	⋮	⋮	⋮	⋮	⋮
6/3/79	7	317	221	1:00	40	40	40	0.00	0.00
			TOTALS =		$550	$400	$400	$0.00	$150.00

(Adapted from William Underhill)

Figure 6. Example of a Client Event File

FISCAL SOLVENCY

Potential balances provide a basis for discussion with program funding agencies and third-party payors. (The numbers are from the example.)

— (Charge − Paid) = Amount to be collected ($0.00)
— (Costs − Charges) = Net costs beyond or over charges ($150)
— (Costs − Paid) = Net costs relative to amount paid ($150)

UTILIZATION REVIEW

Cost outcome analysis for the individual client.

— By episode, sum costs over episode and list entry and termination level of functioning (Entry Level 4, Termination at 7, costs $550)
— Over course of episode or for any time period during the course of service

PROGRAM ANALYSIS

Cost outcome analysis for groups of clients or services.

— Utilization and review
— Client care evaluation studies

Management Functions and the Use of Data

The most impressive aspect of a client-oriented system is the clear statement of who uses what data and for what purposes. In order to specify these uses, job descriptions must identify staff responsibilities in client-oriented terms. Specifically, the position is described by questions and issues addressed by the position. ''What questions and issues do you address in support of those who perform the therapeutic process?''

Once responsibilities are identified for all levels of organization, then coordination and authority can be identified:

Lines of Coordination—With whom do you need to coordinate activities in order to address the questions or issues, to make decisions, and to take action?

Lines of Authority—Who sanctions and monitors whom and by what performance criteria? Moreover, will the performance criteria reflect the role responsibilities which support the therapeutic processes?

The organization structure will be clarified from the clients' viewpoint. Rather than examine examples of organization charts, management functions in a client-oriented system may be more easily understood by reviewing how data are used to address questions and issues. Figure 7 presents an example of the managerial uses of data in four parts:

(1) *Question* or *issue* to be addressed.
(2) *Data* summary used to address the question or issue.
(3) *Utility* by staff and management.
(4) *Cautions* pointing out the limitations of data use or possible followup issues that might be addressed.

Management's focus is on the three key elements of a "client-oriented question," i.e., client characteristics, service efforts, with client outcomes. If the question or issue does not include all three elements, a note of caution is inserted to alert the user to a limitation.

Figure 7 provides the greatest detail of management's use of data. Read it through carefully from top to bottom. Note your questions in the margins. As you go through the remainder of the book, check back to see how many of your questions were addressed in detail elsewhere in the book. Hopefully, you will find that all of your questions have been answered satisfactorily.

1) ISSUE: What were the relative cost outcome episode results for the outpatient program when comparing clients with prior or no prior hospitalization history?
2) DATA: For a 5-month period, each cell provides % of group in row, number, and average costs.

Prior Hospit. History	CLIENTS STARTED DYSFUNCTIONAL				CLIENTS STARTED FUNCTIONAL			
			IMPROVED		REGRESSED			
	Regressed	Maintained	Still Dysf.	To Funct.	To Dysf.	Still Funct.	Maintained	Improved
YES N = 20		5% 1 $1365.90	10% 2 $374.11	5% 1 $422.79	5% 1 $ 965.46	10% 2 $755.86	35% 7 $1238.76	30% 6 $694.13
NO N = 57		5.3% 3 $ 327.38			5.3% 3 $1027.59	12.3% 7 $474.62	42.1% 24 $ 537.54	35% 20 $661.09

(From: Paul Sherman, Ravenswood Hospital, CMHC, Chicago)

3) UTILITY: a) *For Clinicians:* How do my results compare with the whole outpatient program?
b) *For the Utilization Review Committee:* Were there differences in resource utilization and outcome for these two groups?
c) *For Quality Assurance and Supervision:* What followup activities took place for discontinued clients who regressed to the dysfunctional level or who were maintained at the dysfunctional level?
d) *For Service-Program Managers:* What changes in available resources might improve the cost-outcome picture?
e) *For Policy Levels:* Could policy changes affect differences in resource allocation and outcomes?

4) CAUTIONS: —Are these data supported by what is in the clinical records? (Check by inspecting a random sample.)
—Are these results consistent with other past time periods? (Check by performing a retrospective study.)
—Would these results also be true in the future? (Check by running a prospective study.)

Figure 7. Client Oriented Question-Data-Utility-Caution

IN SUMMARY

Six major components of the Client-Oriented Cost-Outcome System have been described:

(A) *Program Design.* Relates program goals for consumers to services.
(B) *Clinical Process Design.* Describes the concerns and decisions of clients and staff during client entry, service planning and delivery, and termination from a service program.
(C) *Visible Evidence.* Records and supports clinical communication; creating such evidence should include procedures to help staff develop dependable clinical data.
(D) *Fiscal System.* Formulates cost-finding procedures to relate costs and clinical efforts.
(E) *Management Support.* Describes the supporting roles of staff in relationship to the therapeutic/service process.
(F) *Information Systems.* Provides the links among clients, staff, and managers in providing and managing service delivery.

Two major products can be expected:

(1) Staff will be able to raise questions and review data relating
- — Client characteristics,
- — Service efforts, with
- — Client outcomes;

(2) Data will be available for tne ongoıng ıssues tacıng program management.

Chapter 2
Program Design

What Are Your Program Goals?
How Do Services Relate to These Goals?
How Do the Program Services Relate to and Complement Other Available Community Services?

The first major step in the development of a client-oriented system is to produce a clear statement of who are the consumers of your services, what your program can do for them, and how your services are designed to achieve these goals. Chapter 2 has six major components:

(1) *Identifying Client-oriented Program Goals and Services:* An introductory discussion and example are provided to describe how a program's goals and services can be directly linked to patterns of client behaviors, specifically, the clients' problems, strengths, and community circumstances.

(2) *Relating Program Goals to Service Design and Coordination:* An outline and examples are provided for you to design (or redesign) your own services in terms of client-oriented goals.

(3) *Identifying Potential Concerns:* The procedures outlined have advantages and disadvantages within different social, economic, and political settings. A self-study exercise is provided to help specify the potential products and pitfalls of the proposed procedures for your situation. The purpose is to identify these potential products as positive objectives and criteria for implementing a customized client-oriented system. The pitfalls represent a potential guide for system implementation by avoiding the pitfalls, dealing positively with them, or stopping the implementation.

(4) *Assuring Dependable and Useful Measures of Client Behaviors and Service Goals:* What is needed to assure that you have dependable (reliable) and useful (valid) measures of program performance? A brief overview identifies the operating components of clinical service management needed to assure clinical data are dependable and useful.

(5) *Relating Internal Program Management Measures to External Reporting and Monitoring:* A client-oriented system develops measures of program performance uniquely suitable to your clients, community, and service efforts *and* still permits reporting to external regulatory and funding agencies. An outline is provided on how to design a system of services suited to unique circumstances.

(6) *Appendix: Examples of Global and Multifactored Scales*

1. IDENTIFYING CLIENT-ORIENTED PROGRAM GOALS AND SERVICES

A client-oriented system draws clear lines connecting program goals for client-consumers with service design, process, and management activities. Moreover, the program can be uniquely tailored to a specific community's circumstances. This introductory chapter draws the connecting themes between your program's goals and service design. Subsequent chapters will describe the connections of goals with the clinical process and with management.

Connecting clients with services flows in two directions. One is establishing the overall purpose and goals of your program and the other is the design and coordination of the clinical process. Four major clinical process design issues are identified below and will be addressed in Chapter 3.

Issues	Stage of Process
1. Who is the client? Is the client at the right place?	1. ENTRY
2. What are the issues? What events are to happen?	2. SERVICE PLANNING
3. Are events occurring as planned? What changes are needed?	3. REVIEW
4. Were goals met? Is followup required?	4. TERMINATION AND FOLLOWUP

Now consider an example of a program goal. Many mental-health programs with client-oriented systems have adopted a goal for adult citizens in their community similar to the following:

> To provide services for the purpose of helping citizens attain the highest level of psychosocial functioning in their ordinary community setting.

These programs use the goal statement to serve as a basis for defining a level of functioning scale and for describing the intended impact of their program of services and clinical processes on client functioning. The diagrams in Figures 1 and 2 show how one Pennsylvania program envisioned its services.

In the upper half of Figure 1 is the basis for a program's definition of psychosocial functioning. The lower half of Figure 1 identifies the three major categories of service activities related to the activity's goals. Psychosocial functioning is based on the behavior patterns of both an individual (client/consumer) and the community in which the individual resides. In viewing the behavior patterns of an individual, psychosocial functioning is the degree a person is operating independently, productively, and at a satisfactory level of personal well-being. Personal well-being can be described in terms of levels of health and emotional distress. For the community in which the individual resides, the individual's psychosocial functioning is the degree of community responsibility, expense, and control exerted on behalf of the individual. Thus, as the individual operates at a decreased level of functioning (i.e., decreased independence, productivity, and personal well-being), the community tends to increase its level of responsibility, expense, or control. Two examples would be extensive alcohol abuse, or a broken family with teenage children who are disruptive in school and community.

Service activities can be described by their goals for client/community level of functioning.

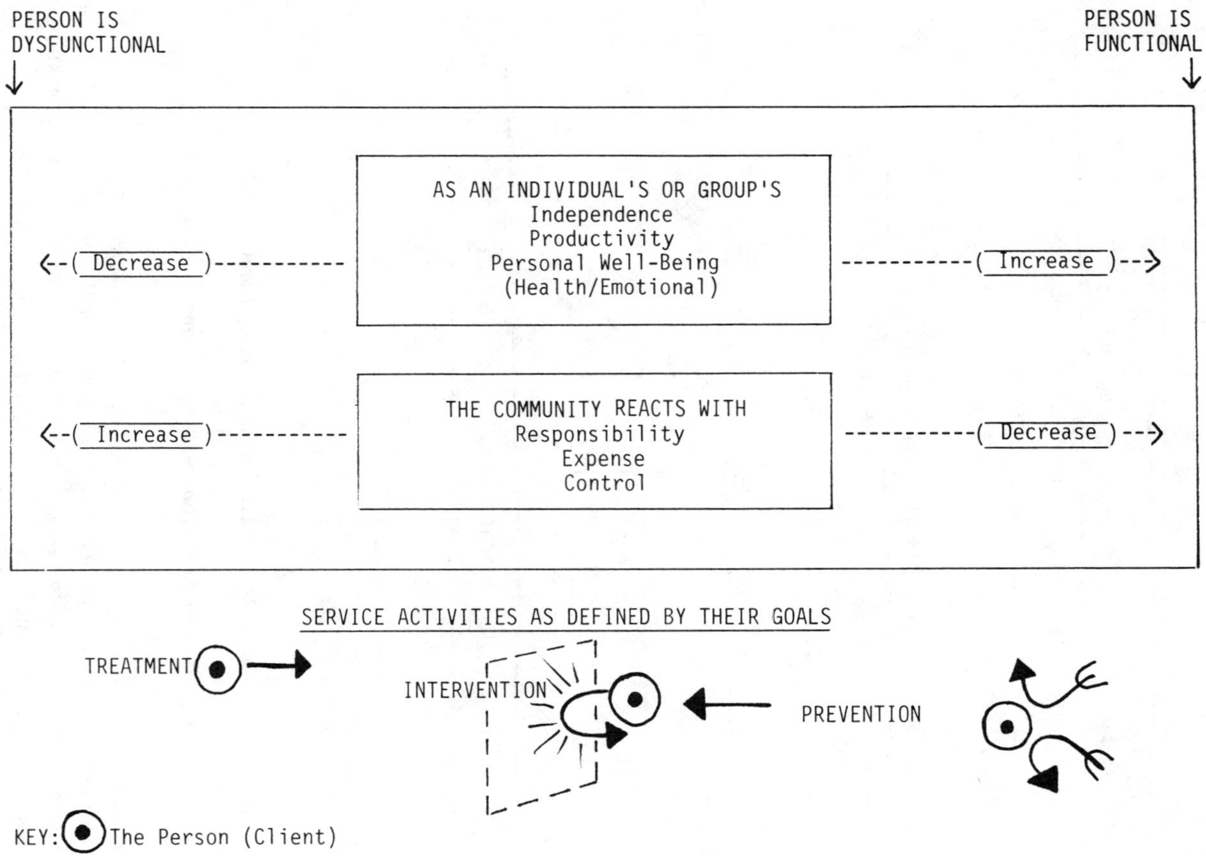

Figure 1. Relationships Among Individual and Community Behaviors and Service Activity Goals

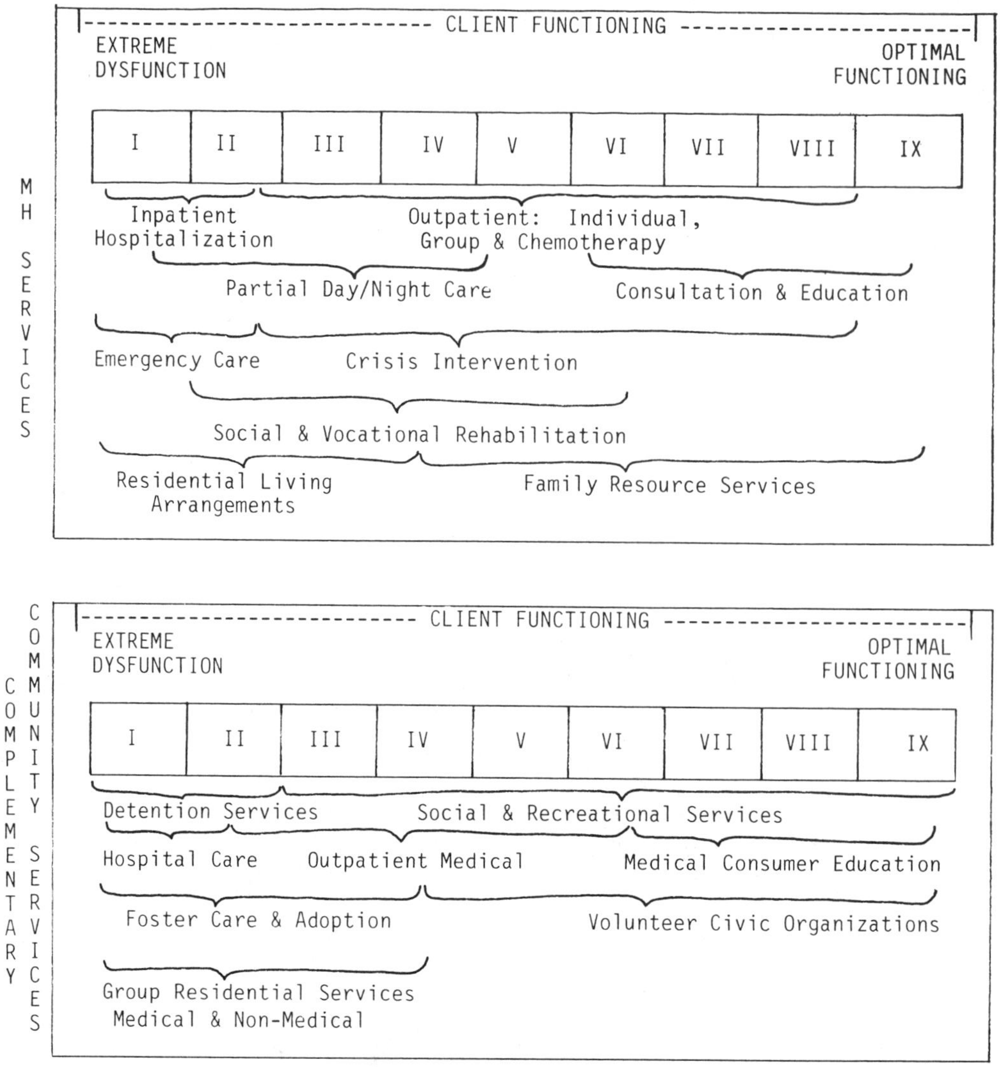

Figure 2. Designing the Array of Mental Health (upper panel) and Complementary Community (lower panel) Services (This figure was adapted from Nelson, Newman, & Hinkle, 1975)

Treatment is an activity to *increase* the client's level of functioning.
Intervention is any activity to *retard* or *stop* negative movement in level of functioning.
Prevention is any activity to *increase* an individual's *resistance* to any factor(s) producing a decrease in level of functioning. For example, job or family stresses can lower the individual's level of functioning while health and skill development can help an individual withstand some stresses.

Most services, e.g., counseling or medication, have elements with all three kinds of goals: treatment, intervention, and prevention. A service is usually defined by its predominant goals and by its intended range of impact along the level of functioning continuum, e.g., psychotherapy is considered to be predominantly a treatment activity.

In Figure 2, a sample program of services describes how these services are expected to affect clients at various levels of functioning. The upper half of Figure 2 describes the array of mental-health services offered by the sample program. The intensive-care services assist the clients at the lower functioning levels (on the left-hand side of the figure). The bottom half of Figure 2 describes the array of complementary nonmental health services for clients at various levels of functioning. Again, the intensive-care services provide assistance to those at the lower levels of functioning.

Figures 1 and 2 link a program of services to program goals and the potential impact on clients. Knowing the kinds of client and community behaviors to be reviewed helps determine current and future service needs. Potential impact on client functioning is specified as well as the relationships among other mental-health services and complementary nonmental-health services. The framework provides the basis for planning, evaluating, and managing an entire program of services.

Flexibility is a key concept and asset of client-oriented systems by tailoring program goals and services to suit clients, community, and available resources. A program of services need not adopt the same level of functioning concept described earlier. Any integrating concept describing the overriding goals of a program will work. Here are other examples:

(a) *Alcohol or Drug Abuse.* To provide services for those abusing alcohol or drugs to reduce the risk (frequency) of such abuse.
(b) *Developmental Disability.* To provide services so developmentally disabled citizens fully utilize the potential of their skills and available resources.
(c) *Children Mental Health.* To provide services to help children achieve optimal functioning and growth in their ordinary family, community, and educational settings.
(d) *Geriatric.* To provide services to help older adults function and adapt to the physical and social changes which accompany the aging process.
(e) *Health Services.* To provide services to help citizens attain the highest level of physical well-being possible given their age and circumstances.
(f) *Environmental Health.* To provide services to help individual citizens, as well as public and private industries and services, to support the community's highest standards of physical, social, and economic well-being.

Another example of flexibility is seeing how services provide coverage at each level of client functioning (or level of alcohol abuse or developmental disability). For example, if strong partial hospitalization and family support services exist, then a lower level of client functioning could be served by these less expensive services instead of inpatient services. The necessary requirement in a client-oriented system is a clear link between client/consumer behaviors and service goals—the bottom line measures if a program works.

A Note on Self-Study Exercises

The Exercises are designed to achieve two purposes: First, to assure yourself you understand the concepts; and second, to extend the text by providing different views of the concepts. We suggest that you always read through each exercise set and review the answers provided. We have tried to provide sufficient introductory comments for each exercise so the exercise's objectives will be clear.

A Self-Study Exercise on Figures 1 and 2

Figures 1 and 2 provided an example of how a program of mental-health services relates to client behaviors and to other community services. This exercise will help you understand some of the applications of these concepts for program design and provides a foundation for the next portion of Chapter 2. In reviewing the Figures, assume the Program's goal is to "help citizens attain their highest level of psychosocial functioning in their ordinary community setting," and the program has adapted the global scale described in the chapter's Appendix, Example 2. Be sure to call upon your own experiences to answer the questions and not just the text materials.

(1) Could a client receiving services from the partial hospitalization program partake of activities available in the other programs? If so, which ones, and how could this view of services be useful in treatment planning? ____________________

____

____

____

(2) What is the difference in coverage between MH *Emergency* and MH *Crisis Intervention*, and what is the relationship of these services to medical services? ____________

____

____

____

(3) Both the MH services and other community services sponsor *residential* services covering the same functioning levels. What two issues might you or a Health Service Agency (HSA) raise?

(a) ____

____

(b) ____

____

(4) Identify advantages of describing services in terms of the services potential impact on the client from the viewpoint of each of the following:

	Advantages (List one or more)
The Client	
Clinical Staff	
Clinical Supervisor	
Administrator	
Citizen Board	
Regulatory Agency	

Suggested Answers to Self-Study Exercise on Figures 1 and 2

(1) Yes, social and vocational rehabilitation, family resource services, and community social and recreational services. In treatment planning, counseling, and case management with clients at levels II–IV, these other services should be used to the extent that they are suitable to the client's goals. This view of available services can, therefore, serve as a guide for treatment planning, counseling, and case management. Would this way of viewing services be helpful in your situation?

(2) The crisis intervention services are designed to intervene with clients before they go charging into the lowest levels of functioning (II or I). Once clients are at the lowest levels, then emergency care or general hospital care services are used to stabilize the clients' behavior. Once stabilized, either inpatient, partial hospitalization or even outpatient services could be used, depending upon the client's network of family and social supports.

(3) (a) Are both needed as separate programs, or could they be integrated into a single service?
(b) What lines of communication and guidelines for coordination are needed to make optimal use of both services as separate entities or as a combined service?

(4) The advantages given below represent only one of many examples which could be provided, so let your own experiences be your guide here.
The Client: Addresses how the services they receive relate to each other and to their own behaviors.
Clinical Staff: Assists in treatment planning, review, and communicating with other services.
Clinical Supervisor: To help clinical staff understand the impact of their (and other) service efforts on clients.
Administrator: To assist in planning, budgeting, evaluating, and coordinating the management of a program of services.
Citizen Board: To understand the goals of services and setting client and goal-oriented policies.
Regulatory Agencies: To provide the basis for evaluating and monitoring the service program relating regulatory guidelines to local program clients and circumstances.

2. RELATING PROGRAM GOALS TO SERVICE DESIGN AND COORDINATION

Five key steps link overriding program goals to services.

		Adults		
	Children	No Prior Hospital Hist.	Prior Hospital Hist.	Geriatric
MH				
MR				
A & D				

Step I Identify the Major Target Groups the Program Intends to Serve.

This decision, itself, is a statement of policy. Identifying the types of persons served is often prerequisite to receiving state, federal, or other funds. While there probably are as many different ways to describe the categories of clients of mental-health services as there are clients, there are certain guidelines for establishing the criteria by which clients are designated *target populations.*[1]

(a) Criteria should be *mutually exclusive* so that
- — therapists or others responsible for client reports will know the criteria apply to the clients;
- — analysts will be able to compare clients with similar characteristics and contrast clients with different characteristics.

(b) *Limit the number of criteria.* Too many client characteristics may produce more target population definitions than can be managed without confusion.

(c) The criteria should also comply with the requirements of local, state, and federal *categorical funding.*

(d) Finally, the criteria should be *defined* to fit local practice, convention, and resources.

Step II Provide an Integrating Goal Statement for Each Target Group.

The goal statement should:

(II.1) Be measureable and observable by two or more reasonably trained people.

(II.2) Incorporate a global scale which will describe levels of movement toward or away from the program goal.

(II.3) Be defined in terms of three or more underlying factors, e.g., for level of functioning scales, four typical factors employed by programs are:
—Social role functioning
—Personal self-care
—Vocational/educational roles
—Emotional/stress tolerance and symptoms

Scales which incorporate multiple factors are called multifactored scales. Other multifactored scales are given in the Appendix of this unit.

Both a global and a multifactored scale should be used in a client-oriented system. The global scale provides an impressive and useful means of

- — Describing the overall relationships among services and their potential impact on a group of clients, but not the specific areas of problems and supports.
- — Communicating the overall functioning of a client, but not specific factors most critical to the client's particular level of functioning.
- — Coordinating and communicating service efforts among different staff working with the same clients, but focusing on different problem areas.
- — Helping staff to see and appreciate the "whole" client rather than just a person with a particular problem to be treated.

---

[1] Ia-Id adapted from Carter & Newman (1976).

A global scale provides an overall indicator of the client, relative to the specific problems and social circumstances of the client. When properly used, the global scale can help focus management efforts, but once the focus is drawn on a particular client group and service, more detail is needed to solve problems. By analogy, a map to travel between cities and states has much less detail than the map to travel within a city. It is a question of efficiency of effort. Both maps are needed for efficient and effective travel. Both types of scales are discussed later.

Step III Describe the Program of Services for Each Target Group Specifying Intended Impact on the Target Group. For Example:

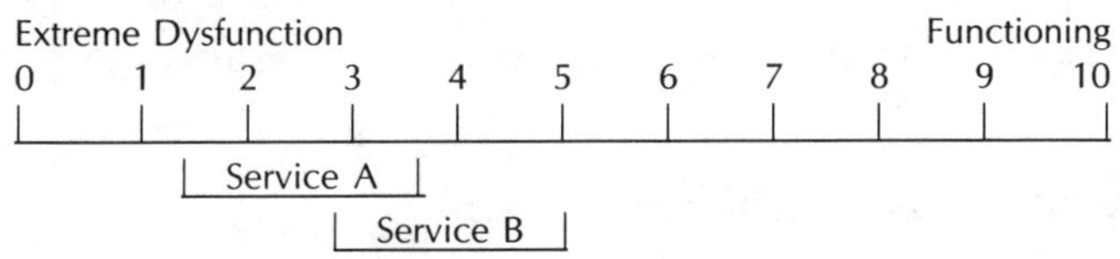

Step IV Describe Other Useful Supporting Services Available in the Community.

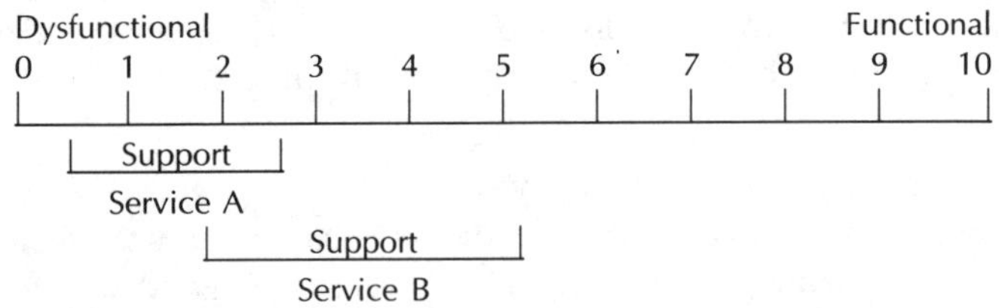

To complete Steps III and IV, consider using the format of Figure 3. Figure 2, shown earlier in the unit, provides an example.

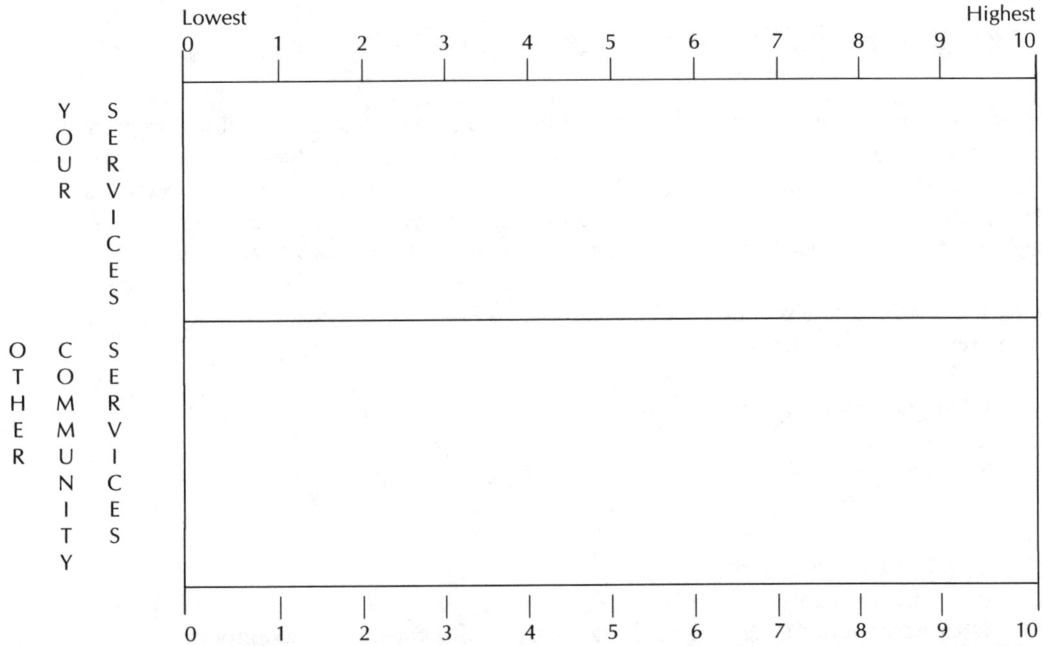

*Note that we are using a 10-point scale. Global scales with fewer than 7–9 points tend to lack the specificity and sensitivity required to be reliable and useful for communicating clinical decisions. We will have more on this later. For now, we suggest you practice with a 10-point scale.

Figure 3. Integrated Service Array*

AGENCY	WHO IS TO COORDINATE	CONSULTATION/EDUCATION & POLITICAL ACTIVITIES

Figure 4. To Describe the Coordination of Responsibilities

Step V Put Steps III and IV Together and Describe:

(V.1) What agencies have to be coordinated?
(V.2) Who in your program should perform the coordinating function?
(V.3) What political, bureaucratic, consultation, and educational activities are needed to achieve the smoothest coordination with optimal impact?

Figure 4 provides a format to complete Step V.

After performing these five steps, the foundation is laid to view the detailed pieces of the clinical process, program management, and clinical records. A good way to understand how these five steps work is to try it in a small subgroup of clients served by your program.

3. IDENTIFYING POTENTIAL CONCERNS

What are the potential products and pitfalls from the 5-step process of describing program goals and services? For example, a useful product results if the behavior scales coordinate services in support of the client's treatment plan. The clinical supervisors and program director may find the approach useful in planning, coordinating, and budgeting resources. But there may be negative factors (pitfalls) such as a tendency to increase paperwork and bureaucratic procedures. These positive and negative issues need to be addressed so procedures can be devised to promote the positive products and to handle the negative events and influences. Specifically there are two sets of questions:

(1) What good products could evolve for
- (a) The client?
- (b) The service staff?
- (c) The clinical supervisors?
- (d) The administration?
- (e) The Citizen Board?
- (f) The regulatory agencies?

(2) What negative influences or products could evolve for these same groups?

These products and pitfalls will become a personalized list of management objectives in the development of your program's client-oriented system.

Self-Study Exercise

(1) Identify at least one positive product and at least one pitfall of the concepts of program design described in this chapter from the viewpoint of each of the six groups listed above, starting with the client. Use Figure 5 to perform this task.

(2) Read the remainder of Chapter 2 and review the example of the client-oriented system described earlier. Then, return to your list of products and pitfalls and place a mark (X) next to those you had listed but were identified in Chapter 2. Ideally most, if not all, of your positive and negative concerns have been taken into account.

TASK: Identify at least one product and one pitfall resulting from the application of the five-step procedure to describe program goals and services.

FROM THE VIEWPOINT OF	POTENTIAL PRODUCTS	POTENTIAL PITFALLS
CLIENT		
SERVICE STAFF		
CLINICAL SUPERVISORS		
ADMINISTRATION		
CITIZEN BOARDS		
REGULATORY AGENCIES County/State/Federal		

Figure 5. Potential Products and Pitfalls for the Program Design Unit

An Example of Potential Products and Pitfalls for the Program Design Unit

From the Viewpoint of	Potential Products	Potential Pitfalls
CLIENT	—I may get a faster & clearer idea of where I should go for specific services —Community agencies may work together more effectively to help me.	—whose "objectives" are being considered: mine or agency's? —will my confidentiality needs be more at risk?
SERVICE STAFF	—clearer understanding of my client's problems, functioning, etc. —presents a way to measure client progress relating to service goals	—may be too restricting, i.e., create barriers to service —will individual client really be described by "grouping"? —too much paperwork

CLINICAL SUPERVISORS	—clearer way to train staff re: their function in relation to overall program —easier way to assign cases, review caseloads, etc.	—necessity for "standardizing" services and training —staff may be threatened, become more resistant
ADMINISTRATION	—clearer way to define both agency purposes and types of clients served —way of tracking clients by severity of problem/need	—could get bogged down in details and run up costs for staff training —information may not help given "politics"
CITIZEN BOARDS	—way to plan for services, examine unmet needs, gaps in services —easier to communicate with community, funders, etc.	—can we trust info. to be "really" reliable, reported honestly —may require too much "expertise" from us to use info.
REGULATORY AGENCIES County/State/Federal	—able to track $ to specific types of clients, services —may be more cost-efficient if number of agencies can plan together	—lack of one standard measure makes comparison more difficult —joint planning may cause more "turf" fights and bad will among agencies

4. ASSURING DEPENDABLE AND USEFUL MEASURES OF CLIENT BEHAVIORS AND SERVICE GOALS

Many questions may emerge about the development, use, and maintenance of dependable measures of client behaviors and service program effectiveness. While the technical issues are addressed in later chapters, the basic ingredients of dependable and valid measures are listed.

(1) The global scale should be:
   (a) Adapted from a scale demonstrated to be reliable and valid elsewhere. (See the Appendix to this chapter for a good starting point.)
   (b) Adapted to local circumstances and mores via active staff involvement to assure both the content and face validity of the scale, i.e., the contents of the scale are related to local clients and circumstances.
   (c) Used regularly by clinical staff at meaningful clinical encounters and for professional communication throughout the service episode. Use helps to assure the predictive validity of the scale, i.e., the scale predicts differences in client behaviors.
   (d) Supported by recorded observations on a multifactor problem or issues list at the time of intake, review, and termination. These data aid in content validity.

(2) Documentation of multiple factors and their relationship to the overall level of functioning must be maintained and reviewed in a clinical record. This documentation lays the basis for both content and construct validity, i.e., that the underlying structure of the scale does what it purports to do.

(3) A review process should exist where three or more staff routinely review:
   (a) A random sample of all cases.
   (b) All cases where goals and outcome standards are not occurring as expected.

   This feature assures the reproducibility of the scale, i.e., that observations will be described with the same scale values by different trained observers.

(4) Staff training procedures on the use of the global scale and multifactor scales should occur 2–3 times per year. Quantitative estimates of reliablity and content validity can be obtained and the statistical procedures employed here are described in Chapter 12.

The rationale for these assertions is provided in Sections III and IV on "Visible Evidence." The series of studies referenced in Newman (1980) suggest global scale reliability will increase under the following circumstances:

(a) Staff were involved in the adaptation and development of the scale. The process of developing the scale forces staff and supervisors to clarify the meaning of the words they use. Clarification often takes the form of examples drawn from actual clients with whom they have had first-hand experience. (These issues underlie the design of the clinical processes in Section II.)
(b) Clinical supervisors have used the scale and its vocabulary in supervision, treatment planning, and review processes. (These issues are discussed in both Sections II and III.)
(c) Staff have compared their independent scale ratings on a common set of case histories. (Chapters 10 and 11 describe the procedures for staff development.)

The validity of the scale is best determined if:

(a) The factors underlying a global scale can be shown to relate to it. The relationship can be demonstrated if there is routine documentation of the multiple factors considered in the global assessment. Since multiple-factor assessment is expensive in time and effort, such assessment is usually confined to intake/service planning, progress review, and termination.
(b) Three or more observers with similar training and experience should compare their observations with the routine observations. A criterion of validity comes directly from the logical basis of a scientific observation. This criterion can be incorporated directly and inexpensively into the review procedures described in Chapters 4 and 5.

In summary, dependable and valid measures of service goals result if there is a:

(a) *Review of the Clinical Process,* particularly judgments of the global and multifactor observations.
(b) *Clinical Record System* routinely documenting global and multifactored observations.
(c) *Frequent use* of the language of the measurement scales by clinical staff in their ordinary communication with clients and one another.
(d) *Routine staff development sessions* (e.g., 2–3 times a year), where staff independently rate brief case histories and compare and discuss their ratings on the same cases.

5. RELATING INTERNAL PROGRAM MANAGEMENT MEASURES TO EXTERNAL REPORTING AND MONITORING

A usual reaction to local program scale flexibility is a concern each program will have different scales of measurement. Regulatory agencies apparently fear chaos and an inability of monitoring and coordinating services on a large scale (e.g., by Health Service Area, state, or federal region). This fear is groundless. Two studies which were reported by Newman and Rinkus

(1978) have shown local programs can develop their own versions of a global scale, yet aggregated outcome data can be compared among programs with as much as 95% accuracy.

First, high behavior scale reliability was found in those programs where four major themes were operating:

— A review process using the language of the scale as a means of communication.
— A clinical record system documenting the client's observable behaviors and situations underlying the global and multifactor ratings.
— Frequent use of global ratings throughout the therapeutic process.
— Routine staff development and training.

Reliability of measures (between .70 and .84) was observed in each program.

Second, each program, as part of their routine staff development sessions (held 2–3 times a year), rated the same set of 10 to 20 case histories using their own global scale. Since their global scale shows reliablity coefficients between .70 and .84 reliablity, the average ratings by clinicians from any two different programs correlated about .975. The average global rating of clinicians in one program predicts the average ratings of clinicians in another program on the same case with better than 95% accuracy.

Thus, if dependable and valid global measures exist within a program, regulatory agencies can convert the outcome data across programs for their own monitoring and planning purposes. Furthermore, this cross-program comparison procedure is minimally obstrusive on the management of local programs. While the procedures developed in this text primarily emphasize local program's management and operation, data can be translated in a comparable fashion for external regulatory and funding agencies.

6. APPENDIX: EXAMPLES OF GLOBAL AND MULTIFACTORED SCALES

Global Scale: Example 1 **Global Assessment Scale (GAS)**

Jean Endicott, Robert L. Spitzer, Robert L. Fleiss, & Jacob Cohen[2]

Rate the subject's lowest level of functioning in the last week by selecting the lowest range which describes his functioning on a hypothetical continuum of mental health-illness. For example, a subject whose "behavior is considerably influenced by delusions" (range 21–30) should be given a rating in that range even though he has "major impairment in several areas" (range 31–40). Use intermediate levels when appropriate (e.g., 35, 58, 63). Rate actual functioning independent of whether or not subject is receiving and may be helped by medication or some other form of treatment.

Name of Patient__________ ID no.__________ Consec. No.__________ Code No.__________

Admission Date__________ Date of Rating__________ Rater__________ Rating__________

91–100 No symptoms, superior functioning in a wide range of activities, life's problems never see to get out of hand, is sought out by others because of his warmth and integrity.

[2] *Archives of General Psychiatry,* 1976, *33,* 766–771.

81–90 Transient symptoms may occur, but good functioning in all areas, interested and involved in a wide range of activities, socially effective, generally satisfied with life, "everyday" worries that only occasionally get out of hand.

71–80 Minimal symptoms may be present but no more than slight impairment in functioning, varying degrees of "everyday" worries and problems that sometimes get out of hand.

61–70 Some mild symptoms (e.g., depressive mood and mild insomnia) OR some difficulty in several areas of functioning, but generally functioning pretty well, has some meaningful interpersonal relationships, and most untrained people would not consider him "sick."

51–60 Moderate symptoms or generally functioning with some difficulty (e.g., few friends and flat affect, depressed mood and pathological self-doubt, euphoric mood and pressure of speech, moderately severe antisocial behavior).

41–50 Any serious symptomatology or impairment in functioning that most clinicians would think obviously requires treatment or attention (e.g., suicidal preoccupation or gesture, severe obsessional rituals, frequent anxiety attacks, serious antisocial behavior, compulsive drinking).

31–40 Major impairment in several areas, such as work, family relations, judgment, thinking, or mood (e.g., depressed woman avoids friends, neglects family, unable to do housework), OR some impairment in reality testing or communication (e.g., speech is at times obscure, illogical or irrelevant), OR single serious suicide attempt.

21–30 Unable to function in almost all areas (e.g., stays in bed all day) OR behavior is considerably influenced by either delusions or hallucinations OR serious impairment in communication (e.g., sometimes incoherent or unresponsive) or judgment (e.g., acts grossly inappropriate).

11–20 Needs some supervision to prevent hurting self or others, or to maintain minimal personal hygiene (e.g., repeated suicide attempts, frequently violent, manic excitement, smears feces), OR gross impairment in communication (e.g., largely incoherent or mute).

1–10 Needs constant supervision for several days to prevent hurting self or others, or makes no attempt to maintain minimal personal hygiene.

Example 2

LEVEL OF FUNCTIONING*

I. Overview of Scale

The scale is used to describe a client's overall ability to function autonomously in the community. A scale rating is assigned at the time of every clinical encounter by balancing the relative contributions of four criteria as they affect a person's overall ability to function autonomously:

* The scale was developed by the Central Montgomery MH/MR Center staff, who adapted the criteria previously developed by the Psychotherapy Research Project of the Menninger Foundation (Health-Sickness Rating Scale, Luborsky, 1962) and the Functional Baseline Scale of the Reading Hospital MH Treatment Center, 1978.

(1) Personal self-care
(2) Social functioning in ordinary social unit and in the general community
(3) Vocational and/or educational productivity
(4) Evidence of emotional stability and stress tolerance

Limited dysfunctioning in any one or more of the four areas could affect a person's overall ability to function.

The time period covered by each rating is the interval immediately surrounding the clinical encounter. This period typically covers an interval between 1 hour to 1 week, shorter time periods for lower functioning clients using emergency or inpatient services. One-week periods would typically be useful for higher functioning clients in outpatient or training program services.

Remember that the scale is designed to describe a person's ability to function autonomously in the community. Factors such as brief situational stresses, isolated physical illness, or injury should not be weighted heavily unless the person's reactions are quite inappropriate and/or the final outcome appears to have permanent or lasting effect.

The balanced weighting of the four criteria must always be considered in terms of the age and circumstances of the individual. The vocational-productivity demands for the head of a household of six are different from those of a single person, and different from the productive criteria of a housewife or retired person. The criteria, when applied to children, are always in terms which are relative to the expectations of children in a given age bracket.

The relationship between level of functioning and degree of therapeutic intervention is often direct. For example, a person who is characterized as totally dysfunctional is usually placed in a setting of intensive care, with chemotherapy and 24-hour supervision. Or, a person at the higher levels of functioning (e.g., level 8) may have only monthly contacts in a group social activities situation. The relationship, however, is not always that direct. A child or even an adult could be at a relatively low level of functioning because of the circumstances of another member of the household. In these cases, therapeutic intervention is less directly related to the client. The most important determinant of treatment for a client is the amount of supportive resources available at home and in the neighboring community and not necessarily the level of functioning.

II. Some Details Describing the Four Criteria

The criteria should always be translated to fit the age bracket and circumstances of the individual. Special notes are indicated below where such considerations may be necessary.

(1) Personal Self-Care (for children, adjust to age level)
   (a) Personal maintenance of washing, dressing, eating, elimination chores.
   (b) Ability to recognize and avoid common dangers.
   (c) Taking responsibility for own maintenance, e.g., caring for own room, personal belongings, daily schedule, personal finances, selecting own clothing and accessories.
(2) Social Functioning (adjust by age, living conditions, and possibly by community)
   (a) *Familiar*—the degree to which those familiar with the person, particularly those in the ordinary social unit (family, roomate, other boarding house residents) can tolerate and interact with the person; i.e., jointly socialize and/or participate in recreational activities with the person.

(b) *Impersonal*—the degree to which relative strangers can interact with the person and vice versa, e.g., store clerks, policemen, or others encountered in ordinary pedestrian, vocational, or recreational activities.

(3) Vocational and/or Educational Functioning

(a) *Working Adults*

(1) The ability to support one's self and one's dependents.

(2) The ability to meet the demands and pressures of one's chosen (or present) vocation, be it lawyer or janitor.

(b) *Homemakers and/or Parents and/or Elderly Persons*

(1) The ability to organize and/or monitor the daily routines of the household, e.g., meals, child care, washing, etc.

(2) The ability to organize, maintain and/or monitor family budgeting, shopping, social and/or recreational activities.

(c) *Children*

(1) Should be considered by general age categories of 0–5, 6–11, 12–14, 15–18.

(2) Play and social activities such that constructive and productive social learning can occur.

(3) Educational activities and performance such as would be expected of that age.

(4) Evidence of Emotional Stability and Stress Tolerance

(a) The degree to which the symptom(s) reflects personality disorganization of such degree that the symptoms and the accompanying disorganization cause discomfort to whomever the person would ordinarily interact with.

(b) The degree to which the person can tolerate the amount of expected daily variation in *present* social, vocational and/or educational realms.

NOTE: There is often an interaction among the social, vocational/educational, and emotional factors such that the strength in one area often compensates for weakness in another. For example, vocational success may come as a result of a person's avoiding or minimizing familiar social encounters at home.

III. Definition of the Nine Scale Levels of Functioning

With regard to the balance of the four criteria (personal self-care, social, vocational/ educational, and emotional symptoms/stress tolerance), the person's ability to function autonomously in the community is at Level X, where X can assume one of the following nine (9) levels:

LEVEL 1: Dysfunctional in all four areas and is almost totally dependent upon others to provide a supportive protective environment.

LEVEL 2: Not working; ordinary social unit cannot or will not tolerate the person; can perform minimal self-care functions but cannot assume most responsibilities or tolerate social encounters beyond restrictive settings (e.g., in group, play, or occupational therapy).

LEVEL 3: Not working; probably living in ordinary social unit but not without considerable strain on the person and/or on others in the household. Symptoms are such that movement in the community should be restricted or supervised.

LEVEL 4: Probably not working, although may be capable of working in a very protective setting; able to live in ordinary social unit and contribute to the daily routine of the household; can assume responsibility for all personal self-care matters; stressful social encounters ought to be avoided or carefully supervised.

NOTE: Levels 5 through 8 describe persons who are usually functioning satisfactorily in the community, but for whom problems in one or more of the criteria areas force some degree of dependency on a form of therapeutic intervention.

LEVEL 5: Emotional stability and stress tolerance are sufficiently low that successful functioning in the social and/or vocational/educational realms is marginal. The person is barely able to hold on to either job or social unit, or both, without direct therapeutic intervention and a diminution of conflicts in either or both realms.

LEVEL 6: The person's vocational and/or social areas of functioning are stabilized, but only because of direct therapeutic intervention. Symptom presence and severity are probably sufficient to be both noticeable and somewhat disconcerting to the client and/or those around the client in daily contact.

LEVEL 7: The person is functioning and coping well socially and vocationally (educationally); however, symptom reoccurrences are sufficiently frequent to maintain a reliance on some sort of regular therapeutic intervention.

LEVEL 8: Functioning well in all areas with little evidence of distress present. However, a history of symptom reoccurrence suggests periodic correspondence with the Center, e.g., a client may receive a medication check from a family physician who then contacts the Center monthly, or the client returns for bi-monthly social activities.

LEVEL 9: The person is functioning well in all areas and no contact with the MH/MR services is recommended.

Example 3: **Global Levels of Functioning Scale***

Cave Run Comprehensive Care Center, Morehead, Kentucky

To function effectively in their ordinary social units, clients must manage their daily living activities and role functions within their circumstances across five areas: PERSONAL SELF-CARE, COGNITIVE, AFFECTIVE, INTERPERSONAL/FAMILIAL, VOCATIONAL/EDUCATIONAL. These five areas are defined below.

DEFINITIONS:

(1) *Daily living activities*—regular, daily activities performed by clients at their expressed level of maturation (e.g., grooming, dressing, feeding oneself, and washing, etc.). It is more *person/individual centered.*

(2) *Role functions*—expected behavior and accompanying obligations in social situations (e.g., housewife caring for children, preparing meals, and shopping, etc. Factory worker operating machinery and using tools, socializing with co-workers, and interacting with foreman, etc.). This is more *social oriented.*

---

* This scale was adapted from and influenced by the levels of functioning scale used at the Reading Hospital Mental Health Treatment Center (L. Rotenberg and M. Gordon), the Menninger Health-Sickness Scale (Luborsky, 1962), the Fayette County MH-MR Scale, and the Central Montgomery MH/MR Scale.

GLOBAL LEVELS OF FUNCTIONING SCALE*

Levels of Functioning

1–10 Danger to self and others. Unable to live in ordinary social units. Unable to carry out daily living activities and role functions without intensive, supervised care.

11–20 Able to maintain minimal self-care. Interpersonally isolated. Difficulty with daily living activities and role functions without supportive supervision.

21–30 Able to work in protective setting; may have difficulty in maintaining a work task. Very limited personal interaction. Able to perform daily living activities and role functions with some supportive services on a more or less regular basis.

31–40 Able to assume self-sufficiency in personal self-care and handle personal needs in social units. Functions in one additional area adequately, but has conflict in other areas. Interpersonally active with familiar people. Requires frequent intervention and support.

41–50 Able to perform living tasks and role functions in social units. Functions in two additional areas, but has conflict in other areas. Is able to identify problems, but has difficulty in resolving them and in decision making. Requires frequent intervention.

51–60 Functions in three areas in addition to personal self-care, but has conflict in one area, which causes evidence of stress in self and others. Has periods of relief, but needs frequent intervention.

61–70 Able to function comfortably in all areas within social units, but experiences conflict in one area. Needs occasional intervention.

71–80 Functions in all areas with little or no conflict; however, due to recurring symptoms, needs occasional help.

81–90 Functions well in all areas in social units and maintains even keel. Does not require services.

CHARACTERISTICS OF THE FIVE AREAS OF EFFECTIVE FUNCTIONING

Personal Self-Care

(1) Personal maintenance of washing, dressing, eating, elimination chores.

(2) Ability to recognize and avoid common dangers and possible self-abuse.

(3) Taking responsibility for own maintenance, e.g., caring for own room, personal belongings, daily schedule, personal finances, selecting own clothing and accessories.

(4) Ability to manage own resources (e.g., funds, family or friend's time).

Cognitive

(1) *Reality orientation.* Person evidences the ability to associate and organize persons and events in time and place. No impairment in recent or remote memory.

(2) *Intellectual and learning capacity.* Person evidences ability to identify, analyze, and solve problems or social situations, and displays the ability to profit from past experiences.

(3) *Train of thought.* Person evidences ability to maintain thoughts on a given topic with little or no diversion.

(4) *Rational thinking.* Person's thoughts are consistent with reality.
(5) *Judgment.* Person is able to organize information and respond with socially appropriate solution to problems or social situations.

Affective

(1) *Appropriate expression of emotion.* Person's *degree* of appropriate expression of emotion is consistent with the expected degree of expressions within his/her culture.
(2) *Feelings appropriate to objective reality.* Person's emotions are consistent with the expected emotional responses to reality of the community.
(3) *Emotional stability.* Person's emotional variance is consistent with reality.

Interpersonal/Familial

(1) *Cope with demands of others.* Person can adequately cope with other's demands.
(2) *Involvement with others.* Person is able to effectively interact and form relationships with others.
(3) *Empathy.* Person is able to describe and demonstrate that he/she feels what others are feeling.
(4) *Functions well in social role(s).* Person adequately carries out cultural expectations implied by the social role which he/she currently fills to the satisfaction of self and/or significant others.

Vocational/Educational

(1) *Working Adults*
  (a) The ability to support one's self and one's dependents.
  (b) The ability to meet the demands and pressures of one's chosen (or present) vocation, be it lawyer or janitor.
(2) *Homemakers and/or Parents and/or Elderly Persons*
  (a) The ability to organize and/or monitor the daily routines of the household, e.g., meals, child care, washing, etc.
  (b) The ability to organize, maintain and/or monitor family budgeting, shopping, social and/or recreational activities.
(3) *Children*
  (a) Should be considered by general age categories of 0–5, 6–11, 12–14, 15–18.
  (b) Play and social activities such that constructive and productive social learning can occur.
  (c) Educational activities and performance such as would be expected of that age.

Rating of Area of Level of Severity at Intake, Review and Termination and Put in Record

Levels 1–3 are difficulties acceptable in community; levels 4–7 are difficulties not acceptable in community.

(1) No apparent difficulty (problem or skill deficit).
(2) Very minor difficulty.

(3) Difficulty of modest proportion.
(4) Relatively severe difficulty (problem or skill deficit).
(5) Severe difficulty.
(6) Extremely severe difficulty.
(7) Difficulty of devasting proportions.

Multifactor List: Example 1: **Standardized Scale Headings for Use in MHS Evaluation with Goal Attainment Scaling***

Standardized Scale Heading	Examples of Content
AGGRESSION	Violence, temper tantrums, fighting, angry outbursts, yelling, screaming, striking out, biting children, injuring others, killing, anger, acting out, hostility, any aggression toward another person(s).
ALCOHOL USE	Drinking, drunkeness, attendance at AA meetings, referral to detoxification center.
ANXIETY	Nervousness, anxious, anxiety attacks, tension.
PSYCHOPATHOLOGICAL SYMPTOMS	Delusions, guilt feelings, obsessions, phobias, compulsiveness, paranoia, suspiciousness, hearing voices, withdrawing into unreal world, hallucinations.
DECISIONS	Decision-making, ambivalence, makes-up mind, acceptance of ______, immobilized by indecision, etc. (any act of acceptance is viewed as decision-making, e.g., "acceptance of self," "acceptance of pregnancy").
DEPRESSION	Crying, sadness, dreams, depressed, apathy.
DRUG USE	(Excluding medications) use of drugs, stoned, trips, addicted, hard drugs, LSD, marijuana, hooked, narcotics.
EDUCATION	School, grades, classes, vocational training, degree, teachers, relationships with other students or professors.
FAMILY/MARITAL	Children, siblings, parents, separation, divorce, wife, husband, marriage, arguments with husband, child-parent relationships, nagging mother, living with children, feelings to children.
FINANCIAL	Welfare, bills, difficulty paying bills, debts, bad checks, money management, finances, bankruptcy.
INTERPERSONAL RELATIONSHIPS AND SOCIAL	Dependency on others, friends, relationships with co-workers, church involvement, movies, hobbies, making new friends, social group involvement, gets along with others, going out socially, talking, communicates, discusses, expresses feelings, receives feedback, withdraws verbally, listening, caring about, social life, seclusion.
LEGAL	Jail, imprisonment, parole violations, felonies, misdemeanors, missed support payments, probation.
LIVING ARRANGEMENTS	Living at home, living independently, living with roommates, staying at a nursing home, living in a hotel, moves to own apartment, finds room.
PHYSICAL COMPLAINTS AND CHARACTERISTICS	Loss of drive, weight gain or loss, loss of ambition, sleep, sleeplessness, headaches, muscle aches, dizziness, shaking, tremors, appetite loss, backaches, tiredness, seizures, physically immobilized, at one with body, physical appearance, clothing.
SELF REFERENCES	Self-image, self-concept, isolation of self, know feelings, working on needs.
SEXUALITY	Sexual identity, sexual deviance, frequency of intercourse, sexual intercourse, sexual responsiveness, relations with boyfriend/girlfriend, dates, affairs, dates married men, homosexuality, pregnancy.

SUICIDE	Self-destructive acts, self-mutilation, suicide, suicidal thoughts, suicide attempts, suicide gestures, aggression toward self.
TREATMENT	Hospitalized, medications, psychiatric hospitalization, therapy, group therapy program, Day Center.
WORK	Employment, job, work performance, supervisors, co-workers, quits work, seeks employment, hired, absenteeism, satisfaction with work, job ambition, housekeeping responsibilities, working at outreach.
MISCELLANEOUS AND THOSE NOT OBVIOUSLY RECOGNIZED AS CATEGORIES	Comfortable, finish what I start, love, material values, material rewards, defensiveness.

*From Kiresuk (1975) Five Year Report on Goal Attainment Scaling to NIMH.

Example 2: **Psychiatric Status Schedule (California's Adaptation)**

Spitzer, Endicott, Feins, & Cohn*

(1) DEPRESSION—Reports of subjective feelings and concerns and psychosocial dysfunctions that may be associated with the depressive symptoms.

(2) ANXIETY—Reports of subjective feelings and concerns, and psychophysiological dysfunctions that may be associated with the anxious, phobic, or obsessive-compulsive syndromes.

(3) INAPPROPRIATE AFFECT, APPEARANCE, OR BEHAVIOR—Appearance, physical behavior, or acts which would be considered odd or inappropriate by most untrained persons.

(4) NEGATIVISM–OBSTINANCY—Refusal to answer questions or cooperate; withholding information.

(5) AGITATION–EXCITEMENT—Overt signs of agitation or excitement (e.g., inability to sit still, pacing, handwringing, accelerated speech, hyperactivity).

(6) MOTOR RETARDATION–LACK OF EMOTION—Visible signs of retardation in speech and movement, a tendency to ignore the surroundings, and flattening of affect or general lack of emotional expression.

(7) SPEECH DISORDERS—Impairment in the form or organization of speech (e.g., blocks, rambles, is incoherent, stutters, ''babytalks'').

(8) SUSPICION–PERSECUTION–HALLUCINATIONS—Distrustfulness; feelings of having been mistreated, taken advantage of, tricked, or pushed around; ideas of reference; various paranoid delusions; auditory hallucinations which mock, threaten, or command.

(9) GRANDIOSITY—Inflated appraisal of self-worth, contacts, power, or knowledge; boasting; sensational plans; delusions of power, status, knowledge, or contacts; and hallucinations with a grandiose connotation.

(10) SUICIDE–SELF-MUTILATION—Suicidal thoughts, preoccupation, threats, gestures, or attempts, and thoughts or acts of self-mutilation.

(11) SOMATIC CONCERN–PHYSICAL PROBLEM—Real or imagined physical complaint or disability; conversion reaction; somatic delusion or hallucinations, hypochondriasis; or body image concern.

* Problem definitions adapted in part from Spitzer, R. L., Endicott, J., et. al. (1970). The Psychiatric Status Schedule, *Arch. Gen. Psychiat.*, *23*, 41–55.

(12) DAILY ROUTINE–LEISURE TIME IMPAIRMENT—The impact of psychopathology on daily routine, on carrying through self-appointed or expected tasks, and on usual leisure time or recreational activities (e.g., difficulty in arising in the morning, getting dressed, and traveling).

(13) REPORTED OVERT ANGER—Reported or observed overt anger or belligerence; shouting, temper tantrums.

(14) DISORIENTATION–MEMORY IMPAIRMENT—Visible signs of disorientation as to time, place, and persons, and impairment in recent or remote memory.

(15) SOCIAL ISOLATION—Lack of friends; avoidance of contact or involvement with others, and feelings of isolation, rejection, or discomfort with people.

(16) MATURATIONAL PROBLEMS—Failure to achieve age appropriate interpersonal or family relationships; and/or age appropriate adaptive behavior (e.g., work, school).

(17) DENIAL OF ILLNESS—The extent to which the patient denies, despite the evidence, that his/her current symptoms have psychiatric significance, that he/she is ill or needs psychiatric help or that he/she needs to change his/her attitude in some specific way.

(18) ANTISOCIAL OR ILLEGAL ACTS—Lying; stealing; swindling, conning, commission or involvement in minor or serious illegal or delinquent acts.

(19) ALCOHOL ABUSE—The degree to which use of alcohol is excessive, compulsive, causes physical symptoms or alteration in mood or behavior, or interferes with performance of expected daily routine of duties.

(20) DRUG ABUSE—Excessive self-medication and habituation or addiction to narcotics, barbiturates, stimulants, or consciousness-altering substances.

(21) DANGER TO OTHERS—Has made serious threats of violence or actual assaults against other persons (violence against property not included); child abuse.

(22) IMPULSE CONTROL—Lacks self-discipline; responses to stimuli exceed limits of expected behavior; responses to stimuli are without regard to consequences; or impulses to commit delinquent or illegal acts.

(23) SEXUAL PROBLEMS—Sex role confusion; engages in sexual behavior which is defined as unacceptable by self, family, or society.

(24) PROLONGED EXPOSURE TO POOR ENVIRONMENTAL CONDITIONS—Such as long-term disturbed family relationships, chronic dysfunctioning or absence of a significant other; psychosocial deprivation.

(25) SITUATIONAL CRISIS—A decrease in ablity to cope with actual or threatened loss related to self-image, role mastery, or relationship with a significant other.

(26) HOUSEKEEPER ROLE—Admission of doing a poor job as a housekeeper, no pleasure or satisfaction in any aspect of household duties; marked discomfort or difficulty with, or refusal to carry out, one or more expected household tasks.

(27) WAGE EARNER ROLE—No interest or satisfaction in one's job; dread of one's work; failure to meet task standards; need for constant supervision; psychopathology interferes with work; excessive job changes; or limiting oneself to part-time, temporary, or transient work because of psychopathology.

(28) STUDENT OR TRAINEE ROLE—Poor motivation; avoidance of available extracurricular activities; missing classes; difficulty doing homework or assignments; poor grades; need for extensive help; or, conflict with teachers or administration.

(29) MATE ROLE–MARITAL PROBLEMS—Affectionate feelings rarely experienced or expressed; many quarrels; little or no sexual activity; few shared friends or social activities.

(30) PARENT ROLE—Inability to carry out important child-care tasks; requiring considerable help to manage child; morbid fears of child being injured or ill.

SECTION II

DESIGNING THE CLINICAL PROCESS AND PROCEDURES

Chapter 3
Design of the Clinical Service Process

> What Happens to Clients?
> Who Does What? Why? With What Outcomes?

Section II is designed to help describe the client's entry, service planning, review, and termination processes to clearly show the relationships among:

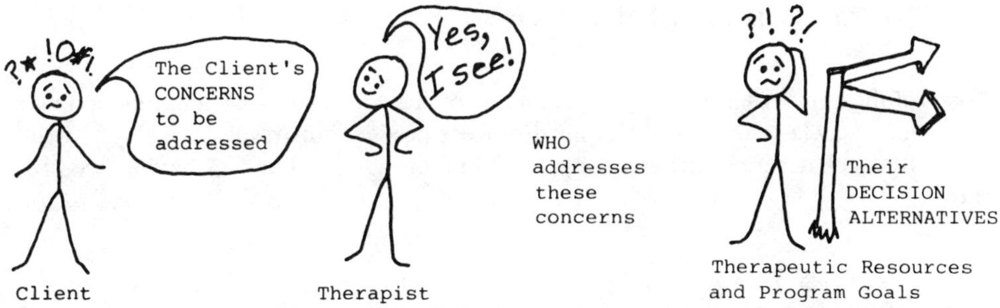

The Client's CONCERNS to be addressed
Yes, I see!
WHO addresses these concerns
Their DECISION ALTERNATIVES
Client
Therapist
Therapeutic Resources and Program Goals

Clear design of how clinical services assist clients enhances control of both service quality and costs. Designing (or redesigning) an existing service system involves identifying the four stages and eight questions of the clinical process:

	STAGE	QUESTION
Chapter 4	CLIENT ENTRY	Who is the client?
		Is the client at the right place?
Chapter 5	SERVICE PLANNING	What are the issues?
		What events are to happen?
Chapter 6	REVIEW	Are the events occurring as planned?
		What changes are needed?
Chapter 7	TERMINATION AND FOLLOWUP	Were goals met?
		Is followup required?

Section II addresses a series of questions and issues about how services support the client/consumer in achieving their service goals. During this process it is likely that you will discover your present system of services is not ideally designed to help the client/consumer with available resources—thereby giving rise to anxious concerns. The underlying problem rests in the chaotic way most service programs have grown during the last decade. The problem is a classic case of the tail wagging the dog. Expanding and contracting funding for specific target groups of clients, along with the growth of standards and regulations from different agencies and professional organizations, have promoted chaotic service-system designs. The resulting system looks like the product of the famous committee setting out to construct a horse and producing a camel instead.

Sometimes external forces can be disruptive. The next self-study exercise is a tongue-in-cheek quiz to highlight the chaos faced by managers of service programs. Your concerns are the same as those of the people who influence the flow of money and standards and regulations. The issue is whether the description of the clinical process relates program-service design and procedures to program goals and to client/consumer outcomes. If you can provide an understandable description to a typical client/consumer, to staff, and to Citizen Board members, the demands of the regulatory agencies and accreditation organizations will also be satisfied.

A potential cure for concerns about existing service-system design can come from designing and documenting your clinical service system to clarify the relationships among clinical processes, services, and program goals. If problems exist in achieving program goals, there ought to be clear procedures for surfacing and correcting the problem.

THE CLIENT-FOCUSED CLINICAL PROCESS

The focus of the clinical service process should be on the consumer—a client functioning at the highest level possible. How can the clinical process produce this result?

The first step describes the clinical process in four major stages each having two principal questions.

Stage of Process	Questions Addressed
ENTRY	Who is the client? Is the client at the right place?
SERVICE PLANNING	What are the issues? What events are to happen?
REVIEW	Are the events occurring as planned? What changes are needed in the service plan?
TERMINATION AND FOLLOWUP	Were goals met? Is followup required?

Addressing the two principal questions at each stage requires identification of the characteristics at each stage:

(1) CONCERNS relevant to the stage?
(2) WHO should address the concerns?
(3) WHAT DECISIONS can be made?

A TONGUE-IN-CHEEK TEST OF REALITY

ANXIETY ATTACKS CAN ARISE WHEN . . .

(rate each of the following on a 0–10 scale, with 0 = No Problem in Your Program, 5 = Some Concern But We Can Cover Ourselves, and 10 = Oh, My God!)

____ a) New funding sources start, old sources cut back, and the same clients are coming to your door.

____ b) Major intake and service planning decisions are being made by the receptionist, and by an intake worker fresh out of undergraduate school, both with little training or supervision.

____ c) The service planning process for some clients involves up to ten staff before formal treatment begins.

____ d) 70% of your staff have less than three years of supervised clinical experience and require more supervision and review of their clinical efforts—but where are the supervisory resources to come from?

e) Treatment planning and review process are the same for:

____ Suicidal and mid-life crisis patients

____ Families with child abuse and those with life adjustment reactions

f) Clinical staff have different frames of reference, standards, and service planning decisions for:

____ Preserving or dissolving a marriage

____ Recommending an abortion as a therapeutic solution to a crisis

____ The relationship of being "capable of working" and "actually employed" to the definition of role functioning

____ Medication usage

( ) TOTAL SCORE

SCORING KEY

0–30	30–60	60–100
10 20 30	40 50 60	70 80 90 100
YOU ARE GREAT! OR YOU'RE NOT FACING REALITY,	NEED SOME WORK OR PARTIAL REALITY FACED,	OH, MY GOD! OR WELCOME TO REALITY!

These four stages and three characteristics provide an outline for designing the clinical process and setting procedures and standards for clinical practice and program service goals.

Examine Table 1 to see how the four stages and three characteristics come together. Reading the cell entries from left to right produces an outline of the major issues, persons involved, and their decisions for each of the four clinical processes. After reading Table 1, answer the three following questions:

(1) Is the general outline in Table 1 a basis for
   (a) A procedures manual (Yes or No and Why?) ______
   (b) Staff training guide (Yes or No and Why?) ______
   (c) Setting standards for policy or regulations (Yes, or No and Why?) ______

Table 1. A General Outline for Designing Clinical Process, Procedures and Standards

Stage of Process	Characteristics at Each Stage		
	Concerns?	Who?	Decisions?
ENTRY Who is the client? Is the client at the right place?	Age, Family, Address? Major problems and supports?	Client/Family Receptionist Intake Worker (Crisis team on call)	Appropriate client here? Immediate action? Refer elsewhere? Regular intake?
SERVICE PLANNING What are the issues? What events are to happen?	Problems and supports? Goals? Expense? Potential income?	Client/Family Therapist/Case Manager Supervisor or Treatment Team Fiscal/Billing	Problems to be treated? Activities which may produce goals? Services providing the activities? Review strategy of what, why, who, and when?
REVIEW Are events occuring as planned? What changes are needed?	Problems and supports? Efforts, progress, and goals? Expense and income?	Client/Family Therapist/Case Manager Supervisor or Treatment Team Fiscal/Billing	Are changes in service plan needed? If so, what change? Have standards been met?
TERMINATION AND FOLLOWUP Were goals met? Is followup required?	Problems and supports? Efforts, progress, and goals? Expense and income? Client/consumer satisfaction?	Client/Family Therapist/Case Manager Supervisor or Treatment Team Fiscal/Billing	Is referral needed? Is followup needed? —Clinically? —Fiscally/bills? If so, when and how?

(2) Does the general outline of all entries change according to different client characteristics, e.g., age, level of risk to self and others, family or social supports, willingness to participate in treatment, etc.?
(Yes or No and Why?) ______________________

(3) Are the criteria for making the decisions clear? (Yes or No and Why?) ______________

____

Recommended answers are:

(1) The outline is not quite complete. While the example provides a good general framework, the outline should be individually tailored to suit your program, your program's service goals, and your clients/consumers.

(2) Yes; the outline does change according to major client characteristics. Major groups of clients for whom the clinical process is similar should be identified as distinct groups:
— For children and youth, categories by levels of family and social support
— For adults, example categories could be
  Type of commitment and cooperation
  Level of family/social support

Level of risk to self and others
Goals of sustenance or growth

(3) No; decision criteria should be specified if the outline is a basis for staff training, supervision, and justification to funding and accreditation agencies.

Table 1 can serve as a guide to document the major components of the clinical process. Potential products include:

— *A basis for staff training and supervision:* Usually between 60% and 80% of service program staff have less than 3 years of supervised clinical experience and suffer from insufficient experience about the major concerns and decisions in the wide variety of circumstances.
— *A set of clinical practice standards to align program goals:* Service staff should have a clear idea of the relationships between service activities and the program's goals. Without drawing this connection for staff, their job descriptions, service activities, and outcomes will not necessarily relate to program goals.
— *Descriptive evidence of service activities and standards for funding sources and accreditation agencies:* In an era of tight money, funding and licensing agencies want to have visible evidence of program procedures and standards.
— *The data base for information system development and program evaluation procedures:* When Table 1 is clearly developed, an information system specialist and a program evaluator can help set up a clinical record and information system as well as provide program cost outcome evaluations.

WHAT IS A STANDARD AND A CLINICAL POLICY?

The procedure outlined develops standards relating clinical practice activities to program goals and, in effect, sets clinical policies.

Will these standards serve as a basis for meeting the standards set by funding and accreditation agencies? Yes! The process has been the basis for the development of standards in many accreditation agencies since it is a systems approach of relating service activities and program goals.

Return to the outline (Table 1) and see how explicit standards can be developed:

CONCERNS focuses on the general issue requiring a standard.
WHO focuses on who should be involved; what qualifications they should have; the lines of responsibility and authority; the needed training, supervision, and review processes.
DECISIONS focuses on the information to be considered in making decisions, e.g., immediate emergency or regular intake procedures.

Policies on standards and clinical procedure assure alignment with program goals. The most important product in using Table 1 could be a set of clinical standards and policies, aligned with program goals, to serve as a basis for staff training and supervision as well as program evaluation.

THE PRODUCTS OF SECTION II

The answers generated in Section II and in the Section IV on management will structure the clinical records, fiscal data, and the information system for an integrated clinical and fiscal management system. Section II provides an outline for establishing and reviewing clinical standards as well as providing the basis for clinical supervision and staff development. With this outline, foundation program analysis and planning can be evaluated by costs and outcomes. Finally, Section II provides a basis for relating the clinical process to the standards and regulations imposed by funding and accreditation agencies.

Beware: Consciousness can induce anxiety attacks! When describing the details of your program's clinical processes as prescribed in Section 1, you may realize there is discontinuity of care or poor communication among clients and staff. If this happens, use the exercises to diagnose the problems and to create a better system. If your clinical procedures are in good order, then the exercises will be helpful later in understanding how the clinical and fiscal procedures can be integrated.

Documenting the Clinical Process

At each of the four stages of the clinical process the objective is to diagram the CONCERNS of the client, WHO addresses these concerns, and their DECISION ALTERNATIVES. Diagramming the flow of the process (a "flow diagram") may appear awkward at first. Use stick figures rather than the formal, systems flowcharting approach to symbolize the people involved in the therapeutic process. Experience using stick figures as a preliminary step in designing the clinical intervention system has helped many programs save dollars and avoid clinical disaster. The simplicity of stick figures helps service staff understand the overall process, clinical standards, and encourages them to contribute ideas for better ways to design the system and improve current standards. The technique helps focus on the human interactions necessary for the therapeutic process to have impact on the client's concerns instead of just documenting the paper and forms flow.

The formal systems approach, appropriate when designing the clinical record and information systems, should wait until after documenting the clinical concerns, human interactions, and decisions necessary for the therapeutic process.

A Hint for Self-Study—Do Not Bog Down!

Because Section II is so basic to the entire client-oriented system, it is necessarily thorough and rather lengthy. Do not become bogged down in detail. Remember, the goal as a program director is to oversee the development of the design of a service system. You are not trying to design it yourself. To assist you in your self-learning experience, each of the next 5 chapters is organized on 2 levels.

The first level is geared toward your self-study of the concepts. The second level provides recommendations for general implementation of the concepts in your service program. Brief outlines are provided to describe how you might organize an implementation strategy. Don't get bogged down on your first pass through Section II. Only work each exercise until you see how the entire developmental process evolves and then move on.

Chapter 4
Client Entry Process and Admission Criteria

> Who Is the Client?
> Is the Client at the Right Place?

Four critical questions are addressed in the design of the client entry process: (a) Who is the client? (b) Is the client at the right place? (c) Who asks these questions? (d) What decisions should they make? The three principal objectives of Chapter 4 are to:

— identify the steps involved in the client entry process;
— identify how information is provided and collected to decide if the program (or some other program) is suitable to the person's needs;
— assess the adequacy of and refine the entry process.

Two major products of Chapter 4 will be the establishment of *Admission Criteria* and *Admission Review Procedures* to assure the initial intake continuity and quality of care.

Chapter 4 outlines the major concerns to be documented and reviewed routinely in the design and management of the client entry process. Most service programs have more than one or two points of entry. Moreover, each point of entry requires a different set of concerns and procedures. The steps in identifying the concerns for each type of entry should, however, fall within the following outline:

(1) WHO is the first staff person a client would contact?
(2) WHAT information is gathered at that time?
(3) WHAT decisions are to be made by this person?
(4) WHO works with the client to identify:
    (a) Demographic information?
    (b) Problems and supports?
    (c) Goals?
(5) WHAT decisions does the person in 4, above, need to make?
(6) WHAT are the terminal (final) points of the entry process?

At initial contact (often by phone), all information is preliminary and the primary tasks are information collection and some client ventilation. Sufficient data should be collected to determine if the person is an appropriate client for the program or should be referred to another agency.

AN EXAMPLE OF CLIENT ENTRY

To illustrate the approach, review the example client entry process in Table 1 and the "flow diagram" in Figure 1. Assure an understanding by answering the questions in the Self-Study on Client Entry 1.

Self-Study on Client Entry 1

(1) To whom does the client talk initially ______________________________?

(2) What is discussed ______________________________
______________________________?

Table 1. Example of Client Entry: Who Is the Client? Is the Client at the Right Place?

Category of Client: Walk-In Adults, Mid- and Upper Level of Functioning			
	Concerns	Who	Decisions
CLINICAL	Wants attention as client?	Client and receptionist	If mid-level functioning, explain intake process? If low functioning, call Intake Worker immediately
	Basic demographics? Present problems and supports? What does client expect to happen with service? Health review? Prior psychiatric history?	Client and intake worker on call	Appropriate client, or refer elsewhere? Type of intake process, e.g., —Short term ventilation and then release —Schedule service planning appointment —Immediate therapy and service planning
ADMINISTRATIVE	Detailed information	Client and receptionist or intake worker	Do we have the information needed for the prescribed decisions given above?
	Financial information	Client and fiscal officer or intake worker on call	Do we have the data needed to determine first and third party liability?

SUPERVISION RESPONSIBILITY: Adult outpatient supervisor and outpatient unit director are to assure that the staff involved here understand the process, the information needed, and the criteria for making decisions. This is to be accomplished by staff training and review of a random sample of cases.

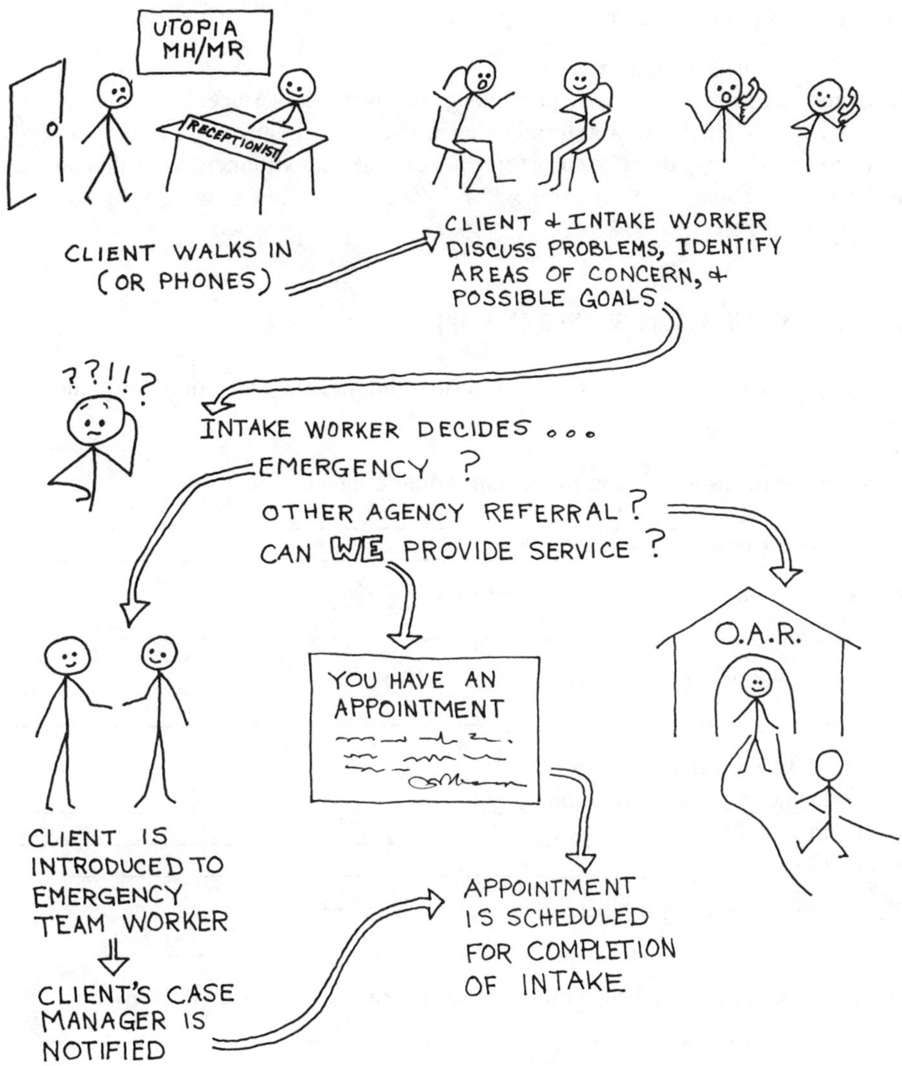
UTOPIA MH/MR
RECEPTIONIST
CLIENT WALKS IN (OR PHONES)
CLIENT & INTAKE WORKER DISCUSS PROBLEMS, IDENTIFY AREAS OF CONCERN, & POSSIBLE GOALS
??!!?
INTAKE WORKER DECIDES ...
EMERGENCY ?
OTHER AGENCY REFERRAL ?
CAN WE PROVIDE SERVICE ?
O.A.R.
YOU HAVE AN APPOINTMENT
CLIENT IS INTRODUCED TO EMERGENCY TEAM WORKER
CLIENT'S CASE MANAGER IS NOTIFIED
APPOINTMENT IS SCHEDULED FOR COMPLETION OF INTAKE

Figure 1. Client Entry

(3) What questions are asked ______________________________ ?

(4) What decisions are made? ______________________________ ?

(5) What are the terminal (final) points of the process ____________________ ?

(6) What issues do you feel are not addressed in the flow diagram ________________ ?

Answers to Self-Study Guide 1

(1) Receptionist and then intake worker.
(2) Problems, resources, supports, possible goals, possible services.
(3) Emergency? Other Agency Referral? Can we service client?
(4) Refer to emergency, other agency referral, or make appointment with this agency.
(5) See item #4, above.
(6) Your opinion here!

DEVELOPING YOUR OWN SIMPLE EXAMPLE

Consider your *most typical client* and describe the process by addressing the following questions:

(1) WHO is the first staff person this client would contact
—by phone ____?
—by walking into agency ________________________________?

(2) WHAT information is gathered at that time ________________________
____?

(3) WHAT decisions are to be made by this staff person ____________________
____?

(4) WHO works with the client to identify:
(4.1) Demographic information ______________________________?
(4.2) Problems ____?
(4.3) Goals ____?

(5) WHAT decisions does the person in 4 above need to make at this time? __________
____?

(6) What are the terminal (final) points of the Information and Referral Process ________
____?

(7) Now create a flow diagram to describe your intake process for your most typical clients.

After developing your own example, ask the following questions dealing with staff training, reviewing, and assignment.

(1) Were the staff involved in the Entry Process of limited professional training? If so, what training and supervision ought to be provided for these people? __________________
____

(2) What decisions ought to be routinely reviewed, by whom, and in what manner? ______
____

(3) What staff ought to be assigned to develop the Entry Process for all of the major points of entry? ____
____

Finally, you need to decide whether there are other categories of client entry which require a different set of concerns and decisions. Examples are voluntary/involuntary, English/ non-English speaking, etc.

PROGRAM IMPLEMENTATION STRATEGIES: DEVELOPING ADMISSIONS CRITERIA AND ADMISSIONS CERTIFICATION REVIEW PROCEDURES

After describing the client entry for the most typical clients, and after identifying other categories of client entry, responsibility can be delegated for designing the entry process for each category of clients. Consider assigning two-person teams to draft procedures for each of the major categories of client entry, using the previous outline. The two-person teams ought to consist of one experienced and one inexperienced staff member. The presence of the inexperienced staff person assures the wording is clear enough to be used in staff training and supervision.

Place the procedures developed by the two-person teams together in a training package which identifies role assignments for all staff involved in the client entry process. Specifically, each person should have a written list of

— Questions to be addressed
— Possible responses by clients
— Decision alternatives to be taken independently, and those requiring consultation
— Criteria for selecting among decision alternatives

The written list can become a basis for the program's *admission criteria* required by many third-party payors and regulatory agencies. Moreover, systematically reviewing the intake process, e.g., by a review of a random sample of cases, meets part of the requirement for admissions certification review often required by accreditation and regulatory agencies.

Chapter 5
Service Planning

What Are the Issues? What Events Are to Happen?

The service or treatment plan serves several functions. In its formulation, it assists the client and the service (treatment) staff in deciding upon the client's problems, strengths, supports, possible goals, and what can reasonably be done given available resources. The development of a plan, when coupled with either clinical supervisory procedures or treatment team planning, is also a training device for senior staff to help less experienced staff understand the appropriate concerns and decisions suitable for a type of client. Moreover, the establishment of the service plan also establishes what clinical resources (and costs) are to be allocated to assist the client in moving toward the agreed upon goals. Finally, the service plan will suggest what review procedures appear to be most appropriate for the client. This will minimize the risks of clinical mishap or the risk of providing too much or too expensive a service effort.

Chapter 5 focuses on three objectives of the service (treatment) plan. First is identifying the categories of clients requiring unique concerns and decision alternatives in the service planning process. Second is identifying the CONCERNS of the client, WHO will address those concerns, and their DECISION ALTERNATIVES for each category of service planning. Third is identifying supervisory and review responsibilities in the service planning process.

Chapter 5 is divided into five sections:

(1) IDENTIFYING UNIQUE CLIENT CATEGORIES WITHIN CLIENT TARGET POPULATIONS discusses how service plans need to be tailored to the unique concerns of clients.
(2) CREATING SERVICE PLANNING CATEGORIES discusses how to proceed in creating a category system.
(3) DEVELOPING A SERVICE PLAN OUTLINE reviews a service (treatment) plan through a self-study exercise.
(4) DESIGNING SERVICE PLANS provides an outline for developing customized service plan procedures.
(5) IMPLEMENTATION STRATEGY offers suggestions on how to install service planning.

1. IDENTIFYING UNIQUE CLIENT CATEGORIES WITHIN CLIENT TARGET POPULATIONS

Why identify the unique client groups within each target population for service planning? Treatment plans and review procedures for families involved in child abuse should be different from those for clients with life-adjustment reactions. It is not sufficient to simply identify the client as belonging to the child target population. Distinct client groups and their unique lifestyle and roles will affect their plan of service. Staff must understand (for clinical and fiscal reasons) the need to address two issues: What unique clinical concerns are represented by the clients in each target group? What different sets of service standards should be identified?

But how many unique client groups are there? Too many or too few groups of clients lead to chaos. The major demographic and clinical characteristics for a group of clients need to be established if a unique set of therapeutic or service standards is planned. Some programs will be satisfied by using diagnostic categories. Others might require that other client characteristics ought to be considered. Consider two examples of adult mental-health clients. The first example is shown in Figure 1 where the characteristics distinguishing the client category are delineated by three factors: (a) level of role performance or problem severity; (b) level of family or

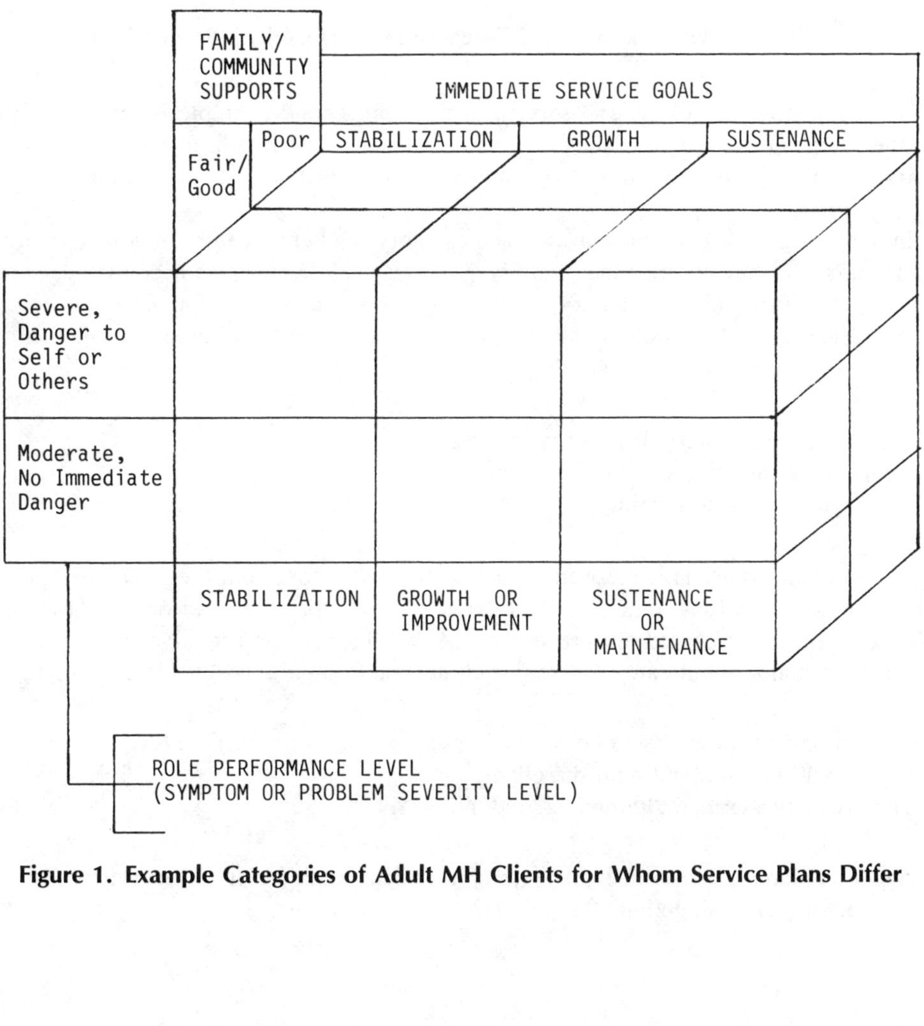

Figure 1. Example Categories of Adult MH Clients for Whom Service Plans Differ

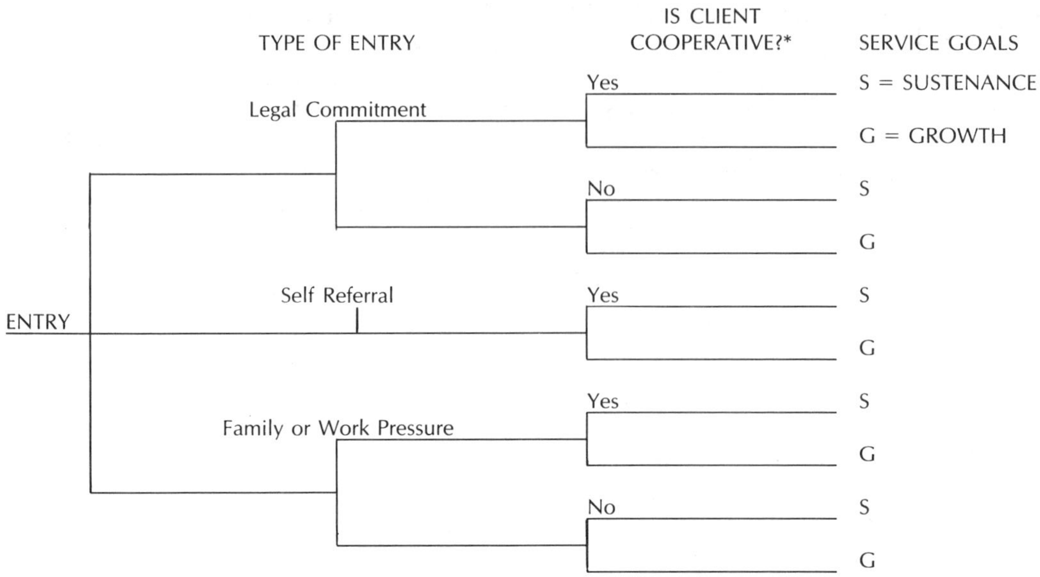

*Other variables can be substituted here, e.g., Prior Hospitalization History or Family/Community Supports.

Figure 2. Example of Client Categories Described by a Branch Diagram

community support; and (c) general service goals. The second example is given in Figure 2 where the characteristics of the client categories are developed in a branching tree process by method of entry (e.g., legal or voluntary commitment), level of client cooperation, and service goals.

In reviewing these examples, ask if each category of clients requires unique concerns and use of resources. If they do, then the category system is useful. Thus, we need to understand the criteria for identifying client category because these criteria will set the stage for admission standards. The principal consideration for establishing the major target groups is whether clients in a particular group would have similar

— Behavior patterns and vulnerability to stress,
— Family or community supports,
— Patterns of service utilization.

If a group of clients does have these three characteristics in common, then treatment planning, case-management activities, quality assurance, and utilization review efforts can be planned, coordinated, and implemented uniformly for better efficiency and effectiveness.

For each major client category, senior clinical staff should establish standards for

— The appropriate questions to be raised,
— Who should be involved with the client,
— What available service alternatives may be useful.

Once these standards are established, there is a clinical basis for staff supervision as well as program planning and budgeting.

2. CREATING SERVICE PLANNING CATEGORIES

Consider a familiar target group of clients, e.g., children, or adult aftercare. Think of one or two *client categories* identifying unique categories of service planning. Each category of client should require a unique consideration in the service planning and implementation process. The primary objective is to create a set of categories that focuses attention on the critical and unique issues needed to help the client with a good service plan, and that provides a guide for staff training and supervision.

In creating a set of client categories two cautions should be noted. First, if there are too many categories, both staff and clients will be confused. Moreover, these will be too difficult and time consuming to develop. Second, too few categories will gloss over the unique concerns of individual clients, thereby raising the risk of clinical mishap or of providing overly expensive services. Between three and twelve categories will suffice for any overall target population, e.g., adults. One final note of caution: do not allow the set of categories to become pigeonholes, where staff treat clients with prescribed solutions. As with any system created for efficiency and effectiveness, it should free staff to focus their attention on the more unique characteristics of the client rather than restrict their view. The set of categories should be considered as guidelines for the development of a service plan, rather than a firm set of rules.

Self-Study on Categories of Clinical and Service Concerns

Task 1. Create a small set of categories for a target group with whom you are most familiar.

Task 2. For at least three of the categories, use Table 1 to identify the unique characteristics of the categories.

Hints

In addition to the categories recommended in Figures 1 and 2, other categories have been designated by:

— Level of affect in a partial hospitalization program, e.g., flat vs. active affect.
— Expected length of service durations in an outpatient setting, e.g.,

Table 1. Outline for Creating Categories of Concern

	Unique Characteristics in One or More Areas:		
Category	Behavior Patterns or Vulnerability to Stress	Family or Community Supports	Patterns of Service Utilization

- Short term, less than 6 to 8 visits
- Long term, more than 6 visits but less than 6 months
- Extended care, more than 6 months.

Once the categories are outlined, the next step is to develop a service planning guide for each category.

3. DEVELOPING A SERVICE PLAN OUTLINE

A service or treatment plan is a reflection of the clinical decision process, i.e., the clinical issues raised and the clinical decisions made. Below is a brief outline identifying the principal clinical issues and decisions.

Issues Raised		Decisions Made
Who is the client and What are the issues?	(1)	With the client or significant other, the clinician or a clinical team identifies: —Problems or skill deficits —Strengths, resources, and support systems
What is to happen?	(2)	Set immediate and long-term goals, identified by problem or groups of problems
	(3)	Design an array of service activities which are: —Goal directed and time limited —Optimize the use of the client's strengths and resources
What services?	(4)	Arrange or contract for personnel or agencies to: Provide (3), the activities, in order to Achieve (2), the goals, to Impact (1), the problems.
How to review to see if the plan is working?	(5)	Describe a review strategy for this client which will minimize the risk of the client not achieving the goals, and will minimize the costs of service efforts.

Three subtle features within the outline deserve further discussion.

ISSUE: How firmly set are the problems and goals at the time of intake?

REPLY: Do not carve a treatment plan in stone. The clinical process is an evolving insight process, unfolding over the course of the therapeutic process. A review strategy should be built into the treatment plan where, at least, the client and principal therapist or treatment team will pause to reflect on "problems, skill deficits, strengths, resources, and goals." More detailed discussion on establishing a review strategy is provided below and in Chapter 6.

ISSUE: Why are separate decisions made for service activity (3) and for service provider (4)?

REPLY: Separate decisions are needed to assure the services are the most appropriate provider of the intended therapeutic activity. Certainly intensive care is needed for a person with severe depression symptoms. In many cases, inpatient care is the best service provider. But in some situations, a combination of family support and day treatment services might be better. Or consider the circumstances of moderate distress symptoms exhibited by someone who expresses feelings of inadequacy as a family bread winner, father, or husband. The choice of individual, group, family, and/or some socioeducational services depends on the specific therapeutic experiences (goals and activities) called for in the plan; e.g., to identify why the client feels inadequate, to enhance self esteem, to listen for positive feedback from family and friends, and to help the family provide more positive feedback. Each of these goals and activities might require a different service approach. Separating the decisions of service activity from the service provider helps staff recognize these as two separate issues in the review of client progress and of service utilization.

ISSUE: Why set a review strategy as part of the treatment plan? Shouldn't review be by some time limit (e.g., every 30 or 90 days), or by a sampling procedure? Review efforts are too expensive to do otherwise.

REPLY: Yes, review procedures, as formatted in many places, are expensive and cannot be applied to all clients as a regular part of the treatment plan. Chapter 6 outlines individual client review techniques meeting professional and federal standards and regulations and yet are in the long run cheaper and more effective. Review strategies for an individual client's treatment plan need to identify:

—What risks for the client are built into the treatment plan and what symptoms or signs would indicate that negative things are occurring?
—Who should be involved in identifying signs or symptoms of risk?
—What stressors are in the client's environment and in the treatment plan which may influence distress and/or negative movement?
—When does the client's treatment plan or the client's ordinary life situation provide stressors on the client?

The issue of identifying what stressors are involved, when they might occur, who should be involved in identifying the stressors, and who should be involved in the review needs elaboration. There are four major kinds of stressors:

—Changes in Location—Moving one's place of residence, office, bedroom, etc. In treatment, for example, moving from home to an inpatient ward to home.
—Changes in Vocation or Role—Shifting one's job, job description, role as a spouse, parent, etc. In treatment, for example, counseling is offered to help people change their jobs or to change their role as spouse or parent. Both of these are stressful.
—Changes in Socialization—Making new friends or acquaintances, or changing the rules of interaction among friends or acquaintances.
—Meeting an Expectation—Setting one's own goal(s) or meeting someone else's goal(s).

At least one, if not all four, of these stressors is common to all treatment plans. The essential elements of a review strategy rest in identifying (a) the stressors, (b) their potential risks to the client, (c) who might help recognize whether the negative impact of these stressors has occurred, and when they are likely to occur. Usually, these issues are raised during the course of the treatment planning and therapeutic process. These features should be identified as part of a review strategy individualized for the client's problems, supports, goals, and service plan. Moreover, the people involved in the individualized review strategy are the client, one or more significant others in the client's life, the therapist, and on occasion, the therapist's supervisor or a knowledgeable colleague. Other types of expensive review procedures are only invoked when:

—Those involved in treatment cannot agree,
—The utilization of available services becomes too expensive,
—The client is deterioriating or not progressing as expected,
—The service utilization or professional standards committees have special studies to be performed.

Self-Study: Developing a Service Plan Outline

Most of these issues of review will be discussed again in Chapter 6, but as a system of review procedures. This Self-Study Exercise on service planning seeks to reinforce critical concepts by reviewing a sample abbreviated service plan.

Review the example of a service plan given in Table 2 and in the flow diagram in Figure 3. It is not a perfectly constructed example. Answer the questions below as a guide for understanding the example along with its good and bad features.

(1) What are the features of the category of concern given in the example?

____

____

(2) Circle the five major elements of the clinical decision process in the example.

Table 2. A Service Planning Outline

CATEGORY OF CLIENT: *ADULT, Mid-Level of Functioning, Some Family/Community Support, Improvement Expected within 6 Months*

	Concerns	Who	Decisions
CLINICAL	Ventilation Problems, Resources & Supports? Possible Goals: Short/Long Term? Possible Service Activities? Possible Service Providers? Possible Review Strategy: What, Why, When, & Who? Client Rights	Client Client's Family or Friends Clinician or Caseworker Treatment Team —Supervisor —Medical —Social Service	Problem to be treated Setting goals Aligning services to activities, resources & goals Setting review strategy: What, Why, When, & Who?
ADMINISTRATIVE	Reimbursement Sources Legal Documentation Required Forms and Documentation	Financial Liability Staff Medical Records Staff	Which 1st and 3rd party payors? Billing procedures & followup strategies? Clinical Record format? Means of coordinating records among service providers & resources?

SUPERVISORY RESPONSIBILITIES (WHO & WHAT): Target/Category group supervisor: (a) Develops service plan outline, (b) Sees that staff are trained in its use, (c) Designs treatment team responsibilities, and (d) Coordinates with fiscal and clinical records staff.

(3) Is it likely there may be a difference between problems identified and problems to be treated? (YES or NO and WHY) ____________________

____

____

(4) Notice that the example separately considers service activities from service providers. This approach suggests that the clinician or clinical team considers alternative service approaches in providing a therapeutic activity. As an example, developing social interactions with mutual positive reinforcement may be a goal with the activity of structured or guided social interactions. Now identify at least three types of services to provide these activities.

____

____

____

____

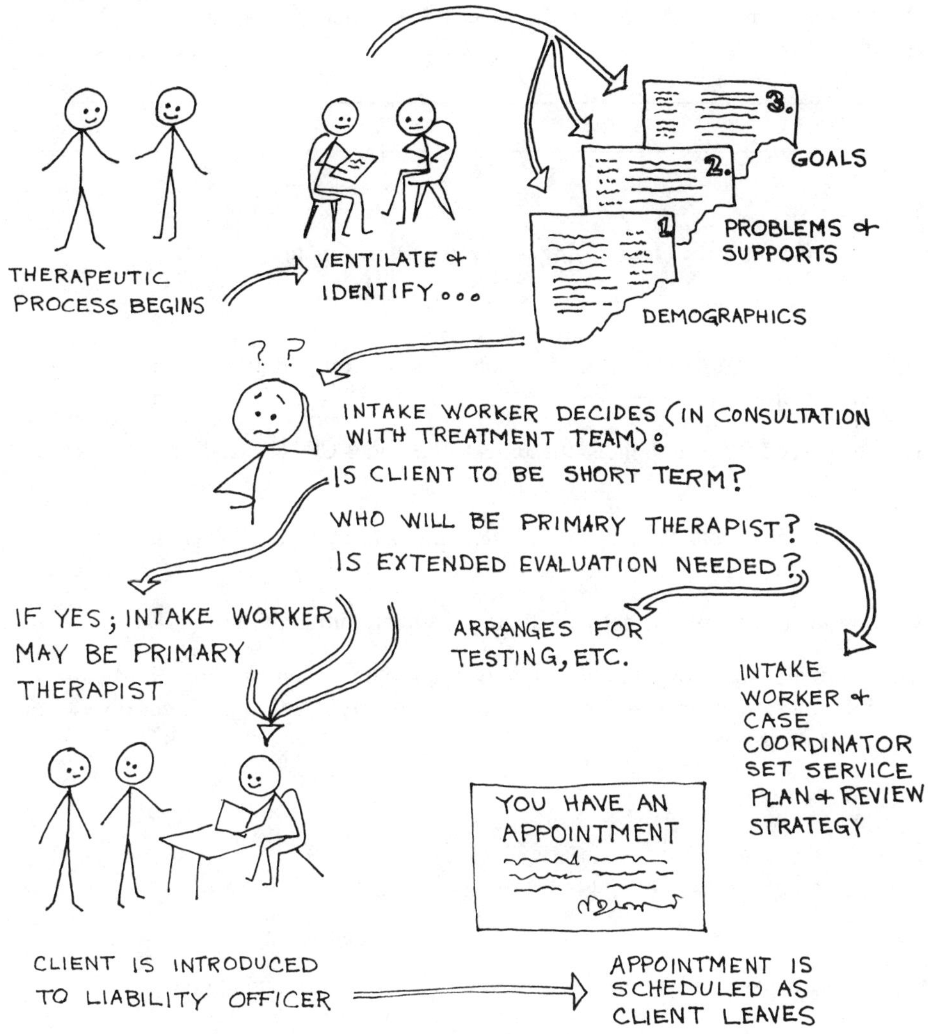
THERAPEUTIC PROCESS BEGINS
VENTILATE + IDENTIFY ...
3.
GOALS
2.
PROBLEMS + SUPPORTS
1
DEMOGRAPHICS
? ?
INTAKE WORKER DECIDES (IN CONSULTATION WITH TREATMENT TEAM):
IS CLIENT TO BE SHORT TERM?
WHO WILL BE PRIMARY THERAPIST?
IS EXTENDED EVALUATION NEEDED?
IF YES; INTAKE WORKER MAY BE PRIMARY THERAPIST
ARRANGES FOR TESTING, ETC.
INTAKE WORKER + CASE COORDINATOR SET SERVICE PLAN + REVIEW STRATEGY
YOU HAVE AN APPOINTMENT
CLIENT IS INTRODUCED TO LIABILITY OFFICER
APPOINTMENT IS SCHEDULED AS CLIENT LEAVES

Figure 3. Service Planning Flow Diagram

(5) Why would you want to have staff distinguish between therapeutic activity and service provider? ______________________________

____

____

(6) Review the supervisory responsibilities. Can you suggest any additional responsibilities?

____

(7) What experience and training would you expect of a supervisor who has these responsibilities? ______________________________

____

(8) Who has what responsibilities in the process? Are there any apparent overlaps or gaps in responsibilities? ____

____

____

Answers to Self-Study on Developing a Service Plan Outline

(1) Adult, mid-level functioning clients, some family/community support, improvement expected in 6 months.

(2) Circle the second through the sixth items listed under CONCERNS in the example as well as all of the clinical DECISIONS.

(3) Yes. Some problems clear up by our dealing with other problems and some we cannot handle.

(4) Group therapy, family or network therapy, social club activities.

(5) To avoid pigeonholing clients, "given X problem, then provide X treatment." It is possible that less restrictive or more "in community" activities might do as well if not better than our services.

(6–8) Your opinion here

4. DESIGNING SERVICE PLANS

Table 3 (see next page) offers an illustrative outline for service planning.

5. IMPLEMENTATION STRATEGY

The strategy here parallels that of Chapter 4. Start small, involving a few supervisors who appear receptive to developing categories of concern and service plans. Then proceed as suggested earlier, i.e.,

(1) Hold a meeting to review the unit and self-study efforts.
(2) Assign two-person teams to work up category systems and service plan outlines.
(3) Develop a consensus on a set of categories for one service program, working with one target group. Then, develop a working draft of service outlines for each category, using the steps described in this unit.
(4) Pilot test the service plan outlines for a 3- to 6-month period.
(5) Evaluate the pilot test and revise as necessary.

Table 3. Sample Outline for Service Planning

CATEGORY OF CONCERN ______________________________

	Concerns	Who	Decisions
C L I N I C A L			
A D M I N I S T R A T I V E			

SUPERVISORY RESPONSIBILITIES (WHO & WHAT?) ______________________________
____
____

IDENTIFY: POTENTIAL OVERLAPS AND GAPS IN RESPONSIBILITIES, CONCERNS AND DECISIONS
____
____

CREATE A FLOW DIAGRAM TO SHOW HOW CLIENT AND STAFF INTERACT IN THE SERVICE PLANNING PROCESS.

Chapter 6
Review and Quality Assurance Procedures

> Are Events Occurring as Planned?
> Are Changes Needed?

The saying "If it ain't broke, don't fix it! If it is, do it now!" is a good operating philosophy. The service or treatment plans in a client-oriented system include a review strategy for each individual client. But the system of review must be client oriented, practical, and cost effective. Skills in designing review systems can be enhanced by critiquing sample systems to see how well they focus attention and correction efforts on client problems of:

— High client risk, i.e., not attaining planned goals;
— High service expense, i.e., requiring more service effort than anticipated;
— Uncertainty, i.e., difficulty defining what are the problems, supports, goals or what are the proper activities, services, or review strategies.

The review procedures described in this chapter have the critical features of being both practical and cost effective, and have been demonstrated to work in a number of different circumstances.

1. THE BASIC CONCEPTS

Definitions

Quality Assurance. The process for systematically reviewing and deciding whether the prescribed services have been helping the client achieve planned goals, or have had impact on the client's problems and circumstances. Less formally, were the clinical decisions made during treatment planning, or during prior review, correct?

There are two focuses to our discussion on progress review and quality assurance. The review procedures should be both individualized to suit the client and cost efficient and effective. The line of discussion will retain the client focus, but will also consider the practical costs and standards set by the major regulatory agencies, e.g., National Institute for Mental Health (NIMH) prior to 1981, Professional Standards Review Organization (PSRO), and the Joint

Table 1. Quality Assurance Process Requirements*

Processes/Requirements For:	NIMH O/P	NIMH I/P	PSRO O/P	PSRO I/P	JCAH O/P	JCAH I/P
UTILIZATION REVIEW	y	y				
admissions certification	?	?	p	y	p	n
continued stay review	?	?	p	y	p	n
concurrent review	?	?	p	p	y	n
PEER REVIEW	y	y	p	y	y	n
CLINICAL CARE EVALUATION STUDIES	y	y	p	y		
retrospective chart audits					y	y
PROFILE MONITORING	n	n	p	y/?	p	p

KEY: O/P = Outpatient, I/P = Inpatient, y = yes, n = no, p = probable, ? = not directly specified as mandatory process/procedure, y/? = yes, but not until some later date

*Developed by Paul Sherman, Ravenswood Hospital CMHC, Chicago, IL, 1978.

Commission on Hospital Accreditation (JCAH). Focusing on the client and the client's risks, service expense, and unresolved issues (puzzles) produces a cost effective means of meeting the recommendations and standards set forth by NIMH, PSRO, and JCAH. A more detailed outline of the standards required by these three agencies is given in Table 1.

2. INDIVIDUALIZED REVIEW STRATEGIES

The plan for reviewing each client's progress should be an integral part of the original treatment plan. The review strategy should specify the four distinct features for each client; i.e., what, why, when, and who. If possible, it should be done with the client, or at least with a supervisor or treatment team. In general, these four review features will be similar for most clients within each major client category and service plan. The four common features of a review strategy are:

WHAT? Aspects of clinical decisions in the treatment plan which should be reviewed, i.e., what changes, if any, are apparent for

① Problems, family, and community supports
"Who is the client and what are the issues?"

② Goals (short and long term)
"What are the desired outcomes?"

③ What Activities —purpose→ ② Goals —impact→ ① Problems?

④ What Services ⟶ ③ ⟶ ② ⟶ ① ?

⑤ What Future Strategy for reviewing ④, ③, ②, and ①?

WHY? To identify instances of high client risk or service expense relative to planned outcomes. (A corollary reason is to identify and compare with successful instances.)

WHEN? At times when the client's treatment plan or life situation places the client under stress, i.e.,
—Changes in Location, Vocation (Role), Socialization
—Meeting Expectations
These stressors will typically show whether treatment plan decisions were proper or not. Thus, reviewing at times of stress will be sensitive to client needs and risks.

WHO? By two and, at times, three people or groups in sequence, on an as-needed basis. Note the qualifier "on an as-needed basis." In general, involve others (thereby adding costs) only if necessary. Another issue, discussed later, is when, why, and how to involve others. The three sequential levels of review are:

① Client and/or significant other, and principal therapist review progress relative to their latest perception of circumstances, problems, goals, and resources.

② Appropriate others, familiar with that category of client, assess progress relative to their own experiences. The appropriate other is someone who is familiar with this type of case and the criteria of high risk and expense.

③ Committee or Supervisor reviews if:
  (3a) The three people in ① and ②, above, seek advice or do not agree
  (3b) Random sample of those cases where there was agreement in Steps ① and ②

3. COST EFFICIENCY-EFFECTIVENESS AND SERVICE REVIEW MANAGEMENT BY EXCEPTION

When initially designing a review strategy, there is a temptation to be expedient. What may be expedient in the short run, however, may be expensive in the long run and vice versa.

Short-Run Cheap and Long-Run Expensive: Two Questionable Review Strategies

Close the Barn Door. No reviews planned, just review when the client is in crisis or the budget limits services. This usually results in both high client risk and excessive service expense for crisis intervention.

By the Numbers. Review on a fixed time schedule (every 30, 60, or 90 days) independent of client problems, supports, goals, and stressors; and independent of budgetary circumstances. Problems of high risk or expense may be missed, or unneeded time is spent in review. In both cases the expenses of review and/or crisis intervention are high.

Short-Run Expensive and Long-Run Cheap: Better Strategies

— Have clinical supervisors (with select staff): (a) develop review strategy standards for each major category of concern, and (b) specify guidelines and criteria for high risk and expense.

— Have staff set individualized review strategies for each client which are
(a) sensitive to that client's individual circumstances and stressors,

(b) sensitive to the established criteria of high risk and expense, and
(c) involve the fewest people possible for that category of case.

— The Quality Assurance Committee should only provide indepth review on
(a) the exceptional problem cases or
(b) a random sample of approved cases stratified by category of concern and therapist.

Self-Study Exercise on Basic Concepts

Because the concepts underlying a client-oriented review system are sufficiently different from many other approaches, there may be benefit in reviewing these concepts by means of an exercise. The answers are provided at the end of the exercise.

(1) Define "Quality Assurance." ____________________
____
____

(2) What are the two focuses of a client-oriented progress review process?
(1) ____________________
(2) ____________________

(3) What is meant by:
"High Risk?" ____________________
____
"High Expense?" ____________________
____

(4) WHEN TO REVIEW? An individualized review strategy is described by stressors which either occur in a person's life or are built into the service plan. For each of the four major types of stressors, give one example of how such a stressor might occur in a treatment plan.
Change in Location ____________________
____
Change in Role or Vocation ____________________
____
Change in Socialization ____________________
____
Meeting an Expectation ____________________
____

(5) Give examples to describe why each of the two following review strategies is questionable in terms of long-run expense.
By the Numbers ____________________
____
____
Close the Barn Door ____________________
____
____

(6) What are the key responsibilities of staff and supervisors in developing cost effective review strategies?

Clinical Supervisors should
(a) ____________________
(b) ____________________
Staff should
(a) ____________________
(b) ____________________

(7) If proper review strategies and criteria are developed, then what is the basis for
(a) Selecting the appropriate other? ____________________
____
____
(b) Referring a case to the quality assurance committee? ____________________
____
____

Answers to Self-Study Exercise on Basic Concepts

(1) Are services moving clients toward goals as expected and at what risk and expense?

(2) Individualized and cost effective.

(3) High Risk: Not achieving agreed upon goals.
High Expense: More effort than anticipated.

(4) Location: Move from inpatient to partial or from individual to group.
Role or Vocation: Changing job status or rolc in family from passive to active (as done in assertiveness training or as in directive to nondirective therapy).
Socialization: Who interacts with whom as in group or family therapy.
Expectation: Any behavioral goals or length of treatment expectations.

(5) By the Numbers: Review every 30, 60, or 90 days; Review every 5 or 10 visits.
Close the Barn Door: Review any dropouts and suicide attempts.

(6) Supervisor: (a) Develop and maintain review process
(b) Set criteria for high risk and expense
Staff should be sensitive to:
(a) Individual client's concerns, stressors
(b) Criteria and standards for that category of client
(c) Involving the fewest people possible in the case and still move toward goals.

(7) (a) Select appropriate other by experience and knowledge of that type of case
(b) Only if the people involved in parts 1 and 2 do not agree or by random sampling selections.

4. AN EXAMPLE OF A COST EFFECTIVE REVIEW COMMITTEE—ONE INSTEAD OF FOUR

There are four types of review mechanisms now recommended by professional and government agencies:

— Utilization Review
— Peer Review
— Clinical Care Evaluation Studies
— Profile Monitoring

Table 1 summarizes how these review functions relate to regulations by different organizations. This portion of the chapter describes a system of review originally designed for a rural program with no federal funding. The design has since been implemented in a number of other settings because of its cost efficiency and client focus.

Separate committees for each four types of review mechanism can be costly in both time and effort. Each time a group of 8–10 professionals meets for 1.5 hours to perform any one of these review functions, the expense can run over $1,000 in time cost and professional time taken away from direct client services.

Instead of having separate committees, consider creating a single committee fulfilling all types of review. A typical committee meeting may function as follows:

The primary role of the committee would be to discuss quality of care for the exceptional cases. Specifically:

> *Exceptional Case Quality Assurance*—Discussion on the exceptional cases referred to the committee by the client/therapist/appropriate other.

During such discussion, the meeting is chaired by the chairperson on quality assurance, with notes on this portion of the meeting kept in the Quality Assurance Notebook. But this represents only one objective of the meeting.

When the meeting inevitably digresses toward a discussion of how a particular service provides for a particular category of clients, e.g., partial hospitalization for low role performance sustenance clients, then the group can officially consent to review the utilization of that service for that category of client. Specifically:

> *Utilization Review*—Periodic discussion of a program's service components in terms of the data on types of clients served, amount and costs of services provided, and outcomes.

During the discussion of service utilization, the meeting is turned over temporarily to the utilization review subcommittee chairperson.

When the group reviews the randomly sampled cases, the session then becomes a

> *Peer Review*—if the cases were randomly selected by staff, and if the discussion of each case is led by a professional of the appropriate discipline.

Of course, the standards for the peer review should also meet the standards recommended by the professional disciplines involved. If cases selected in peer review are also judged in terms of the standards and criteria established for each client category, you also have the basis for *Profile Monitoring,* i.e., reviewing cases in light of some standard profile.

Any one of the three review mechanisms can trigger a call for a "clinical care evaluation study." These are special studies requiring either a retrospective audit of clinical records (charts) or a controlled evaluation research study on a specific client group or service unit. According to most regulatory guidelines, at least two clinical care evaluation studies should be performed each year.

If, over the course of a year, all services and all staff are incidentally reviewed in conjunction with the committee's primary focus on the exceptional cases of high risk or expense, a cost-effective review system is in effect. Moreover, the review system covers all required review activities.

But what about the *concurrent review* process? The concurrent review process is built into the first two phases of the review process, i.e., when

(1) The client and principal therapist review and document progress, and
(2) The appropriate other and medical staff review the progress.

if

— The criteria for high risk and expense are clearly stated
— The appropriate other is experienced with that type of case and its risks and expense
— The clinical record system efficiently provides visible evidence of:
  (a) Problems and supports
  (b) Goals
  (c) Activities and services
  (d) Progress

This last feature, the visible evidence, is discussed in Sections III and IV.

The flow diagram in Figure 1 describes the process outlined in the example above. Review the example and then address the questions in the Self-Study Exercise on Cost-Effective Review Committees.

(1) In Figure 1, what required features of the review process are being satisfied? ________

____

(2) Under what three conditions should the appropriate other be able to review 10–20 cases in an hour?
  (a) ______________________________
  ____
  (b) ______________________________
  ____
  (c) ______________________________
  ____

(3) What is the most important function, from the client's point of view, of the review committee? ______________________________

____

____

(4) What four regulatory review requirements are fulfilled by the review committee?
  (1) ______________________________
  (2) ______________________________
  (3) ______________________________
  (4) ______________________________

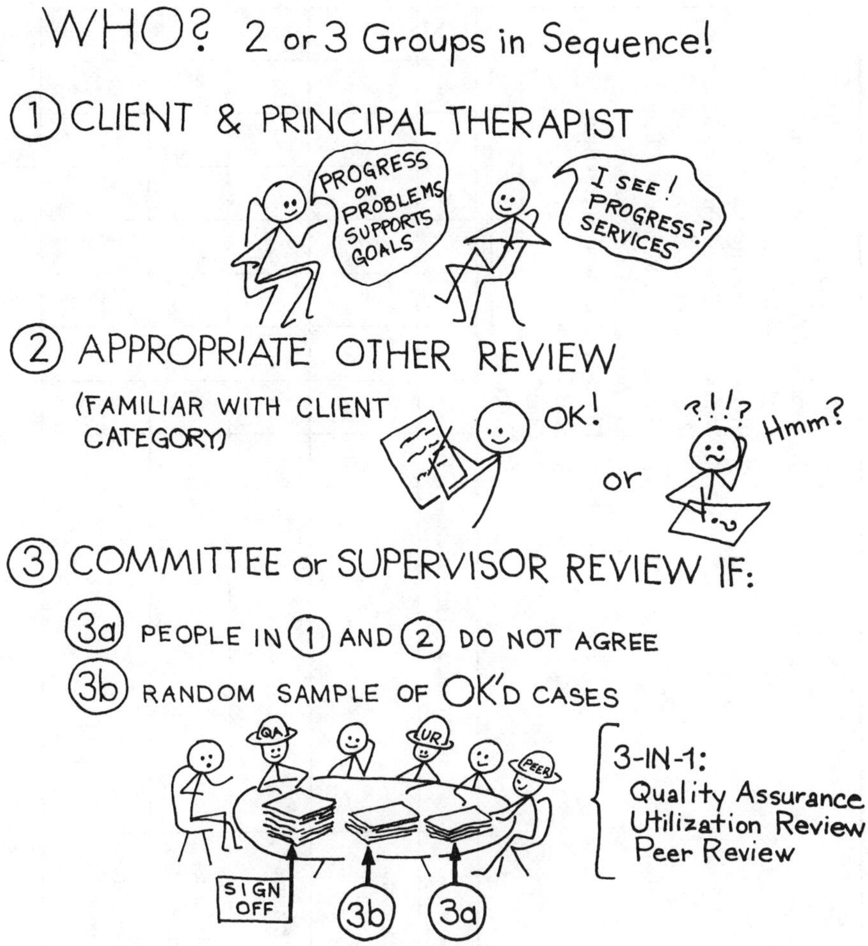

Figure 1. A Sequential Review Procedure Combining Multiple Review Functions in a Cost Effective Fashion

(5) Describe why we might title this example review process "One Out of Four," and in what ways is it cost effective? ______________________________

____

____

____

____

Answers to Self-Study Exercise on Review Committee

(1) Concurrent review, part of peer review, and part of profile monitoring.

(2) (a) Clear criteria for high risk and expense.
(b) Appropriate other has experience with that type of case.
(c) Efficient clinical records system.

Table 2. Defining Review Functions and Roles*

POSSIBLE ROLES AND FUNCTIONS**
1. Treatment Planning with Client
2. Staffing Conference
3. Record Accuracy Review
4. With Client, Review Problems/Resources/Goals, Progress
5. Clinical Record Review of Client's Problems/Resources/Goals/Progess
6. Direct Staff Clinical Supervision
7. Staff Development
8. Other ______
9. Other ______

Title of Role	Textbook Definition	Your Program's Definition	1.	2.	3.	4.	5.	6.	7.	8.	9.
INTAKE WORKER	Clinician making 1st client contact, assists in triage & treatment planning.										
PRINCIPAL THERAPIST	Clinician assigned to set & implement treatment plan.										
TREATMENT TEAM LEADER	Oversees team activities in implementing treatment plan.										
PEER REVIEWER	Clinician in part 2 of review, usually of like training to principal therapist.										
CASE MANAGER	Follows & coordinates execution of treatment plan and review strategy.										

CLIENT ADVOCATE OR OMBUDSMAN	Same as Case Manager, but often independent of service provider.										
TARGET/POPULATION SPECIALIST–REVIEWER	Clinician in part 2 or 3 of review, knowledgeable about client's target group.										
CASE COORDINATOR	Similar to Case Manager, but with power to reallocate staff efforts to clients.										
SUPERVISOR	Similar to Case Coordinator with power to train & direct staff treatment efforts.										
REVIEWING PHYSICIAN	M.D. reviews medical aspects of case, e.g., chemotherapy. Could also be supervisor.										
QUALITY ASSURANCE COMMITTEE	Interdisciplinary team (inc. M.D.) to review all exceptions and random sample of others.										

*Any one staff person can fulfill any one or more roles listed. This is most often an economic necessity.
**POSSIBLE ROLES AND FUNCTIONS

ALL	= All Clients	RAN	= Random Sample of Clients
EXC	= Exceptions	RAN EXC	= Random Sample and Exceptions

(3) Your opinion here, but consider, "Is my therapist using acceptable standards of practice?" and "Am I really getting the best care available?"

(4) Utilization review, peer review, retrospective chart audits for clinical care evaluation studies, and profile monitoring.

(5) See answer to item #4. The single committee serves four committee functions. It is cost effective in that it deals primarily with cases it must deal with to solve tough problems (the exceptions) and also monitors the OK cases.

Self-Study on Creating a Review Strategy

To complete the creation of a personal example of a review strategy, consider using the following outline, using a familiar category of client. If you have difficulty in identifying the WHO and their roles, consider using Table 2 provided for defining review functions and roles.

(a) Category of Client ____________________

	Concerns (by Priority of Concern, Risk & Expense)	Who	Decisions
(b) PART 1: CLIENT & THERAPIST Clinical			
Administrative			
(c) PART 2: APPROPRIATE OTHER Clinical			
Administrative			
(d) PART 3: COMMITTEE Clinical			
Administrative			

(e) What are the supervisory responsibilities for Parts 1 and 2 above? ____________________

(f) For Part 3, what is the committee's organization and lines of responsibility? ____________________

5. IMPLEMENTATION STRATEGY

Have each of your clinical supervisors lead a staff team to develop the three-part review standards for each of the major categories of concern. The development of the standards themselves will serve as the initial part of staff development and supervision. By having staff participate in the developmental process, staff resistance to the review process should diminish. Furthermore, when you have completed these tasks, the basic conditions will be satisfied for both *concurrent review* and *continued stay review* as required by JCAH and PSRO.

Developing the Review Committee

An approach to organizing the review committee is outlined below and was adapted from Dr. Gary Tischler's NIMH Staff College course notebook on Quality Assurance (1977).

I. Tasks and Functioning of Committees and Subcommittees
II. Organization
    A. Structure and composition
    B. Relationship of structure to tasks and functions
    C. Methods of committee selection and term of appointment
    D. Committee chair and subcommittee chair selection and role assignment methods
    E. Committee relationships to other committees and organizational elements within the program, e.g., administration, staff development, clinical records, program evaluation
    F. Frequency of meetings
    G. Types of records kept
III. Process & Methods
    A. Authority of committee
    B. Formal procedures for admissions certification and continued stay review
    C. Methods for case and topic selection
    D. Methods for generating profiles for clinical record audit studies
    E. Methods for developing and revising norms, criteria and standards
IV. Relationship of Quality Assurance Activities to Third Party Claims Review
V. Methods of Providing Feedback of Committee's Review Findings to Administrative and Clinical Staff, Staff Development Program, and the Program's Citizen Board
VI. Method of Followup of Committee's Recommendations

SOME OTHER HELPFUL HINTS FOR IMPLEMENTATION

Random Sampling of Approved Cases

A random sample can be anywhere from 1% to 99% of the cases. There are many rules for random sampling described in elementary statistics books. The essential feature is to attempt to select randomly, i.e., without noticeable bias of selecting one or more subgroups out of proportion to their prevalence in the general population. One suggestion is to add a subjective dimension in determining the size of the random sample. High-risk and high-expense categories should have larger percentages in the sample to assure adequate coverage.

Other general rules of thumb include:

— A minimum of 10 cases per target population or category of concern each 3 to 6 months.
— A minimum of 5 cases per therapist each 3 to 6 months.
— Random selection can be achieved by randomly selecting a sequence of two digits from a

table of random numbers and letting each set of two digits correspond to the last two digits of a client's case number.

Develop a Checklist for Each Category and Part of Review

After outlining the review strategy in terms of ''concerns,'' ''who,'' and ''decisions'' for each category of client, consider converting the outline into a checklist for use in reviewing cases. Such a checklist should help staff focus attention and save time. The items on the checklist should be ordered in a fashion which says, ''If OK, stop reviewing. If not OK, review some more.'' These checklists can become the basis for the *Retrospective Chart Audits* recommended in the guidelines set by NIMH, JCAH, and PSRO.

Chapter 7
Termination and Followup

Were Goals Met?
Is Followup Needed?

The fourth phase of the clinical process is the termination of services. The termination phase needs to address two issues: Were treatment goals achieved? Is followup needed?

The outline of this unit parallels the unit on quality assurance procedures:

(1) Identifying Categories of CONCERNS about termination and followup
(2) Identifying the Roles and Functions of Staff
(3) Identifying the CONCERNS, WHO, and DECISION ALTERNATIVES for each category of concern
(4) Creating a Flow Diagram to Describe the Process

The examples provided in Tables 1, 2, and 3 and in Figure 1 can be used as a guide.

Table 1 provides a convenient outline for developing the definitions of client categories used to describe termination and followup efforts. The categories run from short term, non-critical clients to the serious circumstance of death.

Termination may be conceptualized in many ways. One approach identifies six client categories and definitions:

Client Category	Textbook Definition
Short-Term, Non-Critical	Client terminated in six visits.
Planned Termination	Both client and service staff agreed upon termination.
Drop-out Functional	Client was above the midpoint on a global scale and not heard from in 60 days.
Drop-out Dysfunctional	Client was below the midpoint on the global scale and was not heard from in 20 days.
Death	See local legal precedent.
Other	

Naturally these definitions are merely illustrative, and a given program will have to create its own. After developing definitions, review efforts of each role (e.g., intake worker, principal therapist, treatment team leader, peer reviewer, medical records, etc.) should be identified and linked to the review functions (e.g., treatment planning, staff conferences, record accuracy

Table 1. Termination Review: Roles, Functions and Cases

POSSIBLE REVIEW OF FUNCTIONS AND NUMBER OF CASES**
(KEY TO COLUMNS BELOW)

1. Treatment Planning with Client
2. Staffing Conferences
3. Record Accuracy Review
4. Clinical Record Review of Client's Problems/Resources/Goals/Progress
5. With Client, Review of Problems/Goals/Progress
6. Direct Staff Supervision
7. Staff Development
8. Other ___________

Title of Role*	Your Program's Definition	1.	2.	3.	4.	5.	6.	7.	8.
INTAKE WORKER									
PRINCIPAL THERAPIST									
TREATMENT TEAM LEADER									
PEER REVIEWER									
CASE MANAGER									
CLIENT ADVOCATE OR OMBUDSMAN									
TARGET/POPULATION SPECIALIST/ REVIEWER									
CASE COORDINATOR									
SUPERVISOR									
REVIEWING PHYSICIAN									
QUALITY ASSURANCE COMMITTEE									
MEDICAL RECORDS SEC'T/TECH.									
MEDICAL RECORDS ADMINISTRATOR									
FOLLOWUP COUNSELOR									

*Any one staff person can fulfill any one of rules listed. Feel free to make substitutions.
**Number of Cases Reviewed (to be inserted in appropriate role and column).

ALL = All Clients

RAN = Random Sample of Clients

EXC = Exceptions

RAN EXC = Random Sample and Exceptions

review, clinical record review, reviews with client, staff supervision, etc.). A secondary consideration is the number of cases to be reviewed by each role:

— All clients
— Random sample of clients
— Exceptions
— Random sample and exceptions

Table 1 presents an illustrative matrix combining role, function, and number of cases. Roles are listed as rows and the review functions as columns. At the intersection of the row and column is the number of cases to be reviewed.

Table 2 continues the analysis by linking each role to the categories of concern using the program's own definitions. Rows represent a concern; the columns represent roles and the intersection of rows and columns represent the number of cases reviewed.

Table 2. Categories of Termination Concerns and Review Efforts

REVIEW EFFORTS OF EACH ROLE*
(KEY TO COLUMNS BELOW)

1. Medical Records
2. Peer Colleague
3. Case Manager/Client Advocate
4. Case Coordinator Supervisor
5. Medical Reviewer
6. Target Population Specialist
7. Quality Assurance Committee
8. Utilization Review Committee

Category	Program's Own Definition	1.	2.	3.	4.	5.	6.	7.	8.	9.
SHORT TERM TERMINATION										
PLANNED TERMINATION										
DROP OUT FUNCTIONAL										
DROP OUT DYSFUNCTIONAL										
DEATH										
OTHER										

*Number of Cases Reviewed:

ALL = All Cases

RAN = Random Sample of Cases. Give approximate percent of cases to be sampled.

EXC = Exceptions

RAN EXC = Random Sample and Exceptions. Also give percent for random sample.

Table 3 summarizes the process by examining each termination category. Risk and expense are examined by organizational level (viz., clinical, adminstrative, and supervisory) along with who is involved and their optional decisions.

Table 3. Termination and Followup Review

TERMINATION CATEGORY ______________________________

WHAT AND WHY? Risk & Expense Standards Ordered by Level of Concern		WHO (Describe Characteristics)	Optional Decisions
CLINICAL			
SUPERVISORY			
ADMINISTRATIVE			

Figure 1 presents an example of termination review in "flow diagram" format.

The program implementation strategy recommended here simply parallels that suggested in the previous three chapters.

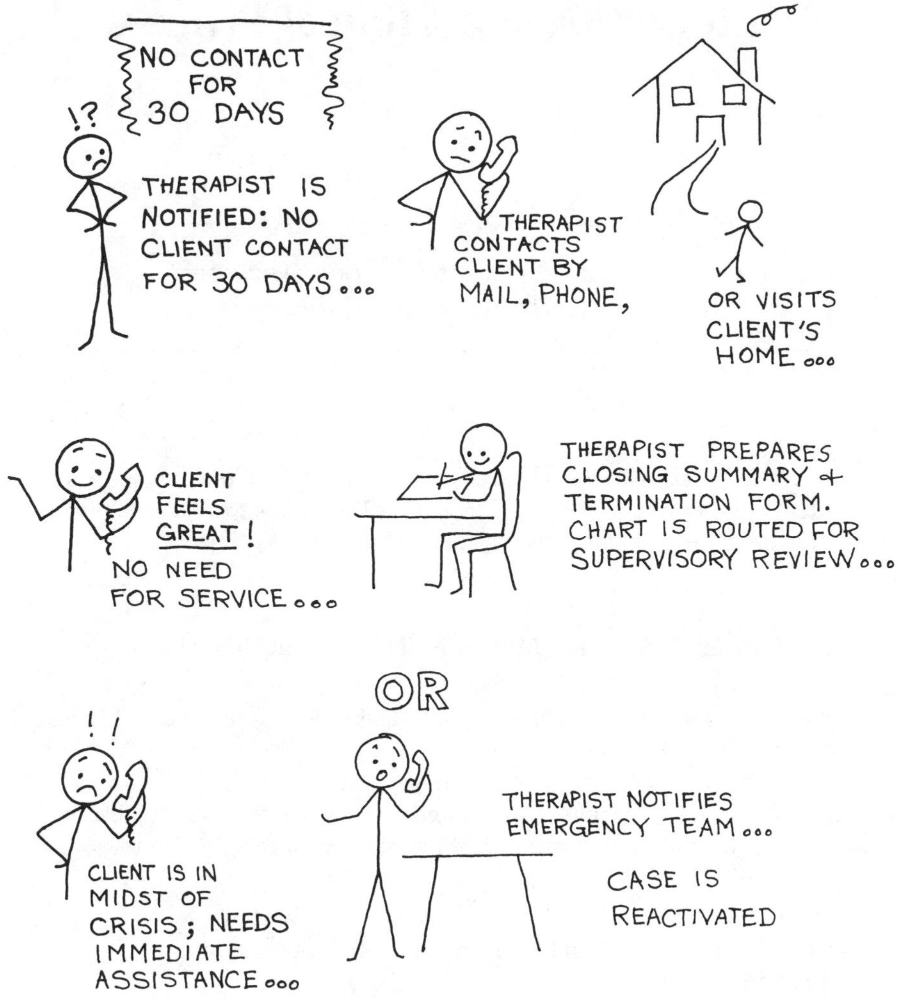
NO CONTACT FOR 30 DAYS
!?
THERAPIST IS NOTIFIED: NO CLIENT CONTACT FOR 30 DAYS ...
THERAPIST CONTACTS CLIENT BY MAIL, PHONE,
OR VISITS CLIENT'S HOME ...
CLIENT FEELS GREAT!
NO NEED FOR SERVICE ...
THERAPIST PREPARES CLOSING SUMMARY + TERMINATION FORM. CHART IS ROUTED FOR SUPERVISORY REVIEW ...
OR
!!
CLIENT IS IN MIDST OF CRISIS; NEEDS IMMEDIATE ASSISTANCE ...
THERAPIST NOTIFIES EMERGENCY TEAM ...
CASE IS REACTIVATED

Figure 1. Example of Termination Review

Chapter 8

Integrating the Clinical Process

How Do the Four Stages Come Together?
Are Modifications for an Integrated Procedure Needed?

The objective here is to design a concise overall summary of the four stages of the clinical process (preferably in a one- or two-page diagram). The product is extremely useful for staff training and for the basis of clinical records and information systems.

REVIEWING CONCEPTS AND EXAMPLE (INCLUDING SELF-STUDY)

Often, the overall picture of the client flow and quality assurance process becomes lost in a tangle of flow diagrams. A simple summary of the entire process can be highly useful. The example provided in Table 1 represents a one-page summary for clients in a rural county alcoholism program. David Glenn, who created the summary, chose to break the clinical process into six stages, rather than four. This diagram becomes the basis for:

— Initial staff orientation and training, particularly for new staff.
— Development of the manual and computerized information system.
— Clinical record management.

A general outline for an integrated summary of the clinical process requires three column headings:

(1) INFORMATION NEEDS AND DOCUMENTS
(2) ACTIVITIES AND PEOPLE INVOLVED
(3) TIMING

The self-study on creating an integrated summary is designed to reinforce the entire chapter.

Table 1. Example Summary of Client Treatment and Quality Assurance Process by David Glenn, Executive Director Counseling Center, Meadville, Pennsylvania

Information Needs	Activity	Time
Intake screening, liability, request for release of/or obtaining information, medical summary, level of functioning chart	Referred Client → Intake Counselor at Center or on Inpatient Unit; Medical Consultant with Medical Exam	As soon as possible
Same as above, plus Treatment Plan recommendations	Intake Review & Assignment → Primary Therapist & CMS*; Inpatient &/or Medical Staff & CMS	As soon as possible
Same as above, plus Progress Notes, and Level of Functioning	Treatment Plan → Primary Therapist; CMS, on call	After two & before four sessions
Level of Functioning Progress Summary, updated medical checkup	Progress Review → Primary Therapist; CMS; Conference with other staff, as needed	Between third and sixth month
Same as above, plus at time of transfer or discharge—a Summary Report	Further Service → Transfer → Discharge Client	At time of Termination
Mailed Followup Questionnaire from Client and Significant Other	Followup Report	Between 2 and 6 months after

*CMS = Case Manager Supervisor

Self-Study on Creating an Integrated Summary

Create an integrated summary for a target client category familiar to you.
NAME THE TARGET CLIENT FOR THE INTEGRATED SUMMARY ____________

____

Information Needs	Activity and People Involved	Timing

Implementation Strategy

After supervisors or service program directors have completed Chapters 3 through 7, have them draft an *Integrated Summary* for their "most familiar target client category." Turn these over to the person who is charged with maintaining your information system. When both the clinical supervisors and the information system person agree on the summary, you can be confident the clinical process is completely designed for the system as it now exists.

SECTION III

THE VISIBLE EVIDENCE—PART I: DESIGNING YOUR CLINICAL RECORDS

Chapter 9

Clinical Record Design: Shaping Records to Your Program Situation

Do the Records Provide Clear Visible Evidence of the Clinical Process?

A well-designed clinical record provides the visible evidence that the clinical service system is working as planned. A clinical record system serves six purposes:

— Communication among client and staff
— Planning continuity and review of care quality
— Staff development in assuring clinical data reliability
— Analyses of service efforts and costs
— Evaluation of process and outcome
— Legal protection and external review

Chapter 9 identifies the major components of a clinical record in two sections:

(1) PURPOSES, USES, AND CHARACTERISTICS OF A CLINICAL RECORD SYSTEM. A clinical record system should be uniquely tailored to clients and programs to support clinical communication. The characteristics of a clinical record system leading to good communication are outlined.
(2) OUTLINE OF A COMMON CLINICAL RECORD AND HOW TO TAILOR RECORDS TO CLIENTS. The approach offered allows flexibility by allowing service managers to design records useful to their own service styles while providing consistency of data across different services.

1. PURPOSES, USES, AND CHARACTERISTICS OF A CLINICAL RECORD SYSTEM

Developing a clinical record system starts with specification of program goals (Chapter 2) and design of the clinical process (Section II). Chapter 9 focuses on the relationships between the design of the clinical record system, program goals, and the design of the clinical process. The emphasis is on the management and policy issues in the design and development of the records, rather than on the detailed elements of the records themselves (which will be covered in Chapters 10 and 11).

The first part of the chapter focuses on two objectives:

— To identify the purposes of clinical record systems;
— To identify the relationships between the clinical process and the visible evidence in the clinical records.

A clinical record provides the *visible evidence* for the *clinical decisions* involved in the therapeutic process. Note the two italicized phrases: *clinical decisions* and *visible evidence*. The records draw a direct relationship to and are supportive of the clinical decision process:

CLINICAL DECISIONS	MUST RELATE TO	CLINICAL RECORDS

If this relationship is not clear to those using the records, the record system can become an empty shell. Since clinical decisions are internal human processes, clinical records can only represent the visible evidence describing the major considerations used in formulating decisions. Figure 1 describes the relationship between the four major parts of the clinical decision process (on the left side) and the visible evidence (on the right side).

Often there is cynicism about viewing clinical records as a useful factor in good clinical practice. A typical comment might be:

> Hog wash! Clinical records are not the handmaiden of the clinical process. They are pieces of paper intruding upon the clinical process to appease the power-trip appetites of the business office, administrators, state and federal regulatory agencies, and JCAH.

Ron Ravneberg (NIMH Staff College Clinical Records Course notebook, 1979) offers a good response to this comment:

> The best first attempt at dealing with regulations might be to completely ignore them! . . . The one thing most sets of regulations have in common is that they are attempting to make sure the clinical services provided are of high quality and effective. Thus, it appears that if one begins by designing a record system *around the clinical process* in such a way that it provides the information necessary for client decision making, one will find that the resultant record will meet most of (if not all) outside recordkeeping requirements.

We will describe how clinical data can be translated into external reporting requirements. Once the records are structured to meet unique program needs, we will suggest ways to demonstrate how the record system does meet formal standards and regulations.

Figure 1 has a number of subtle features. In Chapters 3 through 7, the clinical process was described by Stages of Service (viz., Entry, Planning, Review, Termination) and Characteristics at each stage (viz. Concerns?, Who?, and Decisions). Within each of the four stages of the clinical process are two principal questions. Table 1 sorts the eight basic questions into BASIC DATA and ACTIONS TO BE TAKEN.

The basis for the ACTION in one stage of the process becomes a consideration and DATA for answering questions in the next stage. For example, by reviewing the ''apparent problems

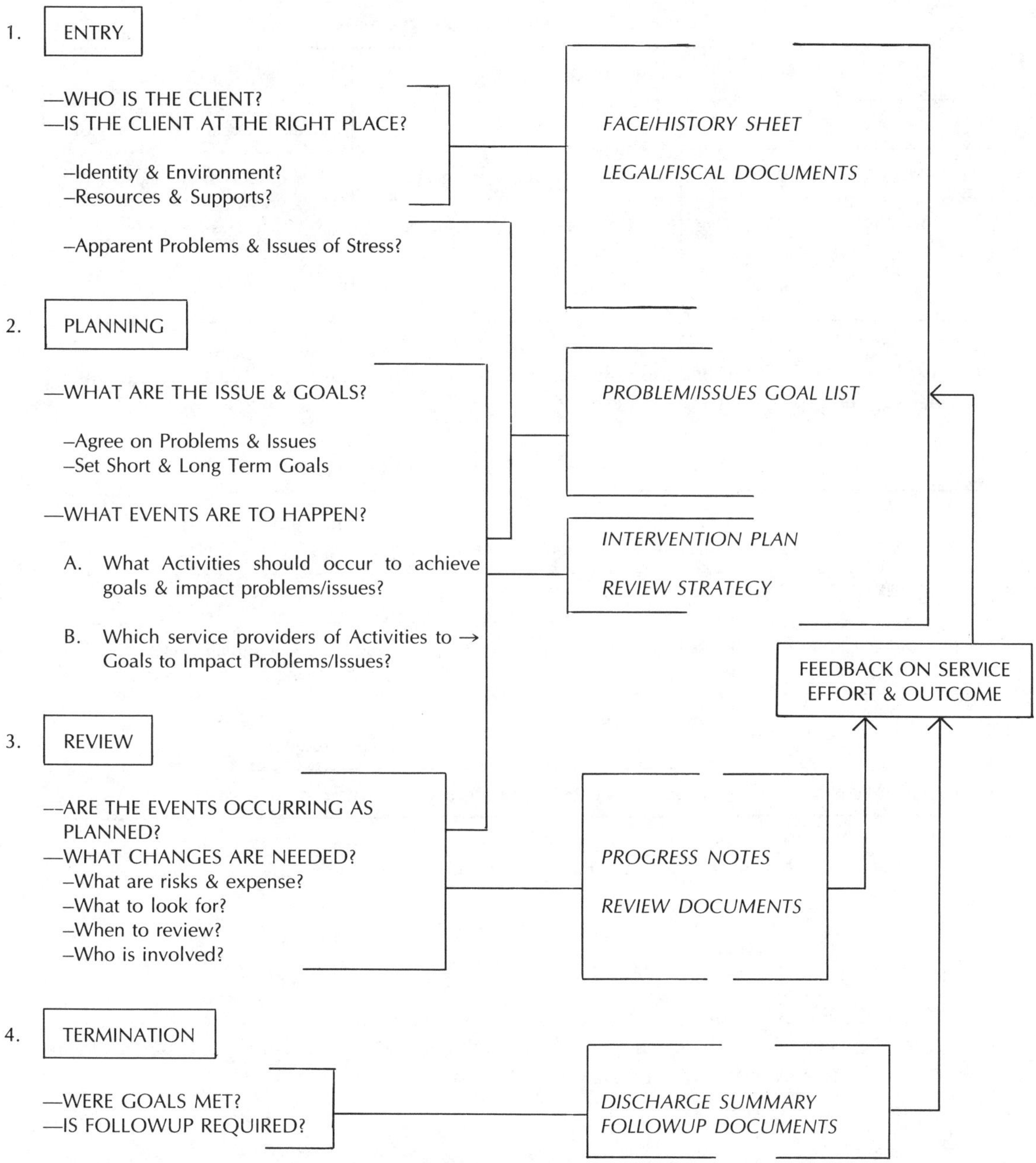

Figure 1. The Relationship of Clinical Decisions and Clinical Records

and issues of stress,'' the intake clinician can decide ''Is the client at the right place?'' Then, in service planning, a more carefully considered review of problems and issues becomes the basis for deciding ''What are the issues and goals?'' ''What events are to happen?'' leads to two more detailed questions: ''What activities can help?'' and ''Which service modality?'' These sub-questions clarify the distinction between an *activity* to achieve a goal and the *provider* of the

Table 1. Data versus Action Questions

Stage of Process	Basic Data Question	Action Question
(a) ENTRY	Who is the client?	Is the client at the right place?
(b) SERVICE PLANNING	What are the issues and goals?	What events are to happen?
(c) REVIEW	Are events occurring as planned?	What changes are needed?
(d) TERMINATION & FOLLOWUP	Were goals met?	Is followup required?

activity. Usually more than one modality can provide an appropriate activity. Table 2 identifies optional service providers for each activity.

Table 2. Activity and Providers of Service

Activity	Example Provider of Service	Alternative Providers (Means) of Service?
a) Intensive Care	Inpatient Unit	Family, Jail
b) Positive Social Interaction	Group Therapy	Social club; card group; athletic activities; music therapy
c) Listening Skills	Group Therapy	Homework assignments recording what other people say
d) Impulse Control	Medication plus Individual Therapy	Social or Network Theory

Clinical records should clearly distinguish between *activities* and *provider of service activities.*

Self-Study Exercise 1

The right side of Figure 1 gives examples of visible evidence documents. Review your own clinical records and decide whether you are addressing each question, and which documents in your record contain the information addressing the question.

QUESTIONS

ENTRY	QUESTION ADDRESSED (Check) Yes	No	DOCUMENTS CONTAINING INFORMATION IN YOUR SYSTEM
—Who is the client?	_____	_____	____________________
—Is this the right place?	_____	_____	____________________
–Identity & Environment?	_____	_____	____________________
–Resources & Supports	_____	_____	____________________
–Apparent Problems?	_____	_____	____________________
–Issues of Stress?	_____	_____	____________________

QUESTIONS

	QUESTION ADDRESSED (Check) Yes	No	DOCUMENTS CONTAINING INFORMATION IN YOUR SYSTEM
PLANNING			
—What are the issues & goals?	____	____	____________
–Activities linked to Goals?	____	____	____________
–Service Providers linked to Activities and Goals?	____	____	____________
—What events are to happen?	____	____	____________
REVIEW			
—Are events occurring as planned?	____	____	____________
—Are changes needed?	____	____	____________
–Potential/Actual Risks for Client?	____	____	____________
–What to, when have Review?	____	____	____________
–Who is involved in Review?	____	____	____________
TERMINATION			
—Were goals met?	____	____	____________
—Is followup required?	____	____	____________
–Problems?	____	____	____________
–Resources & Supports?	____	____	____________
–Followup Plan	____	____	____________
–When? Who?	____	____	____________
–What to look for?	____	____	____________

Records Ought to Read Like a Book. Organization and style of the clinical records will affect the actual use of the records. The following list of Do's and Don'ts are criteria for designing a readable and useable clinical records system. Managers should establish major guidelines prior to design of detailed records by the technical staff. (Other guidelines are discussed the Chapter 10 and 11.) For each of the guidelines given below, review your own records system and subjectively rate the records on each criterion. Let "0" equal "terrible" and "10" equal "perfect."

RATINGS

The records have a *theme* reflecting the clinical process. A clinical record system is not complete until there is a flow of information from problems and supports to documentation of the intervention plan, to the review process, and finally to termination and followup. ______

A professional uninvolved in the case can use the records to *summarize* answers to five major clinical questions within 2 to 3 minutes:

		Check
1.	Who is the client?	____
2.	What are the issues?	____
3.	What is to happen and how will it be reviewed?	____
4.	Who is responsible for treatment and review?	____
5.	What has happened and what followup is needed?	____

______

Information is not categorized by its source, e.g., having MD notes, nurse's notes, fact sheet, and the social history all in separate sections of the folder; the flow of inquiry and communication across the five basic questions is limited if grouped by source. ______

Chronological events are related to the treatment plan. ______

Relationships among problems, issues of stress, and goals are drawn sequentially. ______

Progress on goals should relate directly to problems or issues. ________

Words used to describe clients are reliable and relate to observable behavior patterns, e.g., "apparent anxiety implied by pacing and hand wringing." ________

Out of 70 points possible, a score of 0–28 represents a level of real concern; 29–48 points represents the need for some work; and 49–70 is quite good. Any item lower than 7 should be reviewed and corrected.

2. OUTLINE OF A COMMON RECORD AND HOW TO TAILOR RECORDS TO CLIENTS

In a client-oriented system, service efforts should be tailored to the individual client's problems, supports, and goals. Tailoring clinical records to suit the unique characteristics of clients and services implies potential chaos. The key is maintaining a *common outline* across clients and services, while at the same time encouraging your staff to customize the records to suit *the characteristics of the client, the service goals,* and *the types of service efforts.* Once the common outline is established, the records for different categories of clients and services can be tailored to the individual clients within each service.

Table 3 offers an example to follow in developing a customized outline. The outline links

Table 3. Example of Common Record Outline

1. RELATING CLIENTS TO SERVICES AND PROGRAM GOALS
   - 1.1 *Target Group* (or Category of Concerns) characteristics
   - 1.2 *Program Goal* for this category of client
   - 1.3 *Global Scale* describing overall level of disability, dysfunction, etc.
   - 1.4 *Detailed Factor* (Problem/Issue) *List*
   - 1.5 *Service Array* across levels of the global scale
     - (a) For your services
     - (b) For other community services
2. THE CLINICAL PROCESS FOR EACH CATEGORY OF CLIENT AND SERVICE CONCERN (From Section II)

Stage of Process	Characteristics of Stage			Documents
	Concerns	Who	Decisions	
2.1 ENTRY				
2.2 PLANNING				
2.3 REVIEW				
2.4 TERMINATION & FOLLOWUP				

NOTE the fourth column ("DOCUMENTS") has been added to the clinical process outline to link process with visible evidence.

3. MEANS OF ASSURING DEPENDABLE CLINICAL DATA AND COMMUNICATION (From Sections I and II)
   - 3.1 Review and supervision procedures (Section II)
   - *3.2 Staff development procedures (Section I)
   - *3.3 Scale reliability and validity procedures (Section I)

*These procedures are detailed more completely in the Section IV on Visible Evidence.

services to program goals and provides a means of identifying the vocabulary staff will use to communicate with clients and each other as they assist clients in moving toward their individual goals.

Tailoring Records to Clients and Services

Identifying the major components and outline of a clinical record system is a key initial step. Next, guidelines are needed to specifically deal with: (1) the characteristics of the client population, i.e., their problems, issues and goals; and (2) the characteristics of internal management functions, e.g., case management, service unit, and program management. Shaping the records to external reporting requirements should happen *after* the clinical and internal management needs are satisfied, and not before.

Are clinical staff and clients communicating with each other? Records should encourage and support communication accounting for the unique characteristics of the clients. Consider the lifestyles, expected role performances, and concerns of different groups of clients:

Cultural Circumstances	History/Life Support Circumstances
—A Mormon farmer	—Legal involvement with substance abuse
—A rural Native American male	—Repeated depression episodes
—An urban Black male	—No family supports
—A suburban Anglo female	—Age (youth–geriatric)
—A rural coal miner	

What would be the relative importance of religious influence on each? Of alcohol abuse? Of the cultural acceptance of using public social services? Of the work ethic? What other kinds of influences should be considered, such as psychiatric history or voluntary/involuntary commitment status?

To help focus on your own situation, identify three or more major client groups in your service area for whom the clinical process may be affected by their ethnic identification, lifestyle, chronic behavior patterns, etc.

(A) ______________________ (D) ______________________

(B) ______________________ (E) ______________________

(C) ______________________ (F) ______________________

Focusing on the unique characteristics of clients and service programs does not lead to the chaos of nonstandardized clinical records since all records follow the same outline. But specific sections will be tailored to major client and service categories. Records will be client oriented but structured to meet regulatory standards as well.

Self-Study Exercise 2

To understand how client differences influence clinical records, the following exercise demonstrates how unique client features may require different clinical information. Tables 4 and 5 identify the unique factors which should receive different emphasis in clinical records at the points of entry, service planning, and review. Table 4 shows how client-group characteristics will affect clinical records. Table 5 addresses needs of service-program management.

Table 4. Identifying Unique Client Group Influences on Clinical Records

Instructions: For one or two of the three unique client groups you identify, consider the areas of role performance listed below for different levels of emphasis and detail in entry, service planning, and review.

Use a 0–10 rating scale to assist your efforts, where 0 = No Significant Influence on Role Performance and 10 = The Most Dominant Influence. In each cell, you may enter a number denoting level of influence.

Role Performance Area	Client Group		
	Example: Amish Farmer*	Your Example (A)	Your Example (B)
Vocational Status or Work Ethic	10—Detailed departure from norm		
Family Influence	10—Detailed departure from norm		
Religious Influences	10—Detailed departure from norm		
Emotional Stress Symptoms	5—Same as others		
Personal Self-care	5—Same		
Alcohol or Chemical Abuse	10—Detailed departures		
Involvement with Other MH Services	3—Seldom used		
Involvement with Social Services	5—Check use of private human services		
OTHER ________	5—Amish religious community supports		
________			

*In Pennsylvania, the Amish "Plain People" are a very proud, tightknit group who mainly farm for a living and shun modern conveniences such as automobiles and electricity. Their strong work ethic and sense of community responsibility leads to economic success and relative stability. Yet the effects of inbreeding and the surrounding modern world, along with the common woes of being human, means that they also suffer from mental-health problems. All of the influences cited here would affect the Problem/Issues lists and the review strategy.

Table 5. Support of Clinical Management Functions: Identifying Unique Service-Program Needs

The emphasis and detail of records will be strongly influenced by the management demands of each service program. Consider three services: Inpatient, partial hospitalization, and outpatient. Would the service emphasis and the need for detailed information on the various aspects of lifestyle and role performance be the same for the management of all three services?

Try describing these differences. Indicate the level of emphasis and detail required in a clinical record for the management of each of three services by assigning a number on the scale of 0–10 where 0 = No Emphasis or Detail Needed, and 10 = Highest Level of Emphasis and Detail. Illustrative ratings are provided for a hypothetical inpatient service.

	Service Area			
	Inpatient			
Role Performance Area	Ours*	Yours	Partial Hospitalization	Outpatient
Vocational Status or Work Ethic	3			
Family Influences	5			
Religious Influences	3			
Emotional Stress Symptoms	8			
Personal Self-care	8			
Alcohol or Chemical Abuse	3			
Involvement with Other MH Services	3			
Involvement with Social Services	3			
OTHER ____________				
____________				

*Our Inpatient ratings are based upon the need for detailed information in the planning of services and day-to-day communication within the service.

Table 6. Outline Used to Identify Possible Differential Effects on Clinical Records Due to Unique Client or Service Characteristics*

	Service Area A		Service Area B	
	Client Type		Client Type	
Outline:	(1)	(2)	(1)	(2)
1. REGARDING PROGRAM DESIGNS AND GOALS 1.1 Program Goals				
1.2 Global Scale Language				
1.3 Problem/Issues List				
2. CONCERNS—WHO—DECISIONS at: 2.1 Entry				
2.2 Service Planning				
2.3 Review				
2.4 Termination & Followup				
3. ASSURING DEPENDABLE COMMUNICATION AND DATA 3.1 Review & Supervision Procedures				
3.2 Staff Training & Development				
3.3 Scale Reliability & Validity Procedures				

*You need only make entries in those cells where unique client or service characteristics make a difference.

The unique client or service influences need to be integrated into the general outline of the clinical records. While this task is too difficult to delineate here, the process can be understood by considering two client categories and two service areas from a program. Try to identify one or more effects each of the topics might have on the *common outline* given in Table 6.

3. CREATING YOUR OWN GUIDELINES FOR A CLINICAL RECORDS OUTLINE

There are two general steps in the process of creating your own clinical records guidelines. First, decide upon the *common outline* you are going to use. Second, identify how each combination of client type and service may differentially affect each element in the *common outline*. The three formats given in Table 7 provide you with a guide for creating the common outline and for identifying the unique client and service features which may affect the clinical records. Each of the three formats covers one part of the general outline:

(1) Regarding Program Design and Goals
(2) Clinical Process of Concerns—Who—Decisions
(3) Assuring Dependable Clinical Communications and Data

Table 7. Guide for a Common Clinical Records Outline

PART 1: REGARDING PROGRAM DESIGN AND GOALS	Services					
	(1)			(2)		
Outline*	Client A	B	C	A	B	C

*SUGGESTED COVERAGE: (1.1) Program Goals (1.2) Global Scale Language (1.3) Problem/Issue List (1.4) Service Array

PART 2: CLINICAL PROCESS FOR CONCERNS—WHO—DECISIONS	Services								
	(1)			(2)			(3)		
	Client Type			Client Type			Client Type		
Outline*	A	B	C	A	B	C	A	B	C

*SUGGESTED COVERAGE: (2.1) Entry (2.2) Service Planning (2.3) Review; also see next part of outline (2.4) Termination & Followup

PART 3: ASSURING DEPENDABLE COMMUNICATION AND DATA	Services					
	(1)			(2)		
	Client Type			Client Type		
Outline*	A	B	C	A	B	C

*SUGGESTED COVERAGE: (3.1) Review and supervision procedures and responsibilities (3.2) Staff training and development procedures and responsibilities (3.3) Scale reliability and validity estimation procedures and responsibilities

The footnotes at the bottom of each format provide suggested areas of coverage and the columns on the right permit you to identify the unique characteristics of clients and services.

4. PROGRAM IMPLEMENTATION STRATEGIES

The products of this chapter provide the basis for your entire record system. Thus, drafts of the products should be reviewed and revised with the assistance of all unit directors within your program. It would also be wise to review the results with the Citizen Board. Once an extensive review and a broad base of staff and board consensus is established, then the details of the clinical record system can be developed. The procedures for this development are given in the remaining chapters of this section.

Chapter 10

Technical Chapter
Identifying Data Elements in Clinical Records

> Problem: What Data Elements Do We Need?
> Solution: Plagiarize or Borrow from Others!

The specific elements in the clinical records need to be identified. The following procedure combines two objectives. First, existing records may be evaluated using client-oriented system standards. Second, other records may be assessed to determine what sections and elements to borrow. After some guidelines on how to use the procedures, the outline will follow the basic questions asked in the clinical process:

1.	"WHO IS THE CLIENT?" "IS THE CLIENT AT THE RIGHT PLACE?"	e.g., Face and History Sheet
2.	"WHAT ARE THE ISSUES AND GOALS?" "WHAT EVENTS ARE TO HAPPEN?"	e.g., Problems/Issues/Goals List and Intervention Plan
3.	"ARE EVENTS OCCURRING AS PLANNED?" "WHAT CHANGES ARE NEEDED?"	e.g., Progress Notes and Review Documents
4.	"WERE GOALS MET?" "IS FOLLOWUP REQUIRED?"	Termination and Followup and Documentation

GUIDELINES FOR USING THE CLINICAL RECORD "BORROWING" PROCEDURES

The general procedure for designing the clinical records will take a committee of three or four people about 4–12 hours to complete. The task is not a one-person assignment. For individual study, however, spend about an hour evaluating and redesigning some portion of a clinical record to get a feel for the task. Then, assemble a small group of friendly colleagues from a service unit to use the recommended procedures to redesign the principal components of that service unit's records. When the process makes sense, appoint a program-wide committee to redesign the records for the entire program. Among those appointed should be individuals who will attend compulsively to details and assure the procedures are employed.

STEP 1 To review recommended data capture instruments and data elements useful in addressing each question.

STEP 2 To identify the useful instrument and data elements. Earlier ratings of client and service management demands are needed.

STEP 3 To evaluate existing records by assigning one of three ratings—
0 = Component or element is not present
1 = Component or element present but not formatted properly
2 = Element present and properly formatted

STEP 4 To evaluate one or more sample records from other programs using the same rating scheme (0, 1, 2)

STEP 5 To "borrow" instruments and data elements with ratings higher than existing records.

The Appendix of this chapter has one example for Steps 4 and 5. The Appendix also offers recommendations for encouraging efficient and easy use of a record by clinical staff by constructing a "mini-episode" record section within the overall record. The "mini-episode" section is simply a file within a file that contains the current treatment plans, progress notes, and flow sheet.

EXAMPLE INSTRUMENT AND DATA ELEMENTS

"WHO IS THE CLIENT?"

"IS THE CLIENT AT THE RIGHT PLACE?"

FACE/SOCIAL HISTORY INFORMATION
- Identification
  - Name
  - Address
  - Telephone Number
  - Same for Significant Other
- Entry Condition
  - Date and Time of Entry
  - Legal Status (voluntary–involuntary)
  - Referral Source
  - New or Old Client
- Demographic Information
  - Sex
  - Ethnic Background

Marital Status
Census Tract
Education
Religion
Citizenship
Occupation and Employment Status
Community Situation and Support Systems
Residence
Family, Relatives, or Support in Area
Prior Service History
Dates
Entry/Exit Condition
Services
HEALTH INFORMATION
Seeing, Hearing, Speech
Physical Mobility, Skeletal Structure
Cardiology and Respiratory
Dietary, Digestive, Excrement Behaviors
Sex, Genitals
Historic Ailments
FINANCIAL
Responsible Party (Name, Address, Relatives)
Income
Funding Source (3rd Party Payors)

"WHO IS THE CLIENT?"—"IS THE CLIENT AT THE RIGHT PLACE?"

For these basic questions, identify the major components of the questions and list specific data elements necessary to define those components. Then rate your own record and the sample records in the Appendix.*

What Are the Major Components of This Basic Question?	What Data Elements Are Necessary in a Clinical Record to Adequately Define Each Component of the Basic Question?	Your Record	Example			
			1	2	3	4

*0 = Element not present
1 = Element present but improperly formatted
2 = Element present and properly formatted
N/A = Not applicable

EXAMPLE INSTRUMENT AND DATA ELEMENTS

"WHAT ARE THE ISSUES AND GOALS?"
"WHAT EVENTS ARE TO HAPPEN?"

ISSUE LIST AND INTERVENTION PLAN
PROBLEM/ISSUES LIST (see the Appendix of Chapter 2)
GOALS: Immediate and long term with general timelines
—Relationship of client's resources and support to problem/issues and goals
—Activities which could use resources and support for movement towards goals
—Provider of activities, specifying provider's name, amount, and duration of service
REVIEW STRATEGY
—Danger signals and possible negative impact
—When (timing of stressors may be built into service intervention plan)
—Who involved
—Case management (people and methods)
CLIENT PARTICIPATION
—Evidence of consumers participating and understanding their rights
—Signatures and dates of people involved in constructing the intervention plan and reviews on all forms

"WHAT ARE THE ISSUES AND GOALS?"—"WHAT EVENTS ARE TO HAPPEN?"

For these basic questions, identify the major components of the questions and list specific data elements necessary to define those components. Then rate your own record and the sample records in the Appendix.*

What Are the Major Components of This Basic Question?	What Data Elements Are Necessary in a Clinical Record to Adequately Define Each Component of the Basic Question?	Your Record	Example			
			1	2	3	4

*0 = Element not present
1 = Element present but improperly formatted
2 = Element present and properly formatted
N/A = Not applicable

EXAMPLE OF INSTRUMENT AND DATA ELEMENTS

"ARE THE EVENTS OCCURRING AS PLANNED?"

"WHAT CHANGES ARE NEEDED?"

PROGRESS NOTES
- Who did what, when, and how much?
- Global rating?
- Significant change on any problems or issue relative to goals
- Is a more extensive review needed?
- Will progress notes with review data offer justification for billing for services rendered?

FLOW SHEET
- Chronological index of
- —Services rendered
- —By whom
- —Global rating
- Flow Sheet placed where it can be reviewed easily and quickly

REVIEW DOCUMENTS—1: RECORD AUDIT REVIEW
- Date and who was involved in audit
- Structure and organization
- Completeness
- Accuracy
- Compliance with legal and professional standards

REVIEW DOCUMENTS—2: QUALITY AND UTILIZATION
- Date and who was involved
- Approval or recommended changes in

Problems/issues and global entry	Activities
Resources, supports	Services
Goals	Review strategy in future

"ARE THE EVENTS OCCURRING AS PLANNED?"—"WHAT CHANGES ARE NEEDED?"

For these basic questions, identify the major components of the questions and list specific data elements necessary to define those components. Then rate your own record and the sample records in the Appendix:*

What Are the Major Components of This Basic Question?	What Data Elements Are Necessary in a Clinical Record to Adequately Define Each Component of the Basic Question?	Your Record	Example			
			1	2	3	4

*0 = Element not present
1 = Element present but improperly formatted
2 = Element present and properly formatted
N/A = Not applicable

EXAMPLE INSTRUMENT AND DATA ELEMENTS

"WERE GOALS MET?"

"IS FOLLOWUP REQUIRED?"

TERMINATION/DISCHARGE
- Date
- Functioning status at termination
- Vocational/educational status
- Problems/issues still remaining
- Resources and supports
- Reasons for termination
- Referral
- Followup strategy method and date

CLIENT SATISFACTION
- Date completed (time after discharge)
- Attitudes toward service
- Problems or issues which still persist
- New circumstances for the better and for the worse
- Vocational/educational status
- Family, social-network status

SIGNIFICANT OTHER
- (Same as Client Satisfaction but filled in by a significant other in the Client's family or social network.)

"WERE GOALS MET?"—"IS FOLLOWUP REQUIRED?"

For these basic questions, identify the major components of the questions and list specific data elements necessary to define those components. Then rate your own record and the sample records in the Appendix.*

What Are the Major Components of This Basic Question?	What Data Elements Are Necessary in a Clinical Record to Adequately Define Each Component of the Basic Question?	Your Record	Example			
			1	2	3	4

*0 = Element not present
1 = Element present but improperly formatted
2 = Element present and properly formatted
N/A = Not applicable

APPENDIX: EXAMPLES OF CLINICAL RECORD FORMS

FACE SHEET
(Pennsylvania Intake Form #10)
HEALTH SCREENING
(West Philadelphia Community MH Consortium)
PROBLEM/ISSUES GOAL LIST
(Meadville, Pennsylvania, Counseling Center)
INTERVENTION PLAN
(Meadville, Pennsylvania, Counseling Center)
FLOW SHEET
(Meadville, Pennsylvania, Counseling Center)
REVIEW FORMS:
Record Audit Review and Quality and Utilization Review
(Allegheny County, Pennsylvania)
Case Conference Review Form
(Meadville, Pennsylvania, Counseling Center)
Client Satisfaction Followup
(Langley Porter Institute)
Termination Form
(Chester County, Pennsylvania)
PUTTING THE RECORD TOGETHER:
The Mini-Episode File

Example 1: **Face Sheet**

Facility No: ____________
Case No: ____________
Date of Birth: ____________
Age: ____________
Sex: 1. Male ____ 2. Fem. ____
Census Tract ____________

Target Group ________
1. MH Child
2. MH Youth
3. MH Adult
4. MH Geriatric
5. MR Child
6. MR Youth
7. MR Adult
8. MR Geriatric

Date of Intake ____________
Date of Evaluation ____________
Admission Status ____________

1. New on Unit	4. Re-admiss. 6 mos.
2. Re-admiss. 1 mo.	5. Re-admiss. 1 year
3. Re-admiss. 3 mos.	6. Re-admiss. 1 year+

COMMUNITY OF RESIDENCE □□

01 Aldan
02 Aston
03 Bethel
04 Birmingham
05 Brookhaven
06 Chester City
07 Chester Heights
08 Chester Twp.
09 Clifton Heights
10 Collingdale

ETHNIC □□

01 White Cauc.	04 Asian/Pacific Is.
02 Black/Negro	05 Hispanic (Regardless of race or color)
03 Am. Ind./Alaskan	06 Other

MARITAL STATUS □□

01 Never Married	04 Divorced
02 Married	05 Widowed
03 Separated	06 Unknown

EDUCATION □□

01 Never attended/none	07 8th Grade
02 Special 1–3 years	08 1–3 years HS
03 Special 4–6 years	09 4 yrs. HS
04 Special 7+	10 1–3 years Coll.
05 K–4th year	11 4 yrs. Coll.
06 5th–7th	99 Unknown

OCCUPATION □□

01 Profess. Tech.	08 Farmer/Farm Manager
02 Man./Admin.	09 Farm Laborer/Foreman
03 Sales	10 Service Worker
04 Clerical	11 None (not worked in 5 years)
05 Craftsman	99 Unknown
06 Operative	
07 Laborers	

EMPLOYMENT □□

In Labor Force	Not in Labor Force
01 Full Time	04 School/preschool
02 Part time	05 Homemaker
03 Unemployed	06 Retired
	07 Disabled
	08 Incarcerated
	99 Unknown

LAST MH/MR SERVICE □□

01 PA State Mental Hospital	06 Social Rehab. & Training
02 PA State School & Hospital	07 Interim Care
03 Other Inpatient MH/MR	08 Group Home
04 Partial Hospital	09 Outpatient
05 Vocational Rehabilitation	10 None

PRIOR MH/MR STATE RESIDENTIAL SERVICE □□

01 State Mental Hospital
02 State School and Hospital
03 Both State MH/MR
04 No Prior State MH/MR Service

REFERRAL SOURCE □□

01 Self
02 Family
03 Friend
04 Clergy
05 Private Prac. MH Professional
06 Non Psych. Physician
07 PA State MH/MR Residential facility
08 Other Public MH/MR Residential facility
09 Other MH/MR Facility—Other Private MH/MR Facility both Inpatient/Outpatient
10 Court, Law Enforcement, Correction Agency
11 Medical Facility/Non Psychiatric, Private, Public, Inpatient/Outpatient
12 School System—Public, Private, Special
13 Social or Community Agency not listed above
14 Other
99 Unknown

FAMILY INCOME
Annual Total Gross □□□□□
CLIENT INCOME
Annual Total Gross □□□□□

DEPENDENTS
No. of persons dependent on Family income □□
No. of persons dependent on client income □□

PAYMENT SOURCE (Check all Applicable)

___ 1. No fee Payment	___ 5. Medicare
___ 2. Personal Resource	___ 6. Title XX
___ 3. Medical Assist.	___ 7. V.A.
___ 4. SSI	___ 8. Other Health Ins.

PRINCIPAL PRESENTING PROBLEM □□

01 Anxiety	05 Homicidal	09 Impaired Mental Development
02 Depression	06 Addictive Disease	10 Other ____________
03 Acting Out	07 Marital Difficulty	11 Other Family Disturbance ____
04 Suicidal	08 Dist. School/Work Performance	

APA Code □□□ · □□
Level of Functioning □□

(continued)

Example 1 *Continued*

INITIAL APA PRIMARY DIAGNOSIS ☐☐

01 Mental Retardation (310–315)
02 OBS (not Alcohol or Drug related) (290, 292–294, all 309 except 309.13, 309.14)
03 Schizophrenia—(295)
04 Major Affective Disorder & Other Psychoses (296, 298, 299)
05 Paranoid (297)
06 Neuroses (300)
07 Personality Disorder and Sexual Deviations (301, 302)
08 Alcohol Related Disorders (303, 309.13, 291)
09 Drug Related Diagnosis (303.14, 304)
10 Psychophysical Disorders and Special Symptoms (305.30)
11 Transient Situational Disturbance: conditions w/o manifest psych. disorder Nonspecified condition (307, 316, 317)
12 No Mental Disorders: Nondiagnostic term for administrative use (318, 319)
13 Behavior disorders of childhood and adolescence (308)

Date of Termination ☐☐☐ | Date of Last Service ☐☐☐ | Total No. of Visits ☐☐☐

REASON FOR TERMINATION ☐☐

01 Evaluation only
02 No further Treatment—no referral
03 No further Treatment—referred (Specify)
04 No further treatment—referral needed but not available
05 Treatment needed but rejected
06 Client died
07 Client moved or otherwise unavailable
08 Client lost to contact (include 90 day ruling)

APA Code ☐☐☐ · ☐☐ | Level of Functioning ☐☐

Example 2: **Health Screening Form (West Philadelphia Community Mental Health Consortium, Inc.)**

Health Screening Questionnaire	Yes	No
1. Do you need glasses to read?	....	.....
2. Does your eyesight ever blur?	....	.....
3. Is your eyesight getting worse?	....	.....
4. Do you ever see double?	....	.....
5. Do you often have bad pains in your eyes?	....	.....
6. Are you hard of hearing?	....	.....
7. Have you had any trouble with or discharge from your ears in the last year?	....	.....
8. Do you have any problems with your teeth or gums?	....	.....
9. Do you have any problems with your tongue or mouth?	....	.....
10. Is your nose continually stuffed up?	....	.....
11. Do you have nose bleeds?	....	.....
12. Has your voice become hoarse when you did not have a cold?	....	.....
13. Do you get hay fever?	....	.....
14. Are you bothered by coughing spells?	....	.....
15. Have you ever coughed up blood?	....	.....
16. Do you sometimes have severe, soaking sweats at night?	....	.....
17. Has a doctor ever said your blood pressure was too high?	....	.....
18. Do you have pains or tightness in your chest?	....	.....
19. Do you get out of breath long before anyone else?	....	.....
20. Are your ankles or feet often badly swollen?	....	.....
21. Do you have difficulty breathing in bed when you use less than 2 pillows?	....	.....
22. Are you troubled by heartburn or indigestion?	....	.....
23. Have you ever vomited blood?	....	.....
24. Do you suffer from frequent loose bowel movements?	....	.....
25. Are your bowel movements ever bloody or black?	....	.....
26. Are you badly constipated?	....	.....
27. Have you ever had jaundice (yellow eyes or skin)?	....	.....
28. Are your joints often painfully swollen?	....	.....
29. Are you physically handicapped in any way?	....	.....

(*continued*)

Health Screening Questionnaire	Yes	No
30. Do you have any skin problems?	....	.....
31. Do you suffer badly from frequent, severe headaches?	....	.....
32. Do you have spells of severe dizziness?	....	.....
33. Is any part of your body always numb?	....	.....
34. Have you ever had a fit or convulsion (epilepsy)?	....	.....
35. Have you ever had anything seriously wrong with your genitals (privates, sex organs)?	....	.....
36. Do you have to urinate frequently?	....	.....
37. Do you have a burning sensation when you pass water?	....	.....
38. Has your urine ever been brown, black or bloody?	....	.....
For Men Only:		
39. Do you have a sore on or near your penis?	....	.....
40. Do you have a discharge from your penis?	....	.....
41. Is your urine stream weak and slow?	....	.....
42. Has a doctor told you that you have prostate trouble?	....	.....
For Women Only:		
43. Do you have spotting for 3 or more days between periods?	....	.....
44. Do you have any troubles with your menstrual periods?	....	.....
45. Do you have any sores around your genital area (sex organ)?	....	.....
46. Have you been troubled with a vaginal discharge?	....	.....
47. Do you have lumps in your breast?	....	.....
48. Does working tire you out completely?	....	.....
49. Have you lost 15 or more pounds in weight recently?	....	.....
50. Do you always seem to be hungry?	....	.....
51. Lately are you more thirsty than usual?	....	.....
52. Do you have diabetes (sugar disease)?	....	.....
53. Were you ever treated for severe anemia (thin blood)?	....	.....
54. Were you ever treated for "bad blood" (venereal disease)?	....	.....
55. Have you ever had tuberculosis (TB)?	....	.....
56. Do you have any chronic disease?	....	.....
57. Did you ever have a serious operation?	....	.....
58. Did you ever have a serious injury?	....	.....
59. Have you recently fainted or had a black out spell?	....	.....
60. Do you usually have great difficulty in falling asleep or staying asleep?	....	.....
61. Do you smoke more than 20 cigarettes a day?	....	.....
62. Do you usually take two or more alcoholic drinks a day?	....	.....
63. Has your memory begun to fail you?	....	.....
64. Is there any problem not mentioned you want to discuss with a doctor?	....	.....
Please use this space for any further comments you might want to make about your health.		
Date ____________________		
Reviewed by: ____________________		
Action Taken ____________________		

Example 3: **Problem/Issues/Goals List**

CONTINUUM OF LEVELS OF HUMAN FUNCTIONING:

STEP 1. For each problem confronting a person, circle the level of disability at intake and the intake date (month/date).
STEP 2. Estimate the level of disability expected by circling, also listing date of expected outcome (month/date).
STEP 3. Circle Global Level of Functioning: The person's overall ability to function in their ordinary community setting. Level 6 (Severe Dysfunct.), Level 5, Level 4, Level 3, Level 2, Level 1 (Functions Autonomously).

	6	Date	5	Date	4	Date
Organ damage	a. Extensive system and/or organ damage		a. Continuing minimal system and/or organ damage		a. Arrested system and/or organ deterioration	
Addiction	b. Chronic addiction with extreme withdrawal		b. Physical dependence with tolerable withdrawal		b. Physical dependence with tolerable withdrawal	
Psycho. dependence	c. Chronic debilitating psychological dependence		c. Periodic debilitating psychological dependence		c. Recognition of need for psychological independence	
Self image	d. Undifferentiated self image		d. Distorted self image		d. Recognition of distortions	
Motivation	e. Total lack of motivation		e. Able to articulate some external motivation		e. Able to respond to external motivation	
Anxiety	f. Constant debilitation & unrecognized anxiety		f. Recognition of the sources of anxiety		f. Ability to distinguish between appro. and inappro.	
Reasoning	g. Totally distorted thinking or reasoning		g. Recognition of consequence of rational thought		g. Recognition of distortion in reasoning	
Employment	h. Unemployable		h. Minimally employable & recognized employ. need		h. Seriously seeking employment	
Financial	i. Lack of any financial means		i. Taking steps to alleviate lack of financial means		i. Minimal financial means	
Housing	j. Total lack of housing		j. Taking steps to alleviate lack of housing		j. Finds inadequate housing	
Relationships	k. Inability to form interpersonal relationships		k. Forms superficial relationships		k. Recognizes need for interpersonal relationships	
Rejection	l. Rejection by community		l. Realization of rejection		l. Understanding the rejection	
Social dependence	m. Total dependence on social agencies		m. Partial dependence on social agencies		m. Partial dependence on social agencies	
Behavior	n. Extensive inappropriate behavior		n. Demonstrable discomfort with inappropriate behavior		n. Rejection of some inappropriate behavior	
Abuse	o. Substance abuse daily		o. Substance abuse several times per week		o. Substance abuse once per week	
Intoxication	p. Chronic intoxication		p. Chronic intoxication		p. Periodic intoxication	
Consumption	q. Massive consumption		q. Excessive consumption		q. Reduction of excessive consumption	
Legal	r. Chronic legal involvement		r. Frequent legal involvement		r. Minimal legal involvement	

(*continued*)

Example 4: **Intervention Plan**

Problem Area	Details of Problem	Pred. Outcome	Treatment Activity

Example 3. *(continued)*

		3	Date		2	Date		1	Date
Organ damage	a.	Minimal sys. &/or organ improvement		a.	Significant system &/or organ improvement		a.	Stabilized organ & system use	
Addiction	b.	Nondebilitating physical after effects		b.	Nondebilitating physical after effects		b.	No physical effects	
Psycho. dependence	c.	Minimal development of psychological independence		c.	Extensive establishment of psychological independence		c.	Total psychological independence	
Self image	d.	Elimination of most distortions		d.	Development of realistic self image		d.	Establishment of realistic self image	
Motivation	e.	Beginning to articulate internalized motivation		e.	Able to respond to some internalized motivation		e.	Self motivated and internalized	
Anxiety	f.	Alleviation of inappropriate anxiety		f.	Ability to deal with appropriate anxiety		f.	Constructive use of appro. anxiety with absence of inappro. anxiety	
Reasoning	g.	Rejection in the basic distortions in reasoning		g.	Minimal use of rational thought		g.	Optimum use of thinking or reasoning	
Employment	h.	Employed but dissatisfied with employment		h.	Gainfully employed & accepting of the limits of employment		h.	Satisfied in occupation or preoccupation	
Financial	i.	Beginning of the establishment of financial stability		i.	Financial stability		i.	Financial security	
Housing	j.	Finds adequate temporary housing		j.	Seeks adequate permanent housing		j.	Finds satisfying and secure housing	
Relationships	k.	Initiates authentic interpersonal relations		k.	Establishes authentic interpersonal relationships		k.	Maintains authentic interpersonal relationships	
Rejection	l.	Dealing with the rejection		l.	Overcoming rejection		l.	Acceptancy by community	
Social dependence	m.	Periodic supportive dependence on social agencies		m.	Periodic supportive dependence		m.	Independence regarding social agencies	
Behavior	n.	Substitution of more appropriate behavior		n.	Exercise of more and more appropriate behavior		n.	Practices appropriate behavior	
Abuse	o.	Infrequent abuse		o.	No abuse		o.	Absence of usage	
Intoxication	p.	Infrequent intoxication		p.	No intoxication		p.	No intoxication	
Consumption	q.	Infrequent consumption		q.	Minimal consumption		q.	No consumption	
Legal	r.	Adjustment of legal responsibilities		r.	Demonstrates legal responsibility		r.	Maintains legal responsibility	

Example 4. *(continued)*

Provider	Service	Frequency	Supportive Services	Treatment		Next Reviews			
				Length	Purchase	1	2	3	4

Example 5: **Flow Sheet**

Usually attached to front of file, treatment plan, or an episode mini-file within the larger clinical record file. It serves as a chronological index to the progress notes.

Date	Service	By Whom	Time	Level of Functioning

Example 6: **Record Audit Review and Quality and Utilization Review (Allegheny County, Pennsylvania): Clinical Record Audit and Quality Assurance Review Form***

Hobart Harris
University of Pittsburgh

PROCEDURE

After a random sample of clinical records on a target group is selected, two or more auditors with professional experience review each of the records according to the 16 items given on the following pages. The instrument focuses on two dimensions which can be described as a two dimensional array. The numbers in the cells identify items used in the audit instrument.

	Treatment Concerns				
Treatment States	Medication	Mental Status	Life Status and Goals	Goals/ Services	Breadth or Input
SERVICE PLAN DEVELOPMENT	1	2,3	4,5	6	7, (15)
TREATMENT	8	9	(10)	(10)	11, (15)
TERMINATION	12	(16)	(16)	13	(15)

Items in parentheses cover more than one area.

All 16 items are scored and deficits noted on the scoring summary by both auditors. Discrepancies between auditors are discussed, or a third auditor is asked to also rate the record.

---

* Edited and adapted by F. L. Newman, 8/1/79.

CLINICAL RECORD SCORING FORM

Client I.D. ______________________ Date of Audit ______________
Target Group ______________ Age ________ Agency ______________
Diagnosis ______________________ Prior Hosp. History ______________
Initial Level of Functioning ______________ Last Level of Functioning ______________
Primary Therapist ______________________
Case Manager or Supervisor ______________________

	Item #	Item Description	Score (0)–(4)	Deficiency
SERVICE PLAN DEVELOPMENT	1	Medical History		
	2	Previous Mental Disabilities		
	3	Current Mental Status		
	4	Functional Social & Role Performances		
	5	Immediate Life Management Situation		
	6	Problem/Goal Oriented Treatment Plan		
	7	Breadth of Input, Including Client		
		mean = median =		
TREATMENT	8	Medication Administration		
	9	Mental Status during Treatment		
	10	Treatment Progress & Goals at Review		
	11	Breadth of Input at Review, Including Client		
		mean = median =		
TERMINATION	12	Arranging Client's Medication needs after termination		
	13	Discharge Summary		
	14	Circumstances of Termination		
	15	Release of Acquisition of Client Information		
	16	Degree of Goal Attainment		
		mean = median =		

ITEM SUMMARIES

Medical History Items: 1 ___ + 8 ___ + 12 ___ = ___ ÷ 3 = ___
Mental Status Items: 2 ___ + 3 ___ + 9 ___ = ___ ÷ 3 = ___
Life Status/Problem Items: 4 ___ + 5 ___ = ___________ ÷ 2 = ___
Goal/Services: 6 ___ + 10 ___ + 13 ___ = ___ ÷ 3 = ___
Breadth of Input: 7 ___ + 11 ___ + 15 ___ = ___ ÷ 3 = ___

Service Plan Development	Medication History
Medication	(4) File includes (a) medication history (a) the name of the medication; (b) dosage; (c) route of administration; (d) frequency of administration; (e) adverse reactions
	(3) File includes three or four of the five categories listed above.
1	(2) File includes one or two of the five categories listed above.
	(1) File is missing all of the five categories listed above.
	(0) N/A—To the best of the auditor's knowledge, the client has never had psychoactive medication prescribed previous to entering service in the agency or had it prescribed over three years ago.
	Deficit: ______________________

Service Plan Development	Review of the client's previous mental disabilities and/or services received
Status/Problems	(4) File includes (a) summary records of all previous mental health/health/mental retardation services received; (b) general descriptions (and diagnoses) of previous problems for which the services were received; (c) date of onset of all previous disturbances.
	(3) File includes two of the above three categories of information but is missing one.
2	(2) File includes one of the above categories but is missing two.
	(1) File does not include any of the above information and there is reason to believe that the client has had previous mental disabilities and/or services.
	(0) N/A—To the best of the auditor's knowledge, this client has not had previous mental disabilities and/or services.
	Deficit: ______________________

Service Plan Development	Review of the client's current mental status
Status/Problems	(4) The record includes, where necessary, (a) reports of neurological examinations, (b) discussion of client's affect, (c) description of the client's psychotic symptoms (disorganized speech, hallucinations, appropriate affect, etc.) and (d) descriptions of the client's anxieties, fears, preoccupations.
	(3) Includes discussion of client's symptoms in two or more of the major areas as defined above, but is deficient in at least one *necessary* area.
3	(2) Includes discussion of client's symptoms in one major area but is deficient in at least two others.
	(1) None of the above areas are presented in sufficient detail for the Interviewer to understand the client's mental status.
	Deficit: ______________________

Service Plan Development	Assessment of the client's functional performance, social appropriateness, and role performance.
Status/Problems	(4) The client's ability to function in the folk support system is reviewed sufficiently for the auditor to understand the client's functioning (a) socially, (b) occupationally, and (c) the major external (environmental) stressors affecting the client are described.
	(3) Two of these three areas are sufficiently described; one is not.
4	(2) One of these areas is sufficiently described; two are not.
	(1) None of these areas is reviewed sufficiently for the reviewer.
	Deficit: ______________________

Service Plan Development — Assessment of client's immediate life management situation

Life Situation

5

(4) The record includes, where necessary, an assessment of the client's needs re: (a) housing, (b) income, (c) education, (d) physical health, (e) child or geriatric care, (f) vocational training.
(3) The record does not include an assessment of one of the above areas.
(2) The record does not include an assessment of more than one of the above areas.
(1) The record does not include an assessment of the client's needs in any of the above areas.
(0) N/A—To the best of the auditor's knowledge, the client does not have life management problems.

Deficit: ______________________________

Service Plan Development — Assessment of the client's current problems and construction of goal attainment, problem-oriented, or other objectively-oriented treatment plans based on these problems.

Plans Services

6

(4) (a) The client's problems are listed, (b) specific goals are identified, (c) procedures and/or services are designated to reach each of the goals that are listed, (d) hoped-for levels of functioning are made or a review date specified.
(3) The client's problems are listed and specific goals are identified, but the specific levels of functioning hoped for at the end of treatment are not identified nor is the length of treatment predicted.
(2) The client's problems are listed, but neither goals, nor expected outcomes, nor the expected length of treatment are specified.
(1) The client's problems are not clearly presented, goals are absent or vague, services are not specified, and no expected length of treatment is specified.

Deficit: ______________________________

Service Plan Development — The service plan has been developed by a multidisciplinary team, including the client

Breadth of Input

7

(4) Signatures of (a) the client, (b) the case manager, (c) a supervisor, and (d) a psychologist or psychiatrist appear on the plan.
(3) Three of the required four signatures appear on the service plan.
(2) Two or one of the required signatures appear on the service plan.
(1) None of the required signatures appears on the service plan.
(0) N/A—All signatures but the client's appear on the service plan. The client's does not because the treatment team feels that it is not in the client's best interests to read the service plan, or the client was not competent to understand it, and this is noted.

Deficit: ______________________________

Treatment — Medication Administration

Medication

8

(4) The client's file includes a record of all medications administered during treatment including (a) the name of the medication, (b) dosage, (c) route of administration, (d) frequency of administration, (e) adverse reactions, (f) the prescribing physician's name, and (g) evidence that medication checks are made every 45 days by a physician.
(3) File includes all but one or two of the above seven categories of information.
(2) File is missing three or four of the above categories of information.
(1) File is missing all of the above categories of information.
(0) N/A—To the best of the auditor's knowledge, the client has never used or had psychoactive medication prescribed during treatment.

Deficit: ______________________________

Treatment
Status/Problems

Description of the client's mental status during treatment.

(4) The client's mental status is (a) adequately described in the progress/treatment notes and is related to: (b) the treatment procedures being employed, (c) the client's medication (where necessary), and (d) the external life stresses (interpersonal, legal, or financial) the client is experiencing.
(3) The client's mental status is described but related only to two of the factors listed above.
9 (2) The client's mental status is described but related only to one or none of the factors listed above.
(1) The client's mental status is not described.

Deficit: ______________________________

Treatment
Plans/Services

Description of the client's progress which relates that progress specifically to the client's goals as stated in the service/treatment plan

(4) The client's progress is (a) described adequately enough for the auditor to understand, (b) related to the client's medication (where prescribed), (c) related to the client's external stresses (interpersonal, legal, or financial), and (d) specifically related to the client's treatment goals as stated in the treatment plan.
(3) The client's progress is described in general terms but is not related to one of the categories mentioned above.
10 (2) The client's progress is described in general terms but is not related to two or more of the categories mentioned above.
(1) The client's progress is not described adequately enough to understand.
(0) N/A—The client has left service before receiving service.

Deficit: ______________________________

Treatment
Breadth of Input

The client's treatment progress has periodically been reviewed by individuals of all necessary service specialities at the review date.

(4) Signatures indicate that the client's progress has been reviewed (a) every 50 days by (b) a case manager, (c) the therapist's supervisor, (d) the physician providing medication (if any), (e) the primary therapist.
(3) Signatures indicate that two of the three types of individuals have reviewed the client's progress at appropriately chosen review dates.
11 (2) Signatures indicate that only one of the three types of individuals have reviewed the client's progress.
(1) No evidence is present that the client's progress is reviewed by anyone other than his therapist.
(0) N/A—The client has left treatment before review was appropriate.

Deficit: ______________________________

Discharge
Medication

Arrangements to manage the client's continuing need for medication after discharge have been made.

(4) The client has been given a prescription including (a) dosage, route of administration, etc.; (b) arrangements have been made with a physician to review and update the prescription within 45 days.
(3) The client has received a prescription but no arrangements have been made with a physician to review or update it.
12 (2) The client has been referred to a physician but no prescription has been specified.
(1) No attention has been given to the client's Rx needs following termination from service.
(0) N/A—The client has either never had psychoactive drugs prescribed or stopped using them before termination.

Deficit: ______________________________

Discharge

Status/Problems

13

Discharge Summary

(4) The client's (a) progess towards reaching goals, (b) mental status, (c) capability to function socially and occupationally, and (d) the major external stresses (interpersonal, legal, or financial) affecting the client at discharge are described.
(3) One of the above is missing.
(2) Two or more of the above are missing.
(1) No discharge summary has been written.

Deficit: ______________________________

Discharge

Cause of Discharge

14

Circumstances of Discharge

(4) Both the client and the program agree that discharge is appropriate at this time and neither feels that continued service at this agency is necessary or appropriate.
(3) The client has left the program even though the program feels that continued service at this agency is necessary and appropriate.
(2) The program has discharged the client even though the client feels that continued service at this agency is necessary and appropriate.
(1) Causes other than the desires of both the agency and the client have forced service to cease (i.e., client moves, takes a job, is hospitalized for medical problems, is unable to find transportation; the program loses funds, changes location, etc.).

Deficit: ______________________________

All Stages

Breadth of Input/
Client's Rights

15

Release or acquisition of information about the client

(4) Whenever there is a need to release/obtain information about an active client to/from other agencies, a copy of a form: (a) signed and dated by the client, (b) includes a statement of the client's right to refuse permission, and (c) includes the origin/destination of the information.
(3) Two of the three requirements listed above are present, one is not.
(2) One of the three requirements listed above is present, two are not.
(1) Evidence exists that information was obtained/released without the client's knowledge.
(0) N/A—To the best of the auditor's ability to discover, no data about the client has been released or obtained without the client's knowledge.

Deficit: ______________________________

Other

Goal Attainment

16

Degree of goal attainment at discharge

(4) The client has reached the expected level of functioning on all of treatment goals.
(3) The client has reached the expected level of functioning on more than 50% of treatment goals.
(2) The client has reached the expected level of functioning on less than 50% of treatment goals.
(1) The client has failed to reach the expected level of functioning on any of treatment goals.
(0) N/A—Treatment goals are too ill-defined to evaluate the client's progress.

Goals not attained: ______________________________

Example 7: **Case Conference and Review Form (Meadville, Pa.)**

CASE CONFERENCE AND REVIEW FORM

DATE: ______________________

COUNSELOR: ______________________

NAME OF CLIENT: ______________________ AGE: ______________________

CURRENT EMPLOYMENT: ______________________ MARITAL STATUS: ______________________

CHILDREN: ______________________ AGE: ______________________

______________________ ______________________

______________________ ______________________

DATE OF INITIAL REFERRAL: ______________________ NUMBER OF TIMES SEEN: ______________________

INITIAL CONTINUUM POSITION: Physical ______________________

Psychosocial ______________________

Behavioral ______________________

1. MAJOR PROBLEM AREAS: ______________________

2. PROBLEM AREAS WORKED ON: ______________________

3. BASIC APPROACH TAKEN TO DATE: ______________________

4.* SITUATION AT PRESENT: ______________________

5.* PRESENT CONTINUUM POSITION: ______________________

6.* PROJECTED PROBLEM AREAS: ______________________

SIGNIFICANT DATES: (i.e., hospitalization, jailed, etc.)

*If major changes are called for, a new treatment plan is required (see Examples 3 and 4 of this Appendix).

Example 8: **Client Satisfaction Followup: Service Evaluation Questionnaire***

C. Clifford Attkisson and Tuan D. Nguyen
Department of Psychiatry
University of California, San Francisco

BACKGROUND AND RESEARCH SUMMARY**

The eight-item brief form provided here was tested as part of a 31-item scale, using a sample of 248 mental-health clients in five settings. The results suggested that the 8-item scale could

*Copies of this questionnaire can be obtained from C. C. Attkisson, PhD, LPI Box 4-F, University of California, San Francisco, CA 94143.

**From Larsen, D. L., Attkisson, C. C., Hargreaves, W. A., & Nguyen, T. D. (1979). Assessment of client/patient satisfaction: Development of a general scale. *Evaluation and Program Planning*.

differentiate client satisfaction independent of treatment outcome. Some of the specific findings were low, but there were significant relationships between the total 8-item questionnaire scores and staying in treatment, percent of appointments kept, client's self-report of symptomatology, the client's global improvement rating (but not necessarily the therapists'), and the therapists' satisfaction. While the therapists' assessments of global level of functioning at terminations was not correlated, the total score on the Brief Psychiatric Rating Scale (Overall and Gorham, 1962) was correlated.

GENERAL INTERPRETATION OF SCALE'S TOTAL SCORE

Estimates client satisfaction independent of treatment outcome.

Total Score	Interpretation
8–20	Low Satisfaction
21–26	Medium
27–32	High Satisfaction

FOR STATISTICAL ANALYSIS AND EVALUATION RESEARCH

Contrast client satisfaction ratings by categories of *Background* and *Service* Responses and by total symptom scores.

CLIENT EVALUATION OF SERVICES[1]

Please help us improve our program by answering some questions about the services you have received. We are interested in your honest opinion, whether they are positive or negative. *Please answer all questions.* We also welcome your comments and suggestions. Thank you very much, we really appreciate your help.

CIRCLE YOUR ANSWER

1. How would you rate the quality of service you received?

4	3	2	1
Excellent	Good	Fair	Poor

2. Did you get the kind of service you wanted?

1	2	3	4
No, definitely not	No, not really	Yes, generally	Yes, definitely

3. To what extent has our program met your needs?

4	3	2	1
Almost all of my needs have been met	Most of my needs have been met	Only a few of my needs have been met	None of my needs have been met

4. If a friend were in need of similar help, would you recommend our program to him/her?

1	2	3	4
No, definitely not	No, I don't think so	Yes, I think so	Yes, definitely

5. How satisfied are you with the amount of help you received?

1	2	3	4
Quite dissatisfied	Indifferent or mildly dissatisfied	Mostly satisfied	Very satisfied

6. Have the services you received helped you to deal more effectively with your problems?

4	3	2	1
Yes, they helped a great deal	Yes, they helped somewhat	No, they really didn't help	No, they seemed to make things worse

7. In an overall, general sense, how satisfied are you with the service you received?

4	3	2	1
Very satisfied	Mostly satisfied	Indifferent or mildly dissatisfied	Quite dissatisfied

8. If you were to seek help again, would you come back to our program?

1	2	3	4
No, definitely not	No, I don't think so	Yes, I think so	Yes, definitely

PLEASE WRITE YOUR COMMENTS

The thing I like best about the center is: ______________________

____

____

If I would change one thing about the center, it would be: ______________________

____

____

CLIENT SELF-EVALUATION[2,3]

Below is a list of problems and complaints that people sometimes have. Read each item carefully, and circle one of the answers that best describes HOW MUCH DISCOMFORT THAT PROBLEM HAS CAUSED YOU DURING THE PAST WEEK INCLUDING TODAY. Do not skip any items. If you change your mind, erase your first answer completely. If you have any questions, please ask the questionnaire administrator.

1. How much were you distressed by feeling lonely?

0	1	2	3	4
Not at all	A little bit	Moderately	Quite a bit	Extremely

2. How much were you distressed by feeling no interest in things?

4	3	2	1	0
Extremely	Quite a bit	Moderately	A little bit	Not at all

3. How much were you distressed by feeling afraid in open spaces or on the streets?

0	1	2	3	4
Not at all	A little bit	Moderately	Quite a bit	Extremely

4. How much were you distressed by feeling weak in part of your body?

0	1	2	3	4
Not at all	A little bit	Moderately	Quite a bit	Extremely

5. How much were you distressed by feeling blue?

4	3	2	1	0
Extremely	Quite a bit	Moderately	A little bit	Not at all

6. How much were you distressed by heavy feelings in your arms or legs?

4	3	2	1	0
Extremely	Quite a bit	Moderately	A little bit	Not at all

7. How much were you distressed by feeling afraid to go out of your house alone?

0	1	2	3	4
Not at all	A little bit	Moderately	Quite a bit	Extremely

8. How much were you distressed by feeling tense or keyed up?

4	3	2	1	0
Extremely	Quite a bit	Moderately	A little bit	Not at all

9. How much were you distressed by feelings of worthlessness?

4	3	2	1	0
Extremely	Quite a bit	Moderately	A little bit	Not at all

10. How much were you distressed by feeling lonely even when you are with people?

0	1	2	3	4
Not at all	A little bit	Moderately	Quite a bit	Extremely

SUPPLEMENTARY INFORMATION (FORM A)

BACKGROUND (Please circle or write in appropriate answer)

SEX:
☐ 1. Male
(19) 2. Female

CURRENT AGE:
☐☐ Years
(20–21)

CURRENT EMPLOYMENT:
☐ 1. Employed full-time
(31) 2. Employed part-time
3. Housewife
4. Unemployed
5. Full-time student
6. Part-time student
7. Retired

EDUCATION:
☐ 1. Grade 8 or less
(35) 2. Some high school
3. High school graduate
4. Some college
5. College graduate
6. College past BA or BS

MARITAL STATUS:
☐ 1. Never married
(22) 2. Married
3. Separated
4. Divorced
5. Widowed

YEARLY FAMILY IMCOME:
☐ 1. $2,500 or under
(32) 2. $2,501–$5,000
3. $5,001–$7,500
4. $7,501–$10,000
5. $10,001–$12,500
6. Over $12,500

ETHNOCULTURAL GROUP:
☐ 1. American Indian
(36) 2. Black
3. Chinese
4. Filipino
5. Japanese
6. Mexican American
7. Other Latin or Spanish heritage
8. White
9. Other:

USUAL OCCUPATION: ____________ ☐☐☐ (23–25)

CURRENT OCCUPATION: ☐☐☐ (26–28)

NUMBER OF TIMES RESIDENCE CHANGED IN LAST FIVE YEARS ____________ ☐☐ (29–30)

☐☐ (33–34) NUMBER OF PEOPLE DEPENDENT ON ABOVE INCOME, INCLUDING SELF ____________

SERVICE (Please circle appropriate answer)

I HAVE USUALLY COME TO THIS AGENCY:
☐ (37)
1. Only when I need to.
2. Once every 3–4 months
3. Once or twice a month
4. Once or twice a week
5. More than twice a week
6. I only came here once.

HAVE YOU BEEN CHARGED A FEE FOR THE SERVICES RECEIVED?
☐ (38)
1. Yes, a full fee
2. Yes, a part fee, according to the sliding scale
3. No, I pay no fee

HAVE YOU RECEIVED SERVICES HERE BEFORE?
☐ (39)
1. Yes
2. No

HAVE YOU EVER RECEIVED SIMILAR SERVICES ELSEWHERE?
☐ (40)
1. Yes
2. No

FOR OFFICE USE ONLY (Do not write below this line)

Agency Name ______________________ ☐☐ (42–43)
Respondent Code Number (ID): ☐☐☐☐☐☐ (44–49)
Date Current Service Began: (50–55)
Date Current Service Ended: (56–61)
(Include only where applicable)

Approximate Amount of Services Provided:
Number of Outpatient Visits: ☐☐☐ (70–72)
Number of Partial Care Days: ☐☐☐ (73–75)
Number of Residential or Inpatient Days: ☐☐☐ (76–78)

Major current or most recent service(s) received. (Write in all applicable codes)
1. ☐☐ 2. ☐☐ 3. ☐☐ 4. ☐☐ (62–69)

☐ Previous Psychiatric Hospitalization
(79) 1. Yes 2. No

☐ Did client receive help in completing questionnaire?
(80) 1. Yes 2. No

1. Larsen, D. L., Attkisson, C. C., Hargreaves, W. A., & Nguyen, T. D. (1979). Assessment of client/patient satisfaction in human service programs: Development of a general scale. *Evaluation and Program Planning, 2,* 197–209.

2. Derogatis, L., Lipman, R., & Covi, L. (1973). The SCL–90: An outpatient rating scale (preliminary report). *Psychopharmacology Bulletin, 9,* 13–28.

3. Hoffman, N. G. & Overall, P. B. (1978). Factor structure of the SCL–90 in a psychiatric population. *Journal of Consulting and Clinical Psychology, 46*(6), 1187–1191.

Example 9: **Termination Form (Chester County, Pa.)**

NAME ____________________________ CASE # __________________________
DATE ADMITTED ______ DATE LAST SEEN ______ DATE DISCHARGED ______

DISCONTINUATION INFORMATION

Reason for Discontinuation
______ 1. Client died
______ 2. Evaluation only (client not treated)
______ 3. Client withdrew from treatment—Improved (go to Ques. 1 & 2)
______ 4. Client withdrew from treatment—Not improved (go to Ques. 1 & 2)
______ 5. Family withdrew client—Improved (go to Ques. 1 & 2)
______ 6. Family withdrew client—Not Improved (go to Ques. 1 & 2)
______ 7. Client Transferred—Improved (go to Ques. 3 & 4)
______ 8. Client Transferred—Not Improved (go to Ques. 3 & 4)
______ 9. Client Discharged—Improved (go to Ques. 5)
______ 10. Client Discharged—Not Improved (go to Ques. 5)

1. Reason for Withdrawal:
   ______ (a) Client never returned after initial visit
   ______ (b) Client stopped coming after one or more visits with same therapist
   ______ (c) Client stopped coming after transfer to new therapist
   ______ (d) Discharge demanded by client or family against medical advice
   ______ (e) Other (specify) ______________________________
2. If client withdrew from treatment, was he/she contacted regarding reason for withdrawal?
   ______ Yes ______ No
3. Client transferred to:
   ______ (a) Inpatient
   ______ (b) Community Support Service
   ______ (c) Another BSU
   ______ (d) Partial Hospitalization
   ______ (e) Other (specify) ______________________________

4. Reason for transfer:
   ______ (a) Part of a long-range therapeutic plan
   ______ (b) For short-range therapeutic benefit
   ______ (c) On demand by client or client's family
   ______ (d) Lack of BSU resources
   ______ (e) Other (specify) ______________________________
5. Reason for discharge:
   ______ (a) Maximum benefit derived from BSU (check if applicable in conjunction with another reason
   ______ (b) To go to private care
   ______ (c) Court order
   ______ (d) Moved outside BSU area
   ______ (e) Client was never contacted to continue treatment
   ______ (f) Other (specify) ______________________________

At time of discontinuation, did client need further service? ______ Yes
______ No

DIAGNOSIS AT DISCONTINUATION ______ APA Code ______ Level of Functioning

Comments ______________________________
____
____
____

Signature ______________________________ Date: ____________

Service Record

Each time that client is seen list the service *Type, By Whom, Time,* & Client's *Level of Functioning.*

Date (Mo./Day/Yr.)	Services			Funct. Level
	Type	By	Time	

THE "MINI-EPISODE" FILE: A FILE WITHIN A FILE

The mini-episode file diagrammed below was created to provide a section of the clinical record which is solely concerned with the client's current episode treatment plan and progress. Thus, the clinician, reviewers, and supervisors can go directly to that information which is current.

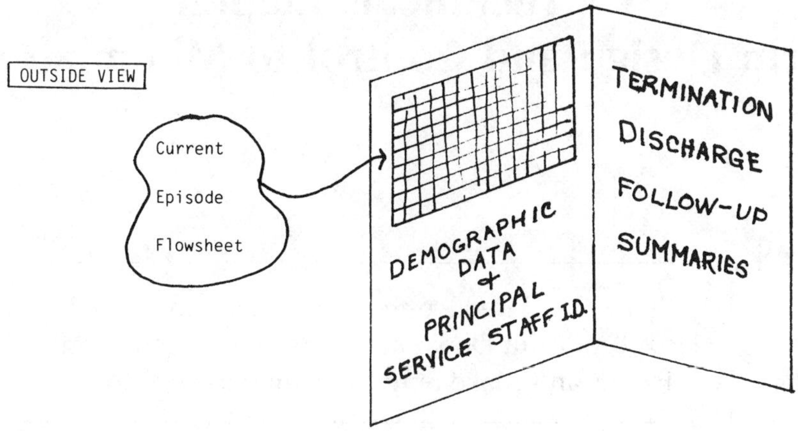

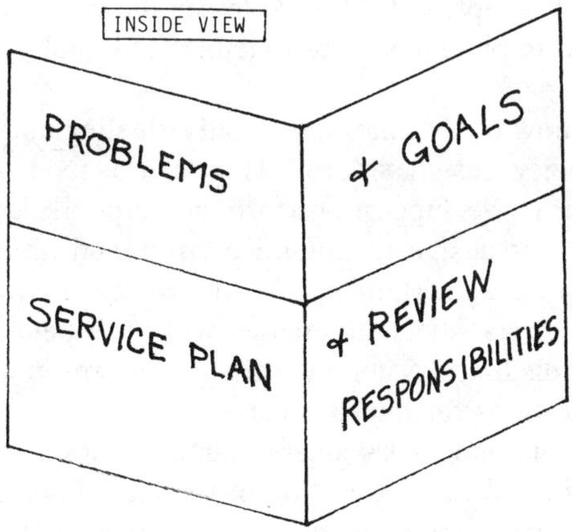

Contents of File

a) Recent Social/Health History

b) Progress Notes

c) Review Summaries

Chapter 11

Technical Chapter
Form Design and Control to Minimize Errors

How Can I Reduce the Time Spent on Forms?
How Can I Cut Down on Staff's Hostility to Forms?
How Can I Make Sure My Numbers Are Right?

There are four critical issues addressed in Chapter 11: How to lessen the time burden of data collection; how to cut down on errors; how to put good forms together; and finally, how to build in controls to assure complete statistical data.

While everyone has to complete forms, how many times are negative feeling and resentment fostered by having staff complete a poorly designed form? How can a good form be distinguished from a bad one? What are constructive suggestions to improve poorly designed forms? What are time-tested approaches in forms design to minimize errors and time costs?

Developing a good form, however, is not enough. Built-in controls are needed to be sure forms are properly completed and processed so statistical summaries will be dependable. A quick checklist will help assure the proper controls in the system, to spot weaknesses in the data-capture process, and to identify positive suggestions for improvement.

Good forms can cut down unwanted errors and save valuable clinician time. Accurate counts feed essential reports for managers and accurate unit costing of services. Poor controls on forms can lead to incomplete reporting and inaccurate costing. Ideally someone should be assigned the design and control responsibilities who has specific training and reviews all forms introduced into the organization. (The Office of Management and Budget [OMB] performs this function for the federal government.)

Chapter 11 identifies the features of good form design, time-tested techniques to evaluate form, and the features of good control over the collection of basic statistical data. The three major sections are:

(1) DESIGN AND FORMAT OF FORMS ease data collection efforts and improve accuracy.
(2) GOOD CONTROLS OVER STATISTICAL DATA CAPTURE assure accurate and useful data.
(3) DESIGN OF THE GENERAL FLOW OF INFORMATION AND DOCUMENTS moves data accurately and in a timely manner through the service system.

1. DESIGN AND FORMAT OF FORMS

If data are being captured for decision making, the quality of the decisions is directly affected by the integrity of the underlying data. If, for example, an item is miscoded or is incomplete for 40% of the clients entering a system, summary data and inferences about the total population may be misleading.

Accuracy and completeness of data are influenced by the form itself. For example, in one system a client release was on the *back* of the form and about 25% of the forms had to be returned because of the omission. Essential information should not be on the back of a form, since most people don't treat forms like pages in a book where both sides of the page are read.

Coding Categories

How many coding categories should be used? Basically, this is a trade-off between precision and reliability. Generally, the more precision of judgment requested, the lower the reliability of the measure (Chapman, page 51).[1] Reliability is affected by the number of categories and the degree to which the categories are mutually exclusive. Simplification is a highly desired objective. Use of relatively simple schemes, or ones whose complications have been demonstrated to be useful by prior investigation (Chapman, page 53), is preferred.

Self-Study Exercise

Let's trace an example of how we could capture data. We could ask, ''Please write your name on the following line.'' (Go ahead and write yours.)

____

Now what if we ask you to do it again, except we give you the following box with ''tick'' marks:

LAST NAME													

What differences do you see between the two writings? List them below.

Difference #1 ____________________________________
____

Difference #2 ____________________________________
____

Did you find, for example, that you printed the second time? Did you put your last name first in your first writing? Is the second writing easier to read? Which way would you like it if you were keying the data into your computer or manual files? Which way is likely to cut down on errors? You're now ready to consider item formats.

---

[1] Chapman, Robert L., PhD, (1976) *The Design of Management Information Systems for Mental Health Organizations: A Primer*, National Institute for Mental Health, DHEW Publication No. (ADM) 76–333, Washington, D.C.: U.S. Government Printing Office.

Item Format

Four major approaches exist (Chapman, page 53).

(1) Write out data in full script and code later:

(first write down) (and then code)

(17) Ethnic Background *White Anglo* [1]

(2) List codes and categories and check:

(17) Ethnic Background

(Item checked) (✓)
(1) ☑ White
(2) ☐ Black
(etc.)

(3) Write in a selected code in a specified box:

(17)	Ethnic Background	1

OR (code goes here)

17. Ethnic Background					1
1.	Wh/Anglo	4. Am. Ind.	7.	Filipino	
2.	Black	5. Chinese	8.	Other N-White	
3.	Wh/Latin	6. Japanese	9.	Unknown	

(4) Blacken code between parallel lines opposite the appropriate digit (optical scan):

(17) Ethnic Background

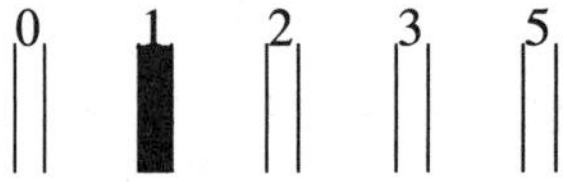

(Mark goes here)

The first three types require keying the data to change it to machine readable form. The last method may be optically scanned, thus eliminating the keying step. The various coding methods have varying effects on the control of errors and cost in time to prepare. Chapman (page 54) advances an evaluation in Table 1.

Table 1.* Control of Errors of Varying Coding Methods

	Control of Errors:					
			In Transcribing:			
Coding Method	In Capturing Data from Client	In Coding Judgments of Person Completing the Form	To Form	To Media (e.g., Cards, Tape)	In Complete Information	Cost in Time to Complete
1. COMPLETE THEN CODE	Excellent(X)	Good	Fair	Poor	Fair	Fair
2. CHECK ITEM	Excellent	Excellent	Good	Fair	Good	Good
3. ENTER NUMBER	Excellent	Excellent	Excellent	Good	Excellent	Excellent
4. OPTICAL SCAN	Excellent	Excellent	Good	Excellent	Good	Good

*Adapted from Robert L. Chapman, op. cit.

The evaluation of error control suggests an interval scale, but is in reality only a rank order. Clearly Method 1 (''Complete Then Code'') is the worst performer. Method 3 (''Enter Number from List'') is rated as the best performer although ''Optical Scan'' is not far behind. There are real differences in error control and time costs of coding methods used on forms.

When data are inserted into a form or record (e.g., name, I.D. number, date) by hand, a major problem is alpha or numeric character recognition by a *subsequent* reader (e.g., keypunch operator or fellow clinician). The place of entry should be clearly delineated by boxes and titles. The internal structure of the box should include ''ticks'' to encourage printing and spreading of letters which enhance legibility and readability.

5. LAST NAME

2. ENTRY DATE
Mo. | Day | Yr.

With these insights in selecting appropriate coding methods, a proposed form and its coding method can be easily reviewed and critiqued quickly and effectively.

Self-Study Exercise

Take one of your current clinical forms and evaluate its coding method:

	Column		
	A	B	C
1. For data to be entered, does it use boxes and ticks?	Yes	No	Not Applicable
2. Does it use more than one coding method (from Table 1)?	No	Yes	Not Applicable
3. Do any of the coding methods used on your form get a ''fair'' or ''poor'' rating on the control of errors?	No	Yes	Not Applicable
4. Is the ''cost in time to complete'' rated ''good'' or better?	Yes	No	Not Applicable

If you circled *any* answer in Column B, you have good reason to consider redesigning your current coding methods. You now could review all of your other forms for the effectiveness of their coding methods.

Coding method isn't the only dimension of forms design. Form layout and combination are two other critical concerns.

Form Layout

Another important feature of any form is its layout. Let the person know what, how, and where information is to be recorded. Figure 1 (from Chapman, page 56) shows two ways that work well. Each form should have a title. Now notice how the layout organizes the data into groups of related questions. Identifier information (e.g., client and therapist) should be at the top. (Note: One good way to get accurate and readable identifier information is by imprinting with plastic cards with raised and preprinted codes, like an American Express card!)

Important items should be asked early on. Less important questions should be at the end, so if fatigue or time constraints set in, essential data will not be missed. Shading on the form can discriminate between absolutely essential and highly desired information. Visual edits of the

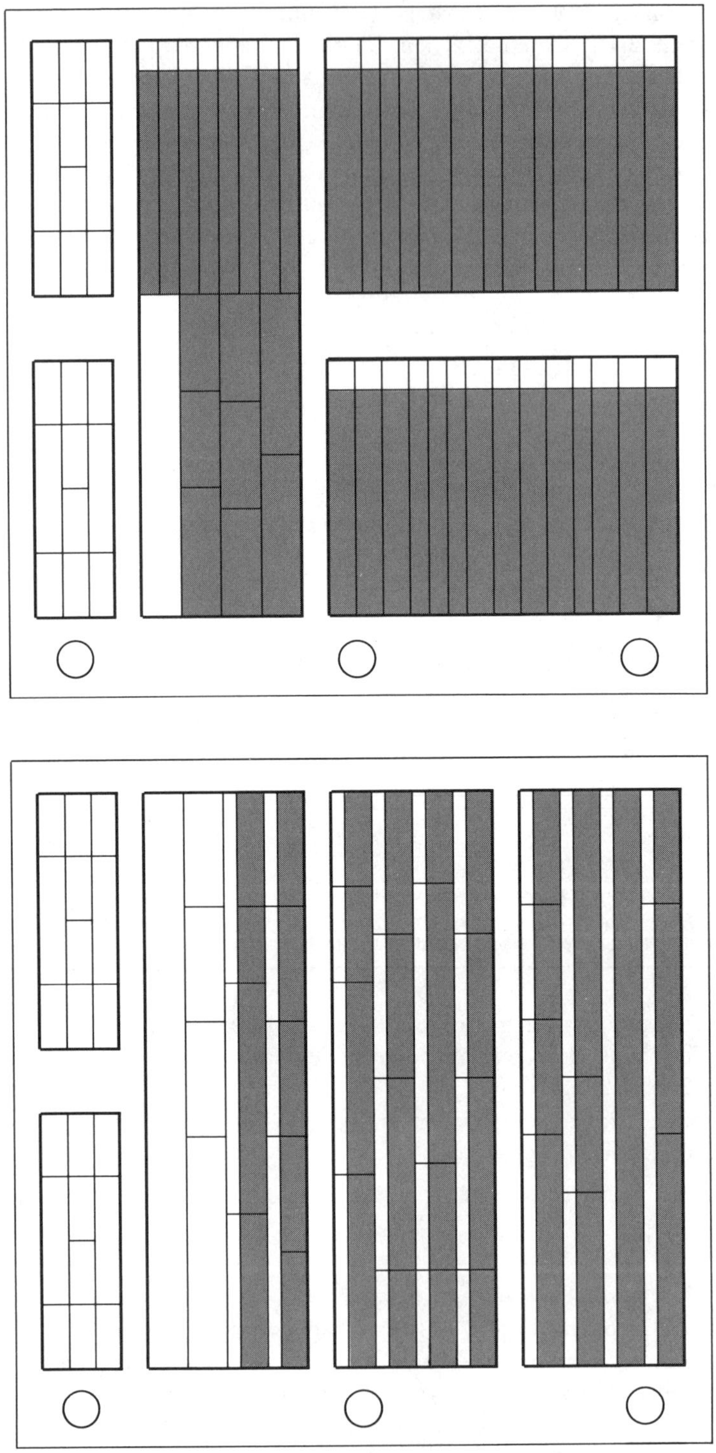

Figure 1. Examples of form layout

form are improved when the essential areas are highlighted so you know where to look for the fatal flaws.

By varying type sizes and using varying colors, the form can become more attractive and easier to read. Each major form should be a different color to enhance its sight recognition. If writing is likely to be in black or blue, then print using a different color to enhance contrasts.

Form Combinations

After deciding on the required forms, consult a firm specializing in business forms. Many standard techniques exist. For example, multiple copies can be separated after common information has been captured on all of the forms. Carbons or no-carbon required (NCR) can be used to get common information on all copies with one writing (up to 10 copies can be prepared if a typewriting instrument is used [Chapman, page 55] such as a typewriter or telewriter) with copies "snapped out" for various users. Different colors should be used to indicate the distribution of the copies (e.g., White = Clinical, Green = Program Evaluation, etc.). An alternative to multiple-copy forms is a multiple-use data base. If a computer is available, a common data base is created and then accessed by varying users (e.g., clinical, fiscal, research and evaluation).

Capturing information from the backs of forms should be avoided. Often the data captured on the back is overlooked. Error rates of data captured on the back of forms are high and will take extra effort to control.

Self-Study Exercise: Layout

Using one of the same forms you used earlier, briefly list up to the first 10 items of information requested.

	Brief Description	Importance	
		A. Essential	B. Desirable
1.	______	☐	☐
2.	______	☐	☐
3.	______	☐	☐
4.	______	☐	☐
5.	______	☐	☐
6.	______	☐	☐
7.	______	☐	☐
8.	______	☐	☐
9.	______	☐	☐
10.	______	☐	☐

Now examine each item in terms of its importance. If it is absolutely essential (e.g., client information), place a check in Column A. If its omission would be undesirable but would not be fatal to the processing of the document, place a check in Column B.

Are all essential items asked before desired ones? Are all essential items highlighted by shading? If not, reordering of the items may be indicated.

2. GOOD CONTROLS OVER STATISTICAL DATA CAPTURE

For a long time, accountants have recognized that the integrity of an agency's accounting system depended on

— The adequacy of the accounting systems to record and document all transactions affecting an agency's assets and equities.
— The adequacy of the internal controls incorporated within an agency's accounting system to promote reliable reporting about operations to ensure stewardship over assets.

However, many times weak internal controls characterize *statistical* data (especially from operations). Often, the controls for petty cash are more rigorous than the controls for accumulating units of service! Internal control developed in accounting because personal owner/manager observation and supervision of employees became impracticable and ineffective. Increasing size, growing complexity, and physical separation were behind the development of these controls. Surrogate control measures have been developed to

— Promote complete and reliable recording, processing, and reporting of authorized transactions (e.g., providing client services).
— Prevent or provide timely detection of errors or irregularities within recorded, processed, and reported statistical data.

At a minimum, statistical internal controls should provide reasonable control over available

— Recording
  - Client Admissions
  - Scheduled Services (e.g., appointments)
  - Disposition of Scheduled, and Unscheduled, Services, (e.g., services rendered, cancelled, no-shows, and walk-ins)
— Processing and Reporting of statistical data.

Transaction Control Procedures

The principal internal control procedures promote accurate and complete data:

— Qualified, well-trained personnel
— Control over and complete accounting for service rendered documents or staff-activity logs (or, in general, ''document'' control)

Acquiring and training individuals for varying statistical data capture is a continuing but essential challenge if statistical data are going to be useable.

Document control is usually done by prenumbering and accounting for the documents evidencing service transactions. If staff logs are used, daily counts should link service personnel accounted for and number of service logs received.

Self-Study Exercise

1.	Does your center or agency have a manual describing how *each* form should be completed?	YES	NO
2.	Is each *new* staff member given a training session on how to complete the forms properly?	YES	NO
3.	If service-rendered documents are used, are all documents prenumbered and systematically accounted for?	YES	NO

Any "NO" answers suggest weakness in the controls affecting complete and accurate data capture.

Assuring Timely Detection of Errors and Irregularities

Two principal internal control procedures can help detect errors and irregularities:

— Separation of Duties — Independent Checks

Separation of duties in statistical data accumulation usually prevents one staff person from fabricating data. For example, separation of duties occurs in the following sequence of events:

(1) Prenumbered service-rendered documents are issued by the accounting department to various receptionists (or service centers.)
(2) Receptionist inserts basic client data and distributes documents to clinicians.
(3) Clinicians insert services provided to clients.
(4) Receptionist collects the documents from clinicians and returns documents to the accounting department along with an account of the number of documents returned.

Contrast the foregoing type of control to an operation where services-rendered documents are distributed in bulk and in advance to clinicians who return them at will (say, once a week). Whose numbers are going to be more complete and more accurate?

Independent checking is the review of one employee's performance by another who has no authority over or contact with the operation being reviewed. Generally this review encourages complete, accurate, and honest reporting as well as timely detection of errors or irregularities. As an example of independent checking, control totals of clients seen from the receptionist should be reconciled with the number of services-rendered documents received by the business office.

Table 2 is for the technically oriented and suggests some minimal statistical internal controls for data arising from admissions and services.

Self-Study Exercise. Does your organization have appropriate internal controls over forms, their completion and processing? Let's examine just a few examples for an outpatient setting:

Objective	What Internal Control Procedures Would You Suggest?	What Would Be the Potential Impact on Dependability of Data?
1. Establishing and controlling authorized transactions for —admissions of new clients —appointments for client services		
2. Recording disposition of authorized transactions for —admissions of new clients —appointments for client services		

Table 2. Minimal Statistical Internal Control Objectives and Procedures Applicable to Admissions and Client Services

<table>
<tr><th>Objectives</th><th>Internal Control Procedures</th></tr>
<tr><td>1. Establishing and controlling authorized transactions
-admissions or new clients
-appointments for client services</td><td>—Enforced check-in with receptionist who confirms name and current address (OP, PC, new admissions)*
—New clients: Complete client information document (OP, PC, IP)*
—Receptionist maintained Master Appointment Schedule (OP, PC)*
—Maintain Master Client File (C & E)*</td></tr>
<tr><td>2. Recording disposition of authorized transactions
-admissions or new clients
-appointments for client services</td><td>—(Enforced check-in with receptionist who makes notation in Master Appointment Schedule)
—"No-Shows" and "Cancellations" noted in Master Appointment Schedule (OP, PC)*
—Utilize "Service Rendered Document" (SRD) which is either
-prenumbered or
-control sheet or "stub" is retained by receptionist to be matched with completed portion to establish accountability for services rendered (OP, PC)*
—Midnight Attendance Form is either
-prenumbered or
-predated
to establish accountability for services rendered (IP)*</td></tr>
<tr><td>3. Controlling processing of established, authorized transactions
-admissions
-appointments for client services</td><td>—Comparison of receptionist's grand control total of clients checked-in with the total of specific control totals for
—admissions or new clients
—appointments for client services

Example:
<table>
<tr><td>Grand control total of clients checked-in for one day</td><td>100</td></tr>
<tr><td>Specific control totals:</td><td></td></tr>
<tr><td>Admissions or new clients</td><td>23</td></tr>
<tr><td>Appointments for client services</td><td>77</td></tr>
<tr><td>Total</td><td>100</td></tr>
</table>
—Comparison of receptionist's grand and specific control totals with corresponding control totals developed by department receiving documents and/or other data from receptionist
-medical records
-business office (e.g., accounting)

Example:
Referring to the preceding example, the control totals of 100, 23, and 77 should be computed by recipient departments based only on documents received from the receptionist. These newly developed control totals, in turn, should be reported back to receptionist to ascertain that all documents have been accounted for.</td></tr>
<tr><td>4. Controlling processing of data relating to disposition of authorized transactions
-no-shows
-cancellations
-services rendered (therapy sessions)</td><td>—Comparison of control totals developed by receptionist or 024 and IP personnel with control totals computed independently by department receiving documents

Example:
<table>
<tr><th></th><th colspan="3">Independently Developed Control Traits</th></tr>
<tr><th>Department</th><th>No Shows</th><th>Cancellations</th><th>Therapy Session</th></tr>
<tr><td>Receptionist</td><td>5</td><td>7</td><td>62</td></tr>
<tr><td>Medical Records</td><td>5</td><td>7</td><td>62</td></tr>
<tr><td>Business Office</td><td>5</td><td>7</td><td>62</td></tr>
</table>
—Review of report containing data on no-shows, cancellations, and sessions by individual therapists
—Statistical sample of clients whose receivables are written off to ensure that services were, in fact, rendered.</td></tr>
</table>

*OP: Outpatient; PC: Partial Hospitalization Care; IP: Inpatient; C & E: Consultation and Education.

Source: James E. Sorensen and Glyn Hanbery (1979). *Using financial management in mental health organizations.* Rockville, MD: National Institute of Mental Health.

The following possible responses are suggestive and illustrative, but they are representative of good practices and likely impacts:

What Internal Control Procedures Would You Suggest?	What Would Be the Potential Impact on Dependability of Data?
1. Everyone checks in with a receptionist who confirms name and current address and makes an entry in the Master Appointment Schedule	—All clients served may not be accurately counted —Billings may be sent to the wrong address
2. (Assuming service-rendered documents)	
—All service-rendered documents to specific client are accounted for by receptionist.	—Counts of services provided may not be accurate —Documents may be retained by clinician or lost
—Are "no-shows" and "cancellations" noted in Master Appointment Schedule?	—Counts of lost hours may be inaccurate.

3. DESIGN OF THE GENERAL FLOW OF INFORMATION AND DOCUMENTS

There are two general designs for the flow of information through your program. Each has its assets and liabilities.

FIGURE 2: The multicopy ticket approach (Cooper, 1975), where four copies of each client-related document are created. Each ticket is numbered for editing control, and copies go to (a) originator at unit creating the document, (b) medical records, (c) accounting, and (d) statistics. This process is shown in Figure 2.

Assets:

–*Speed*—Information goes simultaneously to all four users in the system.

–*Computerized simplicity*—If the documents can be designed for optical scan and computer input, then one recording effort initiates all aspects of the integrated information system.

–*Auditing*—Random samples of documents can be followed through all subsystems of the MIS.

Liabilities:

–*Effect of Errors*—If a mistake in recording is made, the processing may be so fast that the mistake will not be corrected before application, e.g., billing, cost finding, statistical analysis, and management reports.

FIGURE 3: Single line information flow as shown in Chapter 1, where a single copy of a document goes from

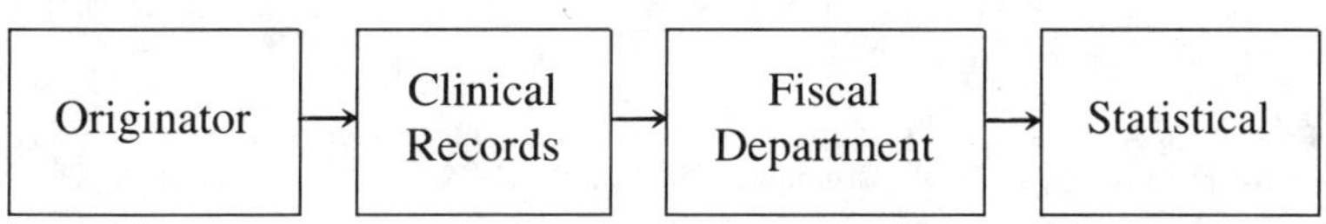

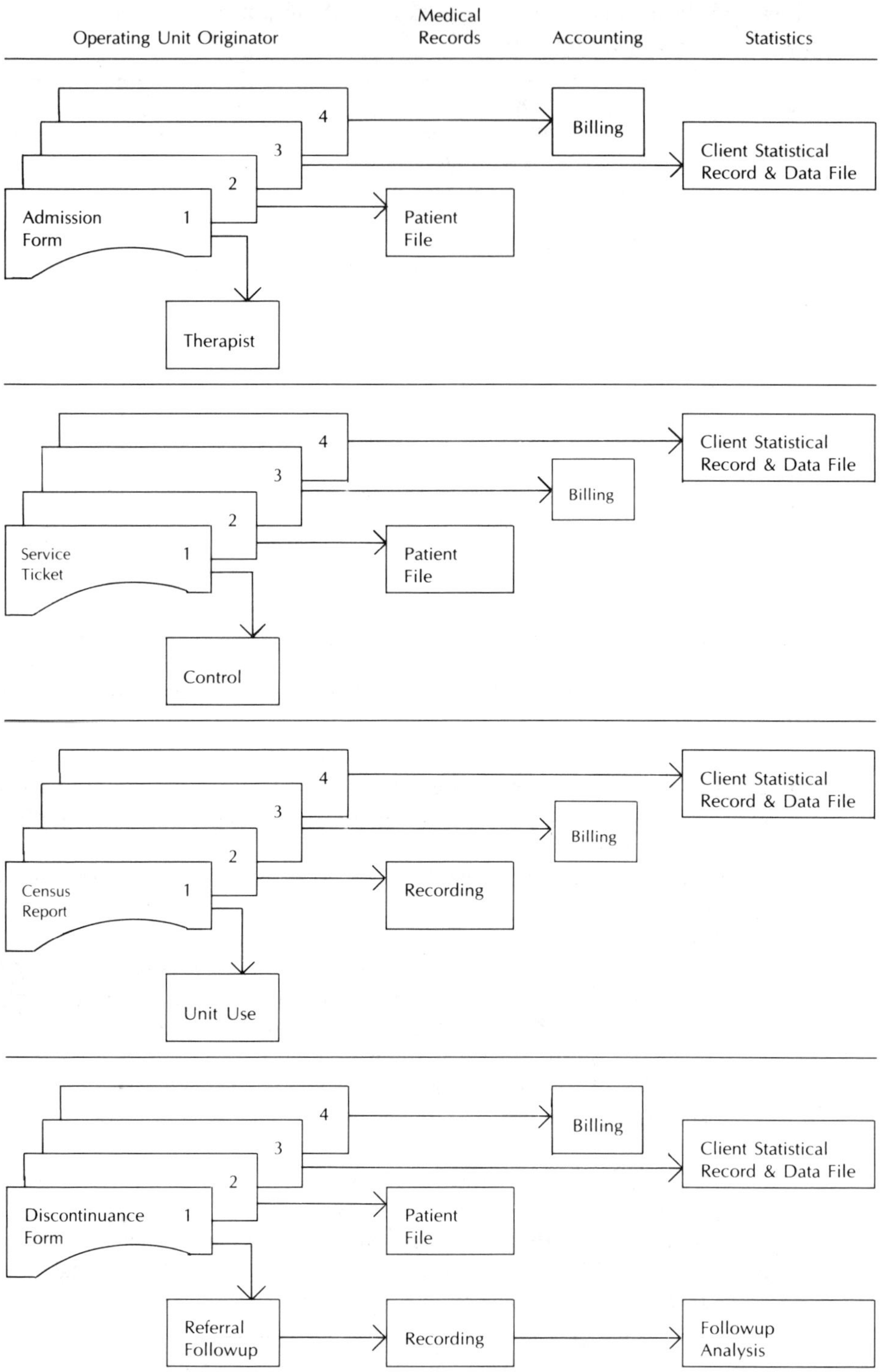

From Cooper, M. E. (1973). *Guidelines for a Minimum Statistical and Accounting System for Community Mental Health Centers* (DHEW Publication No. ADM 77-14). Washington, DC: U.S. Government Printing Office.

Figure 2. The Multicopy Ticket

This technique is also detailed in Figure 3.
Assets: All fiscal, billing, and statistical reports have clinical verification and there is greater accuracy.
Liabilities: Slower process, particularly if medical or clinical records do not have a well-organized problem/goal/service/outcome structure.

The technique chosen will depend greatly upon the structure of the program's organization, what information processing is done mechanically (e.g., by computers), and what is done manually. Once the general design of information flow is selected and developed, then internal controls should be developed for the transactions among people and machines in the general flow of information.

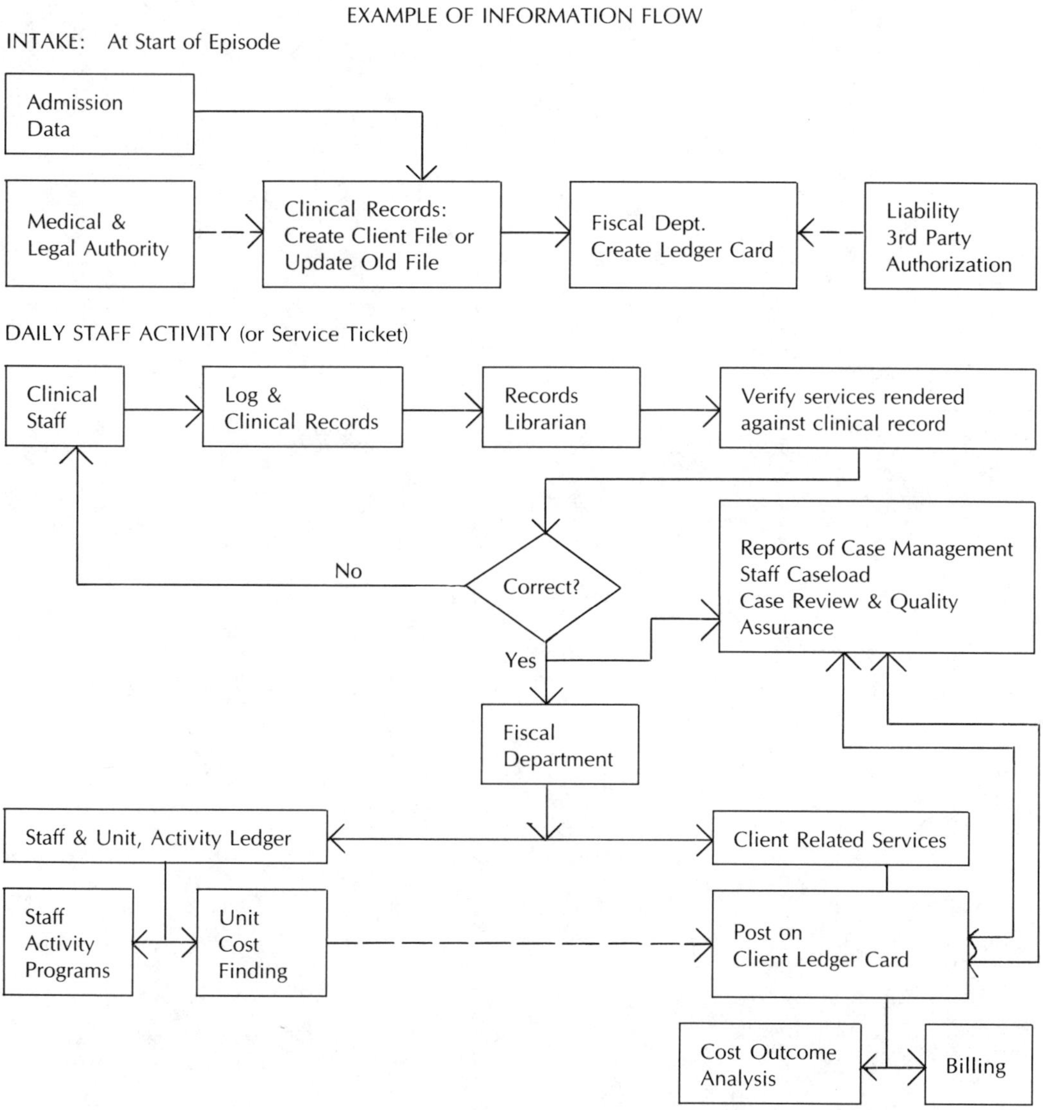

Figure 3. The Single Line Information Flow

SECTION IV

THE VISIBLE EVIDENCE—PART II: CLINICAL DATA DEPENDABILITY

> WHAT ARE DATA SOURCES?
> The systematic observations of clients, clinicians, and significant others.
> ARE THESE OBSERVATIONS DEPENDABLE?
> Yes, if you have procedures which permit your staff to identify and deal with the factors which influence the data.

There are four chapters in Section IV:

— Chapter 12 describes procedures to identify factors influencing the dependability of clinical data.
— Chapter 13 offers a staff development procedure to help staff know how to correct clinical judgment bias affecting dependability of data.
— Chapter 14 provides statistical analysis procedures for evaluators (or part-time consultants) to quantify estimates of clinical data reliability, validity, and the extent to which a given set of factors is influencing clinical observations.
— Chapter 15 provides an outline for creating your own clinical evaluation scales.

Chapters 12 through 14 help staff identify if and when differences in clinical experiences and perceptions are biasing judgments, increasing miscommunication, and contributing to poor treatment outcomes. The approach is a positive one, encouraging staff to work in a constructive, positive manner by showing:

— *Clinicians are typically reasonable and reliable decision makers.* Differences in clinical perceptions, even among the most experienced staff, are a reasonable result of their ordinary clinical practice.
— *The individual clinical decision process can be described* in a manner which can help you and your staff identify factors which may be influencing differences in clinical decisions among your staff.
— *Factors can influence communication among clinicians* in either the coordination of services or in progress review procedures.

Chapter 12

Identifying Factors Influencing Clinical Data Reliability, Validity, and Dependability

UNRELIABLE DATA IN—UNRELIABLE DATA OUT

As we pointed out in Section II, clear and complete records are tremendously valuable tools for the health-care administrator. In practice, you'll find their value greatly enhanced if the staff knows how to use them. This is not a flippant statement; equally competent staff members, but with different backgrounds, will often make very different interpretations and recommendations on the basis of the same set of documents.

This chapter shows how you and your colleagues can spot occurrences of such unintentional bias. It also shows how in the development of your records you can minimize the potential for such bias to skew your clinical data. Moreover—and this is an extraordinary boost to efficiency—at the same time that you are tailoring your records to reflect the needs of your clients and program, you'll be conducting very effective staff-development sessions.

THE CLINICIAN AS A GOOD INFORMATION PROCESSOR

Different prior clinical experiences usually result in different perceptions among clinical staff. In turn, these differences lead to different estimates of symptom severity and treatment planning. This is *not necessarily* a bad situation, but it's a risky one. Uneveness in clinical care and client outcome can result if managers and supervisors are not aware of such differences. An offensive football squad needs both big guards and fleet-wide receivers, but most coaches recognize their differences and assign them different responsibilities.

The following self-study exercise on prior experience and bias shows how the experiences of a practicing clinician can affect clinical judgment. Such diverse influences are common to *all* clinical settings. The trick is not to allow them to become divisive, but to profit from the variety of their experience.

Self-Study Exercise

Effects of Prior Experience. For two of the three categories of clinician listed, identify possible differences influencing their perceptions and decisions.

	A Clinician Who Works Primarily With:		
Experiences	Overactive Children	Chronic Schizophrenics	Marital Conflicts
Success Rate (Give approx. percent success)			
Failure rate (Give approx. percent failure)			
Critical Symptoms most often attended to are:			
Typical Treatment Plans, e.g., Give percent of plans with goals of: Growth/Improvement, Sustenance/Maintenance, Stabilization	______ ______ ______	______ ______ ______	______ ______ ______

After completing the foregoing table, consider what biases might develop.

	A Clinician Who Works Primarily With:		
	Overactive Children	Chronic Schizophrenics	Marital Conflicts
Which Factors or Symptoms may be: (a) Overemphasized:			
(b) Underemphasized?			
Which Treatment Plan Decisions by each clinician may: (a) Be too quickly made but should be more considered?			
(b) Not be typically considered but should be on occasions?			

Obviously, a list of possibly biasing factors could be developed for each of the major categories of client concern you had identified in the clinical process units.

A CHECKLIST FOR DETECTING BIASING FACTORS

One benefit of this exercise is alerting staff and clinical supervisors to the need for review and staff-development activities. The outline for the exercise given can also serve as a checklist for supervisory review with specific types of clients. It may be worth the effort to ask key clinical supervisory staff to use the following outline to review each major category of client:

(A) Typical Success Experiences which may be overemphasized.
(B) Typical Failure Experiences which may be underemphasized.
(C) Symptoms and Circumstances which may be
  (1) Overemphasized
  (2) Underemphasized
(D) Typical Treatment Plan Goals, (e.g., Growth, Sustenance, Stabilization) which are avoided or emphasized.
(E) Treatment Plan Decisions which may be:
  (1) Made too quickly, but should be considered more thoroughly, particularly if certain combinations of circumstances are present; e.g., prescribing certain medications independent of vocational or family supports; using certain behavior techniques with overactive children of single working parents vs. those in two-parent households with just one parent working.
  (2) Not considered typically but should be on occasions, e.g., use or non-use of restraints or multiple medications.

Once these factors are identified for a checklist of cautions, they can be incorporated into any one of a number of review and staff development procedures, e.g.,

— Record audits
— Clinical care evaluations and cost-outcome studies
— Clinical judgment studies to determine what facets are influencing differences in clinical decisions (these are discussed in the next unit).

But before such procedures are implemented, more is needed on how individual clinical decisions are made and how interpersonal (and interprofessional) group interactions can affect the judgments and decisions of individuals.

2. THE INDIVIDUAL CLINICIAN AS A GOOD INFORMATION PROCESSOR

The amount of information actually processed and used is less than the clinician has available. Research has shown that one of the remarkably efficient functions that a clinician performs is to sort all of the available information into a small number of categories. These categories tend to be those which the clinicians consider appropriate for the judgments and decisions they feel ought to be made. As discussed earlier, prior successes and failures influence the clinicians' choice of the categories used for different types of clients.

The number of categories used typically varies from three to nine. If there are fewer than three factors the clinician considers relevant to the judgment, then the clinician will usually express a low degree of confidence in making a judgment. On the other hand, seldom will clinicians actively use or require more than seven to nine factors in their deliberations—not because they are reticent, but rather because they typically feel that there is nothing more to be gained by processing any more "facts." Thus, they stop with three to nine categories and make a judgment or decision.

Since the clinician tends to use from three to nine factors in forming a judgment, it is

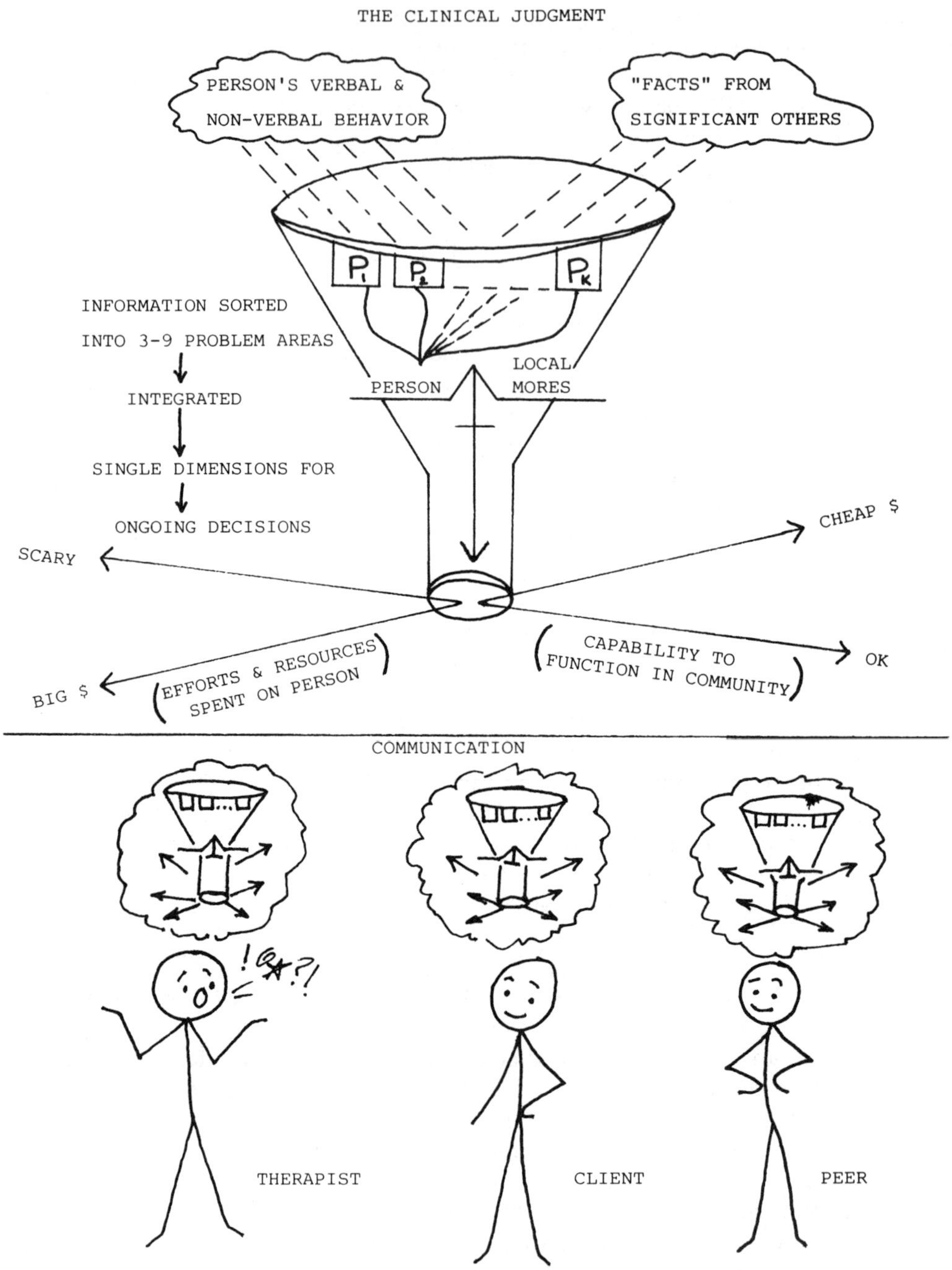

Figure 1. The Clinical Judgment and the Communication Process

therefore wise to systematically document and review these contributing factors. The most appropriate times for such documentation are probably at client entry, treatment planning, progress review, and termination.

An important key to clinical supervision and staff development is to provide a positive framework for a difficult set of tasks of clinical judgment. First, consider the kinds of information which the clinician has available and the kinds of decisions the clinician must make. The clinician obviously has to perform a difficult set of information-processing and problem-solving tasks. The major components of the clinical decision process will be identified and can be readily translated into staff supervision and development procedures.

First, focus attention on the upper panel of Figure 1. This panel shows how the varied kinds of information available to a clinician are:

(a) *Funneled* into a small number of apparently useful categories, usually between 3 and 9, and
(b) *Integrated* in a variety of combinations to formulate different kinds of decisions. (The integration process will be discussed later).

The same categories of information can be used for making different decisions on the same client. Consider an example. Suppose the clinician has estimated that there are three major factors influencing the client's overall level of functioning: (a) mood swings are moderately severe when client is under stress; (b) family support is strained; (c) the client is presently unemployed. Now consider whether these same three categories of information can be used to decide:

(a) What is the level of role performance or functioning in the ordinary community setting?
(b) What are the capabilities of generating third-party revenues?

The simplest answer is "The same information could be used, but in a different manner for each of the two questions."

The lower panel in Figure 1 raises the issue of communication among client, therapist, and peers. While the process for sorting and using information may be similar for all of us, it is unlikely that we would *sort* the same information into exactly the same categories, *identify* the same sets of decisions to be made, *value* the categorical information in the same fashion for each decision, or *integrate* the categorical information in the same manner for any one decision. These issues represent the major stumbling blocks in most communication among people whether they are as close as husband and wife, parent and child, client and therapist, or two professional colleagues. But the stumbling blocks need not be insurmountable. There are staff-development procedures which, when coupled with your clinical progress review procedures, can deal with these issues.

3. INTEGRATING CLINICAL INFORMATION INTO A DECISION

All clinical decisions require judgments which integrate pieces of information. Certainly the clinicians working with overactive children would integrate information differently than clinicians working with autistic children. These integrated judgments can be objective events such as "hand wringing," or a subjective rating such as an "angry reply," or severe depression, or level of functioning. For purposes of discussion here, suppose a clinician were concerned about a client's ability to function in the community. The formulation which could be used to describe the clinician's judgment could be expressed as:

JUDGMENT OF FUNCTIONING	=	INITIAL IMPRESSION	+	3–9 PROBLEMS/ISSUES RELEVANT TO CLIENT'S FUNCTIONING

In more general terms, the formulation for any judgment can be expressed as:

$$\text{JUDGMENT} = \underbrace{\omega_0 I_0} + \underbrace{\omega_1 P_1 + \omega_2 P_2 + \text{----} + \omega_k P_k}$$

WHERE: I_0 = The initial impression
ω_0 = The weighting of credibility of the initial impression
P_i = The severity of one particular problem or issue by itself
ω_i = The relative importance of that problem or issue to the overall judgment

This process is the same one described in the funnel diagram in Figure 1. The process is described again using the foregoing formulation.

A judgment about a client, e.g., function in the community (or level of depression), can be described as a combination of:

(1) *An Initial Impression* of the client at time (I_0) and how much trust can be placed in an initial impression (ω_0) of the type of client.
(2) *The 3–9 Problems/Issues* (P_i) considered to be relevant (ω_i) to the overall judgment, and just how relevant or important the problem or issue is to overall functioning (depression).

Clinical judgment is not merely a matter of adding pieces together to form a whole judgment; it's not that simple. This formulation, however, can be useful for describing the rather complex judgment process when communicating and discussing differences in judgments among clinical colleagues. For example, in the service planning and review procedures, many of the judgments and decisions concern the problems affecting the client's overall role performance or community functioning. Therefore, procedures for treatment planning, progress review, and staff development must have a means for reviewing both the overall level of functioning[1] and the issues relevant to the client's functioning.

Recall the recommendation for a multifactor problem or issue list along with a global scale. Both are crucial for reliable and valid measurement of clinical progress and outcome. The formulation developed above offers a logical basis for this recommendation. In simple terms, if clients and two or more professional colleagues consistently agree upon their observations of problems and overall functioning, then the formulation can be used to show that their judgments are both reliable and valid. When they disagree on their observations, they must have a means of discerning what factors are influencing their disagreement in judgments.

According to the formulation, if the clinicians have clinical records which document both

[1] Remember that you may wish to substitute your own program's global integrating concept for "functioning."

a problem/issue list on a client and a number of global judgments, they can review both sides of the equation in making their judgments. While all those strange little "ω's" will not be in the clinical records, there will be sufficient information on the global judgments and problems/issues for clinicians to determine where are the major areas of disagreement.

Once clinicians have isolated the factors they feel might be leading to differences, they can perform a simple test to see if those factors are indeed the cause. The members of the group should independently write down global ratings for each of a small set (10–12) of brief case histories. The factors in question should vary (none, some, a lot) systematically over the set of case histories. After the group has completed their independent ratings, they should then discuss their ratings together. Usually, independent ratings on 10–12 cases, followed by group discussion, is sufficient to reveal whether a factor is influencing differences in clinical judgments. Two or three such sessions will usually rectify differences in judgments, and produce enough data to estimate scale reliability and validity (see Chapter 14).

The following self-study exercise reviews the clinical information integration process.

Self-Study Exercise

(1) Given the Judgment Formulation,

$$J = \omega_0 I_0 + \omega_1 P_1 + \omega_2 P_2 + \text{- - -} + \omega_3 P_3$$

suppose you were rating an overall level of depression, where "J" = level of depression. Give examples of each of the following which might greatly influence a rating of severe depression:

"$\omega_0 I_0$" ____________________

____

"$\omega_1 P_1$" ____________________

____

(2) Why would the weighting (ω_1) of the same set of problems and issues differ for the two judgments of *Level of Community Functioning* vs. *Level of Psychiatric Impairment*?

____

____

(3) Suppose the review procedures suggested that alcohol abuse symptoms in male and female clients appeared to have different influences on the level of functioning judgments of your outpatient staff. How would you test for this supposition in a staff development training session using brief case histories? ____________________

____

____

Illustrative Answers:

(1) $\omega_0 I_0$ = Initial impression of severe depression because the client is a female of approximately the age of menopause.
$\omega_1 P_1$ = Reactions to sexually loaded questions.

(2) Psychiatric impairment considers the individual independent of the community. Thus, any problem has a different weighting.

(3) Have different degrees of alcohol abuse, in different case histories, rated by the staff.

4. GROUP DYNAMICS INFLUENCING JUDGMENTS

The concepts developed in the first part of this chapter argue strongly for repeated staff interactions and supervision in treatment planning, review, and staff development. But there are pitfalls. The procedures which are sensible for planning, reviewing, and supervising clinical services have a potential negative influence on the judgments and decisions made by individual clinicians, their supervisors, and treatment teams. There is a large body of literature which shows that when a group of two or more people meet to discuss judged attributes—e.g., problems, issues, or level of functioning—the group decision will not be the same as the average of the individual clinician decisions. This discrepancy between group and individual decisions is called the *group polarization and conformity effect.* This polarization effect is not the result of maliciousness or poor clinical leadership. It is a normal and typical result of any group interaction which requires a decision by consensus.

Consider the situation of a treatment team meeting. A front-line clinician describes a client as having four major problems and issues (P_1, P_2, P_3, P_4), leading to a level of functioning judgment of ''5'' on a 10-point scale. Now suppose the clinical team leader suggests that with the available evidence (P_1, P_2, P_3, P_4), the functioning level ought to be lowered to ''4.'' This difference could occur because of differences in the values of ω_1, ω_2, ω_3, or ω_4. As discussion evolves, usually the final group consensus moves toward the group leadership (conformity), provided the direction of the overall group average judgment (if taken privately prior to group discussion) is in the direction of the leadership. The typical group discussion as part of clinical supervision, treatment-team service planning, and review procedures may lead to some biasing of judgments, relative to individual judgments. Most often, the influence is minor and not noticeable. The issue is if it is happening to a notable extent, and counteracting any negative influences or consequences.

Suggestions on Group Dynamics

There are, however, some occasions when ''hot'' issues will arouse strong feelings among staff or supervisors. Under these conditions, strong group polarization and conformity effects may result. When such instances appear to be happening, a straightforward precaution is in order. Obtain independent ratings after a case is presented but *before* discussion of the case begins. If the final decision of the group is markedly different from the average of the prediscussion ratings, then the polarization and conformity effect is evident.

The leader needs to decide whether the result is good or bad. The crucial question is ''Was the polarization effect so serious that no one in the group upon reconsideration would agree privately with the final decision?'' Two options exist. Ask the group members again to give independent ratings after the group discussion has taken place. The degree of difference between the public versus the private ratings should indicate to the leader whether the final group conformity was simply acquiescence to the ''boss.'' A second approach is to introduce the ''hot'' issues into the set of brief case histories used in the periodic staff-development sessions. The polarization and conformity effect is handled as a group problem-solving task. Since these staff-development sessions deal with fictitious example cases, ''strong feelings'' may be better controlled.

5. PROGRAM IMPLEMENTATION STRATEGIES

The program directors and clinical supervisors ought individually to read and complete this chapter prior to meeting and discussing it. A subcommittee should be formed to design a staff development workshop described in Chapter 13. The group should pilot test the workshop with a small group of clinical staff and themselves.

Chapter 13

Staff Training and Development Procedures for Dependable Clinical Data

This chapter will help program directors and clinical supervisors design staff-development procedures to provide: (a) initial staff training in the use of scales to consistently communicate client characteristics; (b) means for detecting and remediating differences in clinical judgments and decisions among staff; (c) a means for identifying issues to be addressed in supervision and review procedures; (d) a basis for client-care evaluation studies recommended by NIMH and required by PSRO and JCAH.

Chapter 13 contains three major sections:

(1) OVERVIEW OF PROCEDURES: Draws a direct relationship between clinical-decision processes and staff-development procedures.

(2) DESIGNING THE GOALS AND OBJECTIVES OF STAFF-DEVELOPMENT SESSIONS:

- (a) Developing initial scales to help staff define the meaning and applications of the scale to their clinical judgments and activities.
- (b) Surfacing influential factors biasing clinical judgments encourages staff to share and work on correcting differences.
- (c) Relating the results of staff development to clinical procedures and cost outcome results clarifies ultimate objectives.

(3) DESIGNING THE PROCEDURES FOR A STAFF-DEVELOPMENT SESSION:

- (a) Constructing case histories to meet goals.
- (b) Reviewing procedural hints for staff-development sessions.

1. OVERVIEW OF PROCEDURES

The guidelines offer a means to design staff-development sessions to constructively address factors influencing the clinician's judgments and decisions. The procedures are designed for direct use by staff and their immediate supervisors.

Staff (who typically work together) independently rate, compare, and discuss their judgments on the same set of abbreviated case histories. The case histories are constructed to differ systematically according to the factors the clinical group (staff and their supervisors) have identified as possibly influencing the judgments communicated among themselves. The theme of the sessions can be set by the staff and their supervisors. To an extent, they dictate the goals of the session and can have a certain degree of ownership of the process. Both the review process and the cost-outcome procedures help to surface the possible influencing factors. Thus, the factors identified come directly from the clinicians' own experiences. Examples of such factors usually include (a) symptoms of emotional distress, social deviancy, or depression; (b) demographic characteristics such as age, sex, socioeconomic class; or (c) prior clinical history, e.g., prior hospitalization or use of antidepressants.

During the initial stages of a session, the staff should understand the cases are specifically constructed to reveal existing differences in their own clinical decisions leading to miscommunication among themselves or with clients. These sessions are to be structured so staff may constructively discuss and correct differences among themselves. Staff often realize that scale ratings are only a means of communicating the "tip" or surface label of a more considered clinical judgment. When differences do occur, the clinical staff, as a group, need to discuss the possible sources of such differences. Here is where the formulation discussed in Chapter 12 becomes useful. The possible sources of differences could be identified as differences in:

(1) Problem or issue definition or severity (P_k)
(2) Weighting the importance of a particular issue or problem (ω_k) in making a particular judgment
(3) Initial impression ($\omega_0 I_0$)

JUDGMENT	=	INITIAL IMPRESSION	+	PROBLEMS/ISSUES RELATED TO JUDGMENT
JUDGMENT	=	$\omega_0 I_0$	+	$\omega_1 P_1 + \omega_2 P_2 + \text{- - -} + \omega_3 P_3$

Usually, two sets of 10–12 abbreviated case histories are rated independently and then discussed in a 3 hour workshop, with about 1½ hours spent on each set of 10–12 cases. The specific procedures, details, and structure of the case histories are tailored to the goals of the staff-development session. The methods for structuring the goals and objectives of a session are provided in section 2; the means for structuring the abbreviated case histories and procedures for the session are described in section 3.

Self-Study Exercise on Staff Development

(1) Identify the three reasons why a clinical supervisor and a program administrator might wish to have staff-development sessions described in section 1.

	Clinical Supervisor	Program Administrator
(1)		
(2)		
(3)		

(2) Identify three factors which you feel may be influencing differences in judgments among your staff.
   (1) ______________________________
   (2) ______________________________
   (3) ______________________________

(3) If differences in ratings do surface in a session, what are some possible influential sources in the judgmental process. (Use the formulation of the clinical judgment process as a guide to your answer here.)
____
____
____
____
____
____

Answers to Self-Study Exercise on Staff Development

(1) For the *Clinical Supervisor* to (1) detect systematic bias in clinical decisions; (2) train staff to communicate consistently; (3) better understand what decisions staff are making. For the *Program Administrator* to increase his/her confidence that (1) clinical data are reliable; (2) staff and supervisors are communicating; (3) judgment biases are being handled in a professional manner.

(2) (1) Prior success/failures history with clients; (2) Types of clients most frequently on caseload; (3) Misperceptions of supervisory direction.

(3) Initial impression (e.g., gender, race, general physical or affect appearance). Problems identified as relevant and the weighting of relative importance to the overall judgment.

2. DESIGNING THE GOALS AND OBJECTIVES OF STAFF-DEVELOPMENT SESSIONS

There are three general purposes for staff development:

— To initially train staff in the use of a scale; adapting or tailoring a standardized scale to a program's social and geographic circumstances can be integrated into the initial training session.
— To reveal differences in the use of an established scale, thereby decreasing miscommunication among staff and increasing the dependability of scale and clinical data.
— To provide a data base (from a staff-development session) leading to designing client-care evaluation studies required by NIMH, PSRO, and JCAH. Are differences in client cost and outcome results because of differences in actual treatment efforts, types of clients involved, or the perceptions of the clinicians? The technical features for designing and performing client-care evaluation studies are given later in the units on cost outcome, cost effectiveness, and evaluation research.

Initial Scale Development starts with the adoption of a programwide policy about overall program goals (see Chapter 2). Once a goal related global concept—e.g., level of functioning—and the principal factors thought to underlie the global concept have been identified, then scale development, staff training, and use of the scale by the staff can start. The following outline identifies the goals and objectives for initial training:

(1) Establish a short-term training goal with a visible product, e.g., to have the clinical staff start using a scale for a 3-month pilot period within 4 to 6 weeks.
(2) Identify the immediate objectives by specifying who is responsible for doing what, when, and with what resources. For example:
   (a) Appoint a committee of three clinicians (one in a supervisory capacity) to select one of three scales developed and tested elsewhere.
   (b) Give the committee one week to modify the wording of the scale to their own liking.
   (c) Distribute the amended scale to staff, asking for their marginal comments on the scale's wording. Comments are to be returned to the committee within one week.
   (d) Hold a staff meeting to deal with the *concerns* of the staff. The format of the meeting will be to surface their concerns about positive and negative features of any scale, and its use in a constructive manner. A recommended format for the meeting is provided in Table 1.
   (e) After the positive and negative features are outlined, the committee should identify to the staff what steps they intend to take to assure attainment of the positive features and deal with the negative features. This can be done either at the meeting, by memo, or at a second meeting. The procedures described in section 3 of this chapter provide the data base for Chapter 14 on scale reliability and validity and Chapter 19 on staff data confidentiality.[1] This will cover most of the concerns staff will have. Since all of the individual staff members' concerns will never be fully satisfied, do not linger at this point.
   (f) Initiate a 3-month pilot test of the scale. The more practice staff has with a scale, the greater the reliability of the scale and the greater the likelihood of uncovering problems. Thus, have the clinicians offer ''quick'' judgments at: each clinician encounter for outpatient clients, each day for partial hospital clients, and each working shift for clients on inpatient units. Do not delay the 3-month pilot test because of differences in viewpoints among staff. The pilot-test period usually helps to iron out such differences.
   (g) Schedule the first staff-development session where two sets of 10–12 case histories are independently rated and then discussed.
   (h) Assign one person to prepare the procedures and materials for the first staff-development session.
(3) Identify the goals for staff-development sessions during the early pilot-testing period. For example, brief bi-weekly or monthly sessions may vary in style and objectives during a 3–4 month pilot period where a scale is in daily use by the staff:

---

[1] In Chapter 19, pay particular attention to the *Rule of 2 and 5* to assure clinical staff that no clinical data will be associated with them personally (by name) more than 2 organizational steps from them. All data which are used more than 2 organizational steps beyond its source will be aggregate over 5 clients and/or staff. This procedure helps the staff feel that their clinical decision data will be reviewed only by professional supervisors with whom they are acquainted. Analyses of program-management decisions in most service organizations have shown that when data have moved more than 2 organizational steps up the hierarchy, there is no need for individual clinician data if intermediate supervisory personnel are doing their jobs. By employing the *Rule of 2 and 5,* you gain a higher degree of ''honest'' clinical data with very little, if any, loss of administratively useful information.

Table 1. Concerns on Scale Development and Use

TASK 1 Starting with the products, identify two ways in which a scale may be useful from the viewpoint of each of the people listed below.
TASK 2 On the pitfall side, identify two features and outcomes you should guard against.
TASK 3 In small groups of 6–8 staff, read positive and then negative features. Have each group offer a brief summary of these.

From the Viewpoint of	Products	Pitfalls*
THE CLIENT		
SERVICE STAFF		
CLINICAL SUPERVISOR		
ADMINISTRATION		
CITIZEN BOARD		
COUNTY/STATE/FEDERAL		

*You will find it a point of interest that most, if not all, "pitfalls" or potentially negative outcomes also exist even without the use of any scales. Often, the use of scales will help systematically surface and address problems.

(3.1) *Amount of Information*—Have staff rate cases differing in the amount of information provided. One benefit is staff recognition of the need for good clinical record information to support good communication among staff working with the same clients.

(3.2) *Change in Behavior and Ratings*—Have staff both rate each case history *and* describe what changes in behavior would lead to their rating that case (a) one level higher and (b) one level lower. Describing changes one level up or down helps staff recognize how sensitive (or insensitive) the scale is to change.

(3.3) *Emotionally Loaded Issues*—Have staff rate cases, half of which contain emotionally loaded issues, e.g., suicide, rape, incest, interracial marriage. Be sure to mix in some straight cases for contrast. Staff will note their own personal fears surfacing and the cathartic effects are typically positive.

(3.4) *Group Discussion Influences*—Have staff rate some cases prior to group discussion about multiple problems and issues and some cases after such discussion. For the "after discussion" case ratings, be sure no ratings are mentioned during the discussion. Let the discussion center on "What are the problems and issues?" Staff should be cautioned to use descriptive adjectives and adverbs rather than numbered ratings during the discussion.

(3.5) *Goal Planning*—Have staff describe the client's current level and what the client's level would be 4–6 weeks from now given reasonable and available services. This is often seen as "impossible" the first time you suggest it. But eventually, the staff usually request such a session at a later date.

(3.6) *Service Planning*—Have staff provide a rating for each case plus the major service activities and modalities of service in conjunction with 3.5 above.

(4) Identify methods to guide and counsel staff on the use of the scale. Examples of these methods were included under items 2 and 3, above. In addition, consider using the committee members who formed the scale as counselors. Above all, insure the staff-development sessions are as supportive as possible. Similarities in judgments do typically occur with good information and an opportunity to discuss observations, while differences in judgment are often the reasonable result of incomplete information, differences in prior success and failure experiences, and amount and type of experience. The ''funnel'' shown in Chapter 12, Figure 1 and the Judgment Formulation integrated initial impression and the weighted importance of problems and issues and should help the staff understand the factors influencing reasonable differences in their ratings.

(5) After the 3-month pilot-test period, obtain recommended changes in scale wording from the staff. The committee should then review the recommendations, agree upon changes, and hold a staff meeting to review the revised scale. Obtaining consensus follows the procedure outlined in Step 2, above. After consensus, implement the revised scale for a year's time.

A Checklist for Staff Development Sessions

(1) Overall goals with visible products and timelines for staff.
(2) Intermediate objectives identifying who, what, when, and resources.
(3) Set of brief objectives for each workshop.
(4) Outline staff feedback and guidance procedures.
(5) Write memo to staff briefly describing the above four items.

3. DESIGNING THE PROCEDURES FOR A STAFF-DEVELOPMENT SESSION

Two issues are addressed in this section: (a) How to construct case histories to suit individualized purposes; and (b) Procedural hints and recommended steps for conducting a staff-development session.

Constructing the Case Histories

Each case history should be responsive to two requirements:

(1) Be *brief and informative*—An average person should be able to read and make a judgment on the case within 2–3 minutes. Usually this is 12–15 lines of type or 100 to 150 words.

(2) Be *constructed to reveal a factor's influence*—Two approaches insure a factor's influence will be shown. First, the case description should be slightly ambiguous to reduce the possibility of complete agreement among raters. This slight degree of ambiguity permits the factors which typically influence judgments to operate. Second, the level of behavioral disability or role performance should be in the mid-range of the rating scale. Methods to estimate mid-range disability will be discussed later.

While there are a number of procedures for constructing case histories, guidelines cut across all of the procedures:

(1) Identify only a small manageable number of factors to be varied in a single session. That is, to vary the level of one or two factors over cases rated in a session, try to keep the other major factors influencing judgments in the middle or upper ranges of disability. Some of the major factor areas which could be varied or held constant over case histories are:
   - — Symptoms of Emotional Stress
   - — Role Performance
   - — Personal Self-Care
   - — Social and Family Support
   - — Psychiatric History
   - — Socioeconomic Status

(2) Try to avoid reference to emotionally loaded issues, e.g., race, suicide, or rape, unless they are factors to be studied in the session.

(3) While you should try to have most of the cases in the mid-range of disability or dysfunction, have a few cases toward the low and high ranges for contrast. Be sure not to make these extreme cases obviously bizarre.

(4) Test the constructed cases on a small group of three to five people.

The three most common procedures for constructing cases are:

Pin a Label on a Person

(1) Create a set of 20–30 case profiles with mid-range levels of role performance by putting together combinations of (a) Mobility, (b) Physical activity, and (c) Social activity. These performance profiles are constructed by using Table 2. The levels of role performance for the various combinations of mobility, physical, and social activity are given in the right-hand column. Mid-range functioning has role performance scores approximately in the range of .52 to .62.

(2) Add the other characteristics (labels) that you wish to vary, e.g.,
—Psychiatric history
—Symptoms
—Socioeconomic status or social/family support
These labels will, of course, raise or lower the overall perception of role performance.

Table 2. Functional Levels: Combinations of Steps on Mobility, Physical Activity, and Social Activity Scales with Associated Levels of Well-being or Role Performance (W_j)*

Numbers in parentheses are step numbers on the three scales.

Function Level Number (L)	Mobility	Physical Activity	Social Activity	Level of Role Performance (W_j)
		NO SYMPTOMS/PROBLEM COMPLEX		
L 43	Drove car and used bus or train without help (5)	Walked without physical problems (4)	Did work, school or housework, and other activities (5)	1.000
		SYMPTOMS/PROBLEM COMPLEX PRESENT		
L 42	Drove car and used bus or train without help (5)	Walked without physical problems (4)	Did work, school or housework, and other activities (5)	0.7433

Table 2. (*Continued*)

Function Level Number (L)	Mobility	Physical Activity	Social Activity	Level of Role Performance (W_j)
L 41	Drove car and used bus or train without help (5)	Walked without physical problems (4)	Did work, school or housework, but other activities limited (4)	0.6855
L 40	Drove car and used bus or train without help (5)	Walked without physical problems (4)	Limited in amount or kind of work, school, or housework (3)	0.6683
L 39	Drove car and used bus or train without help (5)	Walked without physical problems (4)	Performed self-care, but not work, school, or housework (2)	0.6955
L 38	Drove car and used bus or train without help (5)	Walked without physical problems (4)	Had help with self-care activities (1)	0.6370
L 37	Drove car and used bus or train without help (5)	Walked with physical limitations (3)	Did work, school or housework, and other activities (5)	0.6769
L 36	Drove car and used bus or train without help (5)	Walked with physical limitations (3)	Did work, school or housework, but other activities limited (4)	0.6172
L 35	Drove car and used bus or train without help (5)	Walked with physical limitations (3)	Limited in amount or kind of work, school, or housework (3)	0.6020
L 34	Drove car and used bus or train without help (5)	Walked with physical limitations (3)	Performed self-care, but not work, school, or housework (2)	0.6292
L 33	Drove car and used bus or train without help (5)	Walked with physical limitations (3)	Had help with self-care activities (1)	0.5707
L 32	Did not drive, or had help to use bus or train (4)	Walked without physical problems (4)	Did work, school or housework, but other activities limited (4)	0.6065
L 31	Did not drive, or had help to use bus or train (4)	Walked without physical problems (4)	Limited in amount or kind of work, school, or housework (3)	0.5913
L 30	Did not drive, or had help to use bus or train (4)	Walked without physical problems (4)	Performed self-care, but not work, school, or housework (2)	0.6185
L 29	Did not drive, or had help to use bus or train (4)	Walked without physical problems (4)	Had help with self-care activities (1)	0.5800
L 28	Did not drive, or had help to use bus or train (4)	Walked with physical limitations (3)	Did work, school or housework, but other activities limited (4)	0.5402
L 27	Did not drive, or had help to use bus or train (4)	Walked with physical limitations (3)	Limited in amount or kind of work, school, or housework (3)	0.5250
L 26	Did not drive, or had help to use bus or train (4)	Walked with physical limitations (3)	Performed self-care, but not work, school, or housework (2)	0.5523
L 25	Did not drive, or had help to use bus or train (4)	Moved own wheelchair without help (2)	Limited in amount or kind of work, school, or housework (3)	0.5376
L 24	Did not drive, or had help to use bus or train (4)	Moved own wheelchair without help (2)	Performed self-care, but not work, school, or housework (2)	0.5849
L 23	In house (3)	Walked without physical problems (4)	Performed self-care, but not work, school, or housework (2)	0.6488

(*continued*)

Table 2. (*Continued*)

Function Level Number (L)	Mobility	Physical Activity	Social Activity	Level of Role Performance (W_j)
L 22	In house (3)	Walked without physical problems (4)	Had help with self-care activities (1)	0.5002
L 21	In house (3)	Walked with physical limitations (3)	Did work, school or housework, but other activities limited (4)	0.5704
L 20	In house (3)	Walked with physical limitations (3)	Limited in amount or kind of work, school, or housework (3)	0.5552
L 19	In house (3)	Walked with physical limitations (3)	Performed self-care, but not work, school, or housework (2)	0.5824
L 18	In house (3)	Walked with physical limitations (3)	Had help with self-care activities (1)	0.5239
L 17	In house (3)	Moved own wheelchair without help (2)	Performed self-care, but not work, school, or housework (2)	0.5950
L 16	In house (3)	Moved own wheelchair without help (2)	Had help with self-care activities (1)	0.5384
L 15	In house (3)	In bed or chair (1)	Performed self-care, but not work, school, or housework (2)	0.5715
L 14	In house (3)	In bed or chair (1)	Had help with self-care activities (1)	0.5129
L 13	In hospital (2)	Walked without physical problems (4)	Performed self-care, but not work, school, or housework (2)	0.6057
L 12	In hospital (2)	Walked without physical problems (4)	Had help with self-care activities (1)	0.5471
L 11	In hospital (2)	Walked with physical limitations (3)	Performed self-care, but not work, school, or housework (2)	0.5384
L 10	In hospital (2)	Walked with physical limitations (3)	Had help with self-care activities (1)	0.4808
L 9	In hospital (2)	Moved own wheelchair without help (2)	Performed self-care, but not work, school, or housework (2)	0.5520
L 8	In hospital (2)	Moved own wheelchair without help (2)	Had help with self-care activities (1)	0.4934
L 7	In hospital (2)	In bed or chair (1)	Performed self-care, but not work, school, or housework (2)	0.5284
L 6	In hospital (2)	In bed or chair (1)	Had help with self-care activities (1)	0.4099
L 5	In special care unit (1)	Walked without physical problems (4)	Performed self-care, but not work, school, or housework (2)	0.5732
L 4	In special care unit (1)	Walked without physical problems (4)	Had help with self-care activities (1)	0.5147
L 3	In special care unit (1)	Walked with physical limitations (3)	Performed self-care, but not work, school, or housework (2)	0.5070

(*continued*)

Table 2. (*Continued*)

Function Level Number (L)	Mobility	Physical Activity	Social Activity	Level of Role Performance (W_j)
L 2	In special care unit (1)	Walked with physical limitations (3)	Had help with self-care activities (1)	0.4483
L 1	In special care unit (1)	In bed or chair (1)	Had help with self-care activities (1)	0.4374
L 0	Dead (0)	Dead (0)	Dead (0)	0.0000

*Adapted from Kaplan, Robert M., Bush, J. W., & Berry, Charles C. (1976, Winter). Health Status: Types of Validity and the Index of Well-Being. *Health Services Research, 11*(4): 486–488.

Actual Case Adaptation

(1) Identify specific case characteristics to medical records personnel and have them select 20–30 cases.
(2) Have a two-person team review the 20–30 cases and create the brief case histories.
(3) Change sufficient details of the cases to preserve client confidentiality. For example, you may change age, gender, job, or symptoms.
(4) Test the cases on a small group of 3–5 people.

Normal Person Adaptation

(1) Create a normal person in terms of a given age, gender, and socioeconomic class.
  (a) Status and role in family
  (b) Residential situation
  (c) Employment
  (d) Physical history

  In creating the normal person, try not to select characteristics that are too middle class, WASP, ethnic. Don't create a perfectly normal person, but rather one with the average warts, aches, and pains of everyday life.
(2) Create one problem for him or her which is of one of three durations:
  (a) Very recent (within the last 2–3 months)
  (b) Within the last 2–4 years (but more than 3 months)
  (c) Long term
(3) For a problem of long duration, have it surfaced or manifested as a problem either:
  (a) Recent, or
  (b) Recurring
(4) Consider the one problem now; modify the normal life structure to a mid-range of disability. Be careful not to incapacitate the person!

Examples of two case histories which used a combination of all three procedures are given in Table 3.

Procedures for Staff-Development Session

A staff development session involves eleven steps:

STEP (1) Review the concept of clinical judgment as a weighting of specific problems to form an overall global rating.

STEP (2) Review the purpose of the session: to uncover differences in judgments and be sure the stories (cases) are sufficiently ambiguous to promote differing points of view. If specific variables are being studied, inform the participants.

Table 3. Two Example Case Histories

1) Karen is a 24-year old female who was referred to the Center four years ago after an extended psychiatric hospitalization. At that time Karen was unable to dress herself without assistance from her mother. She refused to bathe and spent most of her day in bed. After a year of this behavior, Karen agreed to attend a day treatment program which focused on daily living skills, personal hygiene, and social relationships. After attending the program for a year, she was placed in a sheltered workshop, which she is still attending. She now takes her medication regularly, drives to and from work, and produces satisfactory work. She continues to talk and laugh inappropriately and she needs constant reminders to return to her work station. Her supervisor does not feel that Karen will be employable outside of the sheltered workshop until she is able to control her behavior.
2) David is a 22-year old male living alone in a rented room. He has no family contacts, except for a grandfather. The grandfather is afraid of him and refuses to allow David into the house. David was referred to the Center by a local physician who felt he needed medication and counseling to control his delusions and hallucinations. David is of average intelligence. He has received a GED and has worked at a number of odd jobs. Although he continues to come to the Center, he has stopped his medication and quit his most recent job. The grandfather has called to report that David is hanging around his home, shouting obscenities, and banging on the door.

Take no more than 15 minutes for Steps (1)–(2).

STEP (3) Pass out and describe folders containing the history plus five tables, Tables 4 through 8:
Table:
4—Instructions given participants
5—Response Sheet Part I, characteristics of the workshop participant
6—Response Sheet for each PASS or set of 10–12 cases
7—Group Summary Sheet
8—Followup Questionnaire to obtain participant's insights 24 hours after a session

STEP (4) Instruct group to read the instructions and proceed with the tasks. Up to 30 minutes will be allowed to complete Response Sheet for 10–12 cases.

STEP (5) The leader also should rate the cases.

STEP (6) After about 25 minutes, warn the group only 5 minutes remain.

STEP (7) Starting with leader and moving around the room, each response for each case is read and recorded on the Group Summary Sheet (Table 7).

STEP (8) Review cases where clusters of clinicians differed in their judgments by asking for discussion by those in the different clusters. Caution should be used for the first several times Step (8) is performed.
—Do not let the discussion dwell on "right" vs. "wrong" judgments but rather on differences in attention, perceptions, definitions, and weightings of importance.
—Do not let any one person dominate the session.
—Encourage the "mighty" in clinical leadership roles to be reflective and possibly vulnerable to their own biased judgments or, at least, to differences in judgments. Consider a discussion with the clinical leadership *before* the formal session.

STEP (9) Repeat Steps (4)–(8) on the second set of cases. You have staff offer two ratings, one for "now" and one for 4–6 weeks from "now." The exercise helps staff understand goal planning.

STEP (10) Same as (8).

STEP (11) Collect the folders, with staff keeping the followup questionnaire for submission the next day.

Table 4. Instructions for Staff-Development Sessions

A. *Purpose of the Session*

To identify the major factors which could contribute to the variability in the judgments ______________ among the clinical staff. (e.g., FUNCTIONING)

B. *Instructions*

We will be reading through two sets of abbreviated case histories. In the first set of case histories (PASS I), you are asked to:

—Give a rating judgment on each case, and
—Evalute how "good" the information was for making the judgment, where
0 = terrible 5 = perfectly adequate

After the first set of cases has been rated independently we will

—Compare our responses by listing them on the data summary sheet, and then
—Discuss our differences but not try to resolve or settle the differences.

We will then repeat the process with another set of cases (PASS II). For PASS II you are to give a second rating judgment as to what level you think the client will be at *four weeks from now.*

Note the stories have been constructed to provide information which is short of perfect, but still adequate enough to make a judgment.

C. *The Hypothetical Case History Abstracts*

The hypothetical cases represent all possible levels of functioning, but all levels are not equally represented. Each rating level can have a different number of cases. Thus, do not try to "even out" the number of ratings at each rating level.

For the present attempt at estimating our consistency in ratings, the case histories cover only the _________ target population.
(e.g., adult)

While each of the cases represents a fictitious person, the person presented is a collage (an assemblage) of different cases of real origin. Usually age, gender, occupation, and social conditions were varied sufficiently to obscure any identification with real clients. Hopefully, the cases still retain an air of credibility while guaranteeing client confidentiality.

D. *Staff Confidentiality* (Example for Cross-Program Studies)

The analysis of the data will be so no individual staff person will ever be identified. Specifically, the major identifying sources of differences (variance) will be:

1. Years of experience
2. Professional identification
3. Catchment area
4. County

NOTE: We ask for the last four (4) digits of your social security number on Part I. This is solely for computer analysis. It will allow us to compare responses from one training session to another at each program. This provides a unique confidential identification of the data. No names will ever be attached to this data; in fact, *do not* put your name on any of our materials.

E. *Steps in the Procedure*

Step I Fill in Part I materials as indicated.

Step II Turn to the response sheet of Part II and, in turn, for each case history:

1. Record the code number for that abstract (case history).
2. Read the abstract.
3. Decide upon a rating level for that abstract and record it next to the abstract's code number.
4. Evaluate how "good" the information is and record the appropriate code.
5. Continue the judgment and recording process for each of the case histories. When all participants have completed PASS I, we will discuss our differences. Please do not begin PASS II until told to do so.

Do *not* linger over any one abstract. You should be able to reach a judgment within 2 minutes (most often, in less time).

The abstracts are in a randomized order and you should read them in the order you receive them.

Table 5. Response Sheet—Part 1

A. *Professional Orientation* (Training). If you have training in more than one area, check (X) all areas, but place a number (1) next to your principal area of training.

☐ Clinical Psychiatry ☐ Nursing
☐ Clinical Psychology ☐ Occupational Therapy
☐ Guidance and Counseling ☐ Music, Art, or Activities Therapy
☐ Social Work ☐ Physiotherapy
☐ Sociology ☐ Other ______

B. *Degrees.* Most advanced degree earned. If you are a trainee, intern, or resident, place a (T) next to the appropriate degree category.

☐ High school or less ☐ MS/MA ☐ Ed. ☐ Psych. ☐ Other
☐ Associate general ☐ MSW
☐ Associate MH specialty ☐ EdD
☐ BS/BA ☐ PhD
☐ RN ☐ MD Psychiat., ☐ MD (Other)
☐ OD Psychiat., ☐ OD (Other)

C. *Years of Experience in MH.*

☐ Less than one year ☐ 4 to 10 years
☐ One to three years ☐ Eleven years or more

D. *Current Service* (if employed in more than one, give approximate percent time in each).

☐ Outpatient ☐ Inpatient
☐ Partial Hospitalization ☐ Other ______

E. *Employment Status at Center*

☐ Full time (5 days/week) ☐ Irregular, e.g., Fee-for-Service
☐ 3–4 days/week ☐ Volunteer
☐ 1–2 days/week

F.

Orientation of Therapy	Your Primary Viewpoint	Percent Used in Practice
Psychodynamic		
Gestalt		
Rational/Emotive		
Cognitive/Behavioral		
Behavioral		
Family/Network System		
Other		

G. *Primary Service Activities (Give Percent)*

Individual ______ Medication ______
Group ______ ACTIVITIES (e.g., OT, Music, Art) ______
Family/Network ______ Other ______

H. *Your Socioeconomic Status* during formative years, prior to 21st birthday.

Principal Income provider was

Poverty (primarily living on welfare) ______
Unskilled Labor, unstable employment ______
Unskilled Labor, stable employment ______
Semi-skilled Labor, unstable employment ______
Semi-skilled Labor, stable employment ______
Skilled, unstable employment ______
Skilled, stable employment ______

1. Check one:
☐ Male
☐ Female

H. Last 4 digits of Social Security Number ☐☐☐☐

Table 6. Response Sheet—Part 2

Data Sheet

PASS I Case Code #	Rating Level	Quality of Information

PASS II Case Code #	Rating Level		Quality of Information
	Now	4 Weeks from Now	

Table 7. Summary Sheet

Pass I Case #	Rater										
	You	1	2	3	4	5	6	7	8	9	10
Pass II Case #	**Rater**										
	You	1	2	3	4	5	6	7	8	9	10

Table 8. Staff-Development Session: Followup Questionnaire

DATE OF SESSION (/ /) PROGRAM ____________________

OBJECTIVE: To permit staff to describe the positive and negative outcomes of the staff-development session.

A. COMMUNICATION WITH CLINICAL COLLEAGUES

1. Check (X) the client problem areas where you felt your views differed noticeably from your clinical colleagues. The difference in viewpoint could have been in terms of either problem severity or importance of a problem's overall influence on a client's ability to function in their own community.

____ Aggression
____ Alcohol Use
____ Anxiety (Psychopathological)
____ Symptoms
____ Decisions
____ Depression
____ Drug Use
____ Education
____ Family/Marital
____ Financial
____ Interpersonal Relationships and Social Activities
____ Legal
____ Living Arrangements
____ Physical Complaints and Characteristics
____ Self-References
____ Sexuality
____ Suicide
____ Treatment
____ Work
____ Other (specify):
____
____
____

2. For each of the factors listed below, rate the degree to which each influenced your judgments to differ from your colleagues. Let 0 = No influence on judgments relative to others, and 10 = Extremely influential.

(a) Client characteristics:

____ Age
____ Sex
____ Family Situation
____ Prior Hospital History
____ Socioeconomic Level
____ Other (specify) ____________________

(b) Client behaviors:

Past	Current	
		Dependency on Chemotherapy
		Suicide Attempts
		Other

3. As a result of this session, rate your overall level of communiation with your clinical colleagues:

|—|—|—|—|—|—|—|—|—|—|

Very Much Worse — Very Much Improved

B. CHANGES NEEDED AS A RESULT OF INSIGHTS GAINED DURING THIS STAFF DEVELOPMENT SESSION

1. Clinical intake and treatment planning phases.

____ No opinion
____ Additional information is needed
____
____
____

____ Supervisory staff or case conferences should raise the following issues about client-treatment plans:

TYPE OF CLIENT	ISSUES TO BE RAISED

Table 8 (*Continued*)

2. Clinical review and quality assurance procedures
   ____ No opinion
   ____ Changes

TYPE OF CLIENT	CHANGES OR ISSUES TO BE RAISED

C. Other comments:

D. Name (optional) ____________________

Chapter 14

Technical Chapter
Statistical Analysis Procedures for Estimating Scale Reliability, Validity, and Generalizability*

THREE KEY ISSUES:
How Dependable (Reliable) Are Clinical Data When Influenced
—By Different Clients? —In Different Settings?
When and How Far Can You Generalize the Results of Your Clinical Observations and Data?
How Can You Obtain and Use the Quantitative Estimates of Reliability and Validity in the Management of MH Services?

The Section III discussed how to set up clinical-record systems that meet the needs of your clients and your programs. The next logical step was the training of staff in using those records (Chapters 12 and 13). We're now in a position to look at setting up scales that are appropriate for your clients and the means by which we can measure the validity and reliability of the scales. This, as it turns out, is the first measure of the effectiveness of your staff's diagnostic activities and skills, certainly a cornerstone of your program.

The major emphasis of this chapter is the development of *quantitative* estimates of the dependability of clinical data. In this context, managerial use of such data is stressed and the analysis illustrates how to improve clinical-service planning, periodic review and records procedures.

The chapter does not assume that you are a sophisticated mathematician or that you have

* Some portions of this unit were adapted from the NIMH publication by Carter and Newman (1976). The major influence for the unit's theme, however, comes from Professor Lee Cronbach and his associates. Their recent work on Generalizability Theory (Cronbach et al., 1972) provides a new and rich approach to behavioral measurement. Unfortunately, the recent development of generalizability theory means its concepts and language are foreign to most of our colleagues trained in the language of traditional reliability and validity coefficients as a measure of a scale's reliability. We felt compelled to retain much of the language of classical measurement theory, but we have also attempted to embed the estimates of reliability and validity within the framework of generalizability theory. As familiarity with these concepts increases, more applications will be introduced in the future.

extensive training in statistics. The numerical examples can easily be adapted to a cookbook approach. Most practitioners find that given a day or two of training, the actual computational tasks can be turned over to an administrative assistant.

Some brief sections of the chapter require a working understanding of variance and regression analysis. These passages are technical comments and are *not* necessary for the actual computations and applications of the techniques. Technical comments are offered because some of the procedures are not part of traditional reliability and validity estimation procedures.

On the one hand, Chapter 14 is the logical core of the two sections on "Visible Evidence." On the other hand, its length is that of five chapters. Thus, the outline employed in Chapter 14 covers five subsections:

(1) BUILDING RELIABILITY AND VALIDITY TECHNIQUES INTO YOUR PROGRAM'S SYSTEM: Reliable and valid measures are an integral part of a client-oriented system and Chapter 14 outlines how to obtain and use quantitative estimates of dependability and generalizability.

(2) THE RELIABILITY COEFFICIENT IN ITS SIMPLEST FORM: We start with a procedure for estimating scale consistency for a group of clinicians who regularly work together with clients of similar characteristics in a similar setting, e.g., partial hospitalization service staff, adult outpatient, or children outpatient staff. The applications will be limited to how a clinical supervisor can use the reliability information in staff development, and coordination of the scale's use with other service units serving the same clients. The procedures are unobtrusive to the clinical process and are relatively inexpensive. The data can come from staff-development sessions and a small sample of clinical data.

(3) IDENTIFYING FACETS INFLUENCING SCALE AND COMMUNICATION DEPENDABILITY AND GENERALIZABILITY WITHIN A SERVICE PROGRAM: This is the core of the chapter. The procedures described will permit identification of the principal factors influencing clinical staff perceptions and decisions. The procedures do not intrude on the clinical process; use data for specially designed staff-development sessions based on a sample of clinical records, and, possibly, from cost-outcome data analyses (as described in Chapters 21 through 24).

(4) GENERALIZING RESULTS ACROSS SERVICES AND ACROSS PROGRAMS: Clinical staff must communicate within a program of services in a dependable and accurate fashion. A broader issue needs to be addressed: "Can the clinical data be aggregated to describe differences in client outcome across programs, or across client groups and programs?" (For example, "What is the relative impact on elementary-age children entering service at the mid-range levels of functioning across and among different service programs?")

(5) COMPLETING THE PICTURE: There are a number of traditional validity estimation techniques to be applied either annually or bi-annually to doublecheck that the procedures described in subsections 3 and 4 are working properly.

1. BUILDING RELIABILITY AND VALIDITY INTO YOUR PROGRAM'S SYSTEM

A client-oriented system should build in the means of obtaining and maintaining a high degree of reliability and validity of clinical measures. We start with formal definitions of reliability and validity, then discuss how these definitions relate to each other and to the management of mental health services.

Reliability is the extent to which two or more observers (persons) agree upon how they will label a set of observations, and the extent to which their agreement on applying these labels is consistent over different objects (clients, in our case) over time. As a specific example in mental-health settings, reliability would be the degree of consistency with which a group of clinicians rate a set of clients on a particular scale; e.g., level of functioning, or level of depression, or level of risk of alcohol abuse.

Generalizability is an estimate of the extent to which and under what conditions sets of scale observations, made by two or more people on the same kind of clients, can be discussed. Similar to reliability, generalizability provides a more specific description of the likelihood of generalizing the reliability of data beyond the situation in which the data were collected.

Dependability identifies potential factors influencing the observations of a set of observers (e.g., clinicians, clients, or significant others connected with the client). Dependability as used here is part of generalizability, but with an emphasis on identifying factors influencing clinical observations. Consider two examples: "Will symptoms of social deviancy and depression influence the inpatient clinical staff decisions in the same way as the outpatient staff?" "Will prior history of psychiatric episodes influence the clinical decisions among new or experienced staff in the same manner?"

Validity is the extent to which some external criteria support the conclusion that the reported observations represent what they are supposed to represent. External criteria (verification) are typically sought to establish validity in three ways. One criterion is to show the *contents* of a scale refer directly to the behavior of clients reported to be at that scale level; e.g., low functioning clients should refer to clients not functioning independently or productively, who have emotional stress symptoms that appear to impair their perceptions, problem solving, and/or personal self-care. A second external criterion is the scale's *predictive* capability. For example, persons with certain psychiatric disorders and circumstances are predicted to have a typically lower level of psychosocial functioning with greater fluctuating levels, week by week, than persons with other psychiatric disorders. The third external criterion is *construct* validity, or the relationship of one scale to another scale or set of behavioral observations known to be a "true" measure of the behavior of interest.

Construct validity has historically been considered the most desirable form of external criteria validation. But, recently, there have been some serious issues raised about construct validity's status as a desirable index of the quality of a scale. First, construct validity is the most difficult and elusive to obtain (Nunnally, 1975). Second, construct validity is the notion most vigorously attacked by the proponents of Generalizability Theory (Cronbach, et al., 1972, Chapter 11). The best example of construct validity, used for measures of intelligence, provides an example of its chief problems. Construct validity was thought to exist for some of the measures of intelligence because of a strong relationship to school performance. However, confounding socioeconomic factors have since clouded the validity of tests of intelligence and their relationship to school performance. With studies of generalizability and dependability, better estimates will be obtained for the factors influencing the measures used and the conditions for generalization of results. Thus, the controversy over intelligence testing is directly confronted when approached within the context of Generalizability Theory. For example, the socioeconomic factors can be dealt with directly and the information used to improve upon inferences drawn.

Now these four formal definitions can be integrated and woven into the fabric of a client-oriented system. The basic ingredients of the four definitions can be described by the following human interactions. If two or more people having a common experience use the same language (labels or scale values) to describe that common experience, then their language would be a *reliable* means of communicating that common experience:

> That object is a pen since it has a hard outer surface, a gooey substance on the inside which, when tipped over and pressed across paper, leaves an indelible mark.

But, they would not know whether their experiences and use of the labels are appropriate (real) or whether the percepts are just a unique (fantasy) experience to those involved:

> Gee! I wonder if other people to whom we would only describe the characteristics of a pen would identify the same objects as pens that we did?

To ascertain if the scale is valid, we would need to ask a naive group of observers to use the scale and, if they agreed with the first group on the same objects under the same circumstances, then the scale may be valid:

> Let's ask George to review our definition of a "pen" without showing him a "pen" and then, using only that definition, let him loose in the building to gather up ten examples of a "pen." If all ten objects he gathers are examples of "pens" that you and I previously agreed upon, then maybe our concept (construct) of a "pen" is not just a fantasy, but rather a *valid construct*.

The operations of the preceding example are summarized below in two ways: with stick figure drawings and in a diagram. In Figure 1, we provide a characterization of the concepts of reliability and validity using interactions among people.

In Figure 2, a diagram is used to identify some of the technical features.

Thus, in our earlier example, if George returns with ten out of ten pens which fit our label of "pen" ("having a hard outer surface, a gooey internal substance which, when tipped and pressed across paper, leaves an indelible mark"), perhaps the label is valid. Now suppose one of the ten objects he has, although it meets the criteria, is clearly not a pen but a sealed container of grape juice with a protruding straw. While nine out of ten is a good rate of success, we would still wish to refine our definition of the label. This example provides a good illustration of the operational features to be built into a client-oriented system to insure important clinical data are reliable and valid representations of clinical observations and events. Moreover, we would want to have the means within the system to identify when factors are influencing clinical data, in what ways, and in a fashion which permits us to deal with the influencing factors. The essential components of providing these means of assuring or remediating reliability and validity of clinical data are:

(1) As frequently as is economically feasible, have at least two, and when necessary three, people compare their clinical observations. (See Chapters 4 through 7 for examples of doing this efficiently.)
(2) Establish criteria for systematic communication about each major group of clients.
    (2.1) Adapt global and multifacet scales for use in communication with each major group of clients (see Chapters 2 and 5).
    (2.2) Identify the typical concerns and decisions for each major client group; the *concerns* are the major behavioral and situational characteristics of the client group, and *decisions* are the typical correlated actions suggested by professional experi-

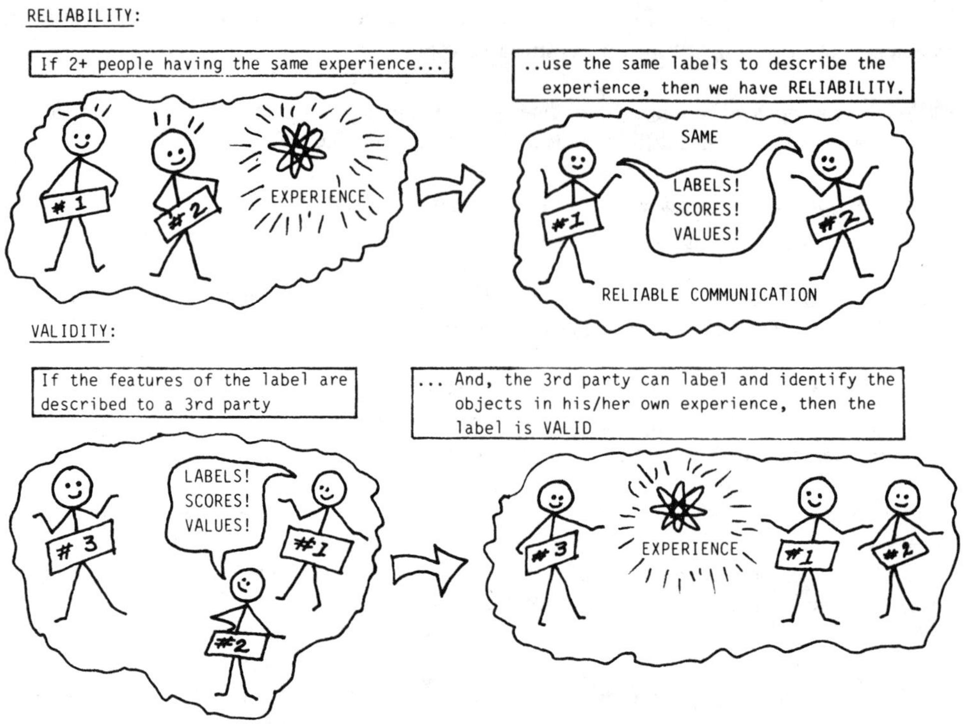
RELIABILITY:
If 2+ people having the same experience...
#1
#2
EXPERIENCE
..use the same labels to describe the experience, then we have RELIABILITY.
SAME
LABELS!
SCORES!
VALUES!
RELIABLE COMMUNICATION
VALIDITY:
If the features of the label are described to a 3rd party
#3
LABELS!
SCORES!
VALUES!
... And, the 3rd party can label and identify the objects in his/her own experience, then the label is VALID
EXPERIENCE

Figure 1. Reliability and Validity among Interactions with People

ences. These criteria become the basis for admissions criteria (Chapter 4), treatment planning (Chapter 5), and both utilization and quality assurance review procedures (Chapter 6). Detailed followup data on a sample of clients can be helpful (see Chapter 7 and the latter part of this chapter). Also external criteria are needed for content and construct validity studies. [Technical note: These criteria can be initially obtained from national norms taken from systematic research studies. Over time, the procedures described in this chapter and in Chapter 23 will permit revisions of the national norms to fit local situations.]

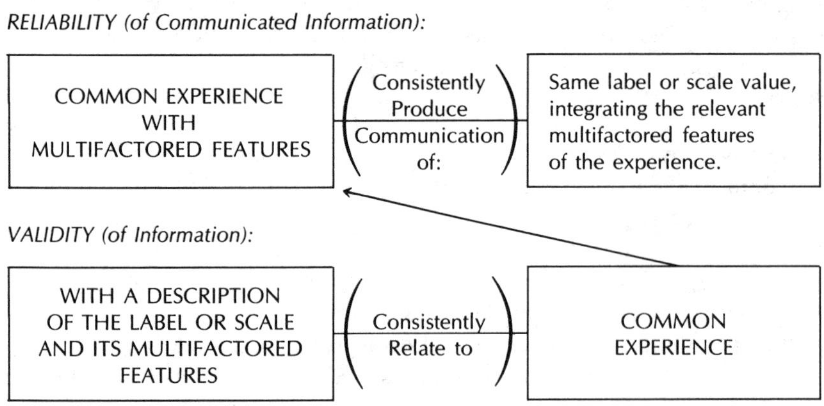

Figure 2. Diagram of Reliability and Validity

(3) Identify factors influencing clinical data by reviewing cost and outcome data.
  (3.1) Cost outcome (Chapters 21 and 22) and cost effectiveness procedures (Chapter 23) can identify factors related to different client outcomes. Weaknesses can result in either reallocation of clinical resource efforts or staff development (see point 3.2).
  (3.2) Manipulating the information in case histories used in staff-development sessions (Chapters 12 and 13) can show whether factors influencing the actual client cost-outcome data may be also influencing clinical judgments. To cross validate the results of factors found to be influencing differences in a staff-development session, randomly sample a small set of clinical records of clients with similar features to those found to be influencing both the client, cost-outcome data, and the clinicians' judgment data.

Together these techniques provide the basis of both generalizability and dependability studies by identifying the situations to which you may generalize the clinical data and the facets which are influencing the data.

There are a number of other control features built into a client oriented system to maintain the reliability and validity of the data.

— Clinical records should be designed to support the communication described in the clinical processes (see Chapters 9 through 11). Many of the control features built into a good record system (Chapter 11) will complement the efforts of clinical review procedures (Chapter 6).
— Management and organizational structures need to be developed so the clinical data support the growth and development of the program. Moreover, Chapters 18 through 20 will describe in detail how clinical data can be used positively and constructively by both clinical staff and management to reallocate clinical efforts or modify clinical procedures to improve upon data accuracy and usefulness.

The likelihood data will be reliable and valid data increases when the program's organization is structured such that the clinical data are useful to both those who generate the data (the clinical staff) and those who manage the program. Obviously, the converse is also true. When "messy" data benefit the clinicians, then it will be difficult to obtain "good" data. Thus, the clinical records need to be both useful to the clinicians and well-managed. The managerial use of clinical data needs to be both constructive and supportive of clinical efforts. All of these components, when operating in a coordinated fashion, can support reliable and valid data. The present chapter provides some quantitative means for ascertaining the degree of data reliability and validity, and helps identify the type and extent of factors influencing this reliability and validity. Other components of a client-oriented system are complemented by the dependability and usefulness of the clinical data.

2. THE RELIABILITY COEFFICIENT IN ITS SIMPLEST FORM

The starting point is to ask about the clinical procedures employed by a group of clinicians who ordinarily work together:

> How consistent are our observations about a given set of clients who are typical of those we serve?

Does an acceptable degree of consistency exist in the communication among clinicians who need to discuss a group of clients served in common? The measure of consistency is called the *reliability coefficient* and has the following interpretations. If the reliability coefficient approaches 0.00, we can conclude that the variability among judgments of clinical staff over cases being judged is vastly greater than the variability among clients (cases) being judged.

If the reliability coefficient approaches 1.00, we can conclude that the variability among judgments of clinicians over cases being judged is practically nil and the differences in the characteristics of cases is the best predictor of the clinical judgment.

In terms of a formula, expressed in words, phrases, and then in symbols,

$$\text{Reliability Coefficient} = \frac{\text{Variability among Cases}}{\text{Sum of} \begin{array}{c}\text{Variability}\\ \text{among Cases}\end{array} + \begin{array}{c}\text{Variability among}\\ \text{Clinicians across Cases}\end{array}}$$

$$\text{Reliability Coefficient} = \frac{\sigma^2_{\text{cases}}}{\sigma^2_{\text{Cases}} + \sigma^2_{\text{Cases} \times \text{Raters}}} = \frac{\sigma^2_{c}}{\sigma^2_{c} + \sigma^2_{c \times r}}$$

If $\sigma^2_{C \times R}$ is very small because of a great deal of judgment consistency over cases, the coefficient becomes

$$\frac{\sigma^2_{c}}{\sigma^2_{c} + 0.0} = 1.00,$$

and there is perfect consistency in ratings over cases.[1]

If σ^2_{CR} is very large—i.e., the variability among clinical raters over cases is very large—there is a great deal of rater inconsistency and

$$\text{The Reliability Coefficient} = \frac{\sigma^2_{c}}{\sigma^2_{c} + \text{A very large number}}$$

$$\text{and Reliability Coefficient} \rightarrow \frac{\text{small number}}{\text{Very small number}} \rightarrow 0.00$$

Let us review this concept by looking at the following two figures representing hypothetical ratings of four judges (1, 2, 3, and 4) on three cases. Figure 3 represents high rater reliability and Figure 4 shows low rater reliability.

When reviewing these two figures, we can see the principal characteristics of high reliability:

— When drawn on a graph, the lines connecting each rater's judgments across cases are nearly parallel. For example, there are only two crossed lines in the high reliability instance and six in the low reliability figure.

— The rank order of ratings across cases is fairly close. For example, in the high reliability

---

[1] *Technical note:* Technically, the interaction of Cases by Raters is an estimate of error of measurement as well, and a more formal representation would be to include σ^2_{error}, i.e., to include both terms as part of a single term: $(\sigma^2_{CR} + \sigma^2_{\text{error}})$ or $(\sigma^2_{CR} + \sigma^2_{e})$.

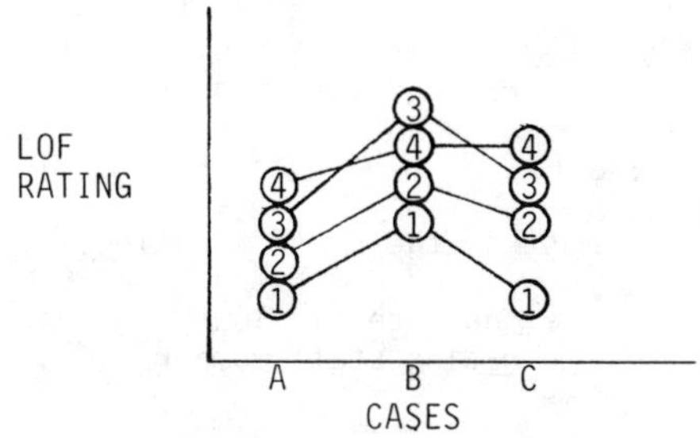

Figure 3. High Reliability

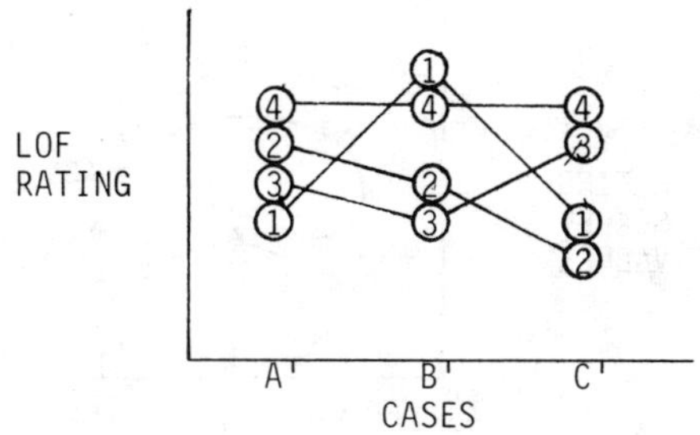

Figure 4. Low Reliability

figure, Cases A and C have the same ranking of clinician judgments. Case B has a changed order of rater rankings, but even here there is only a reversal of one place in the ranking for two individual raters. This is certainly not the situation for the low reliability example. The rank orderings over cases changes markedly in each instance.

The reliability coefficient gives an estimate of the consistency among a group of clinicians. But, the reliability coefficient gives more than a measure of consistency by estimating the *degree of accuracy* of any one clinician compared to the group. A low coefficient value (approaching 0.00) describes little to no similarity of any one clinical rating to the group's typical rating. A high coefficient value (approaching 1.00) describes nearly perfect accuracy of predicting the group's typical rating from any one case rating.

A statistically proper definition to use when interpreting a reliability coefficient is:

> The degree, or proportion, of accuracy of using any one clinical rating to represent the group's rating on these types of clients is *.xx*, where 0.00 is no accuracy and 1.00 is perfect accuracy.

Caution is advised in using a reliability coefficient. The accuracy or consistency of a clinical rating over clinicians rating the same kinds of cases does not mean they will necessarily give the *same* clinical ratings. The coefficient only implies ratings are consistent over cases. For example, one staff person may be consistently lower and another consistently higher in a group of clinicians. The coefficient is simply saying there is a certain degree of consistency among the clinicians and describes the degree of accuracy with which the group's rating can be predicted from a randomly selected individual clinician's rating.

But, to know the accuracy of an individual clinician's ratings requires an inspection of the data of the individual clinician from the staff-development sessions. In most cases, where the ratings of one or two clinicians are consistently different, the consistency of differences is easily seen, as shown in Figure 5.

Use of the Reliability Coefficient

While guidelines exist, no firm rules exist on how reliable a scale should be or how accurate or consistent clinical ratings should be. The quantitative values of the reliability coefficient can provide, however, some guidelines for followup actions by clinical, supervisory or management staff.

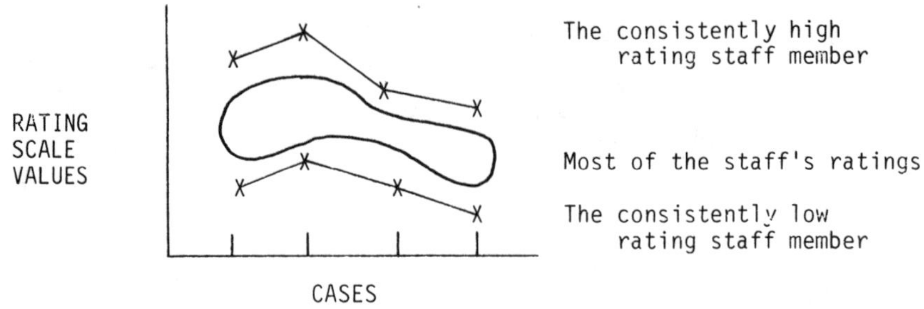

Figure 5. Differences among the Ratings of Clinicians

— Coefficient values 0.70 and higher indicate an acceptable good use of the scale as a communicating technique among the clinicians in a session. (Seldom will values go over 0.85.) Check if any staff were consistently different in their ratings from their colleagues. Usually, these sorts of consistent differences are observed during the actual staff-development sessions, and are handled immediately. A means of dealing with consistent differences can follow three steps:

(1) Discuss possible reasons for the differences either in the group (staff-development) session or individually with the clinical supervisor.

(2) Sample some of the staff person's clinical records to determine if the tendency was pervasive in the person's day-to-day clinical work.

(3) Set up criteria for the clinician's standard review strategy to insure any desired changes in rating style (behavior) are implemented in actual clinical practice.

— Coefficients between 0.50 to 0.70 are acceptable for short periods, but followup efforts should be quickly undertaken to improve these results.

Check the data from the staff-development sessions to identify whether staff or types of cases produced most of the inconsistency. If a small number of staff were highly inconsistent, the effects can be seen on a graph which plots individual staff ratings over cases. The staff with the greatest number of crossed graph lines with other staff are the likely culprits. Individual followup with these staff members would be advisable.

If a small number of cases was used in the session, the type of case may have contributed to the inconsistency. Often controversial topics in cases, such as suicide threats, incest, rape, or financial dependency on public assistance, will lead to greater differences among raters. Here the best course for followup is a threefold process of (a) group discussion of the issues; (b) decisions on what the major concerns are; and (c) after a trial period, another staff-development session focusing on the issues raised. Consider incorporating some of the decisions into the treatment planning and review processes. (Subsection 3 will describe quantitative procedures to test for the influences of certain factors.

Usually, most of the inconsistency can be accounted for by the attention paid to a few staff in need of individual attention, or to a certain subset of cases used in the session. If not, then turn to the scale(s) being used. Have a committee review and revise the scale(s) by the criteria described in Chapter 2 and/or the procedures described in Chapter 15.

— Coefficients below 0.50 indicate either total staff rebellion, lack of any coordinated efforts, or a poorly constructed scale. Even when a scale is poorly constructed (but has apparent face validity) low ratings occur because staff find the clinical situation not conducive to communicating with the scale or to using any scale. In other words, a management or staff

Table 1. Computing a Reliability Coefficient

	No. 1	No. 2	No. 3	No. 4	No. 5	No. 6	No. 7	No. 8	No. 9	T_C = Total Overall Cases
Case 1	7	8	9	9	8	7	7	7	7	69 = T_{C1}
Case 2	7	8	7	8	7	7	8	8	8	68 = T_{C2}
Case 3	4	5	5	5	4	5	5	6	4	43 = T_{C3}
Case 4	7	8	8	9	7	6	5	6	7	63 = T_{C4}
Case 5	4	5	4	5	4	5	4	5	5	41 = T_{C5}
Case 6	8	7	7	9	8	8	8	7	6	68 = T_{C6}
Case 7	5	5	3	5	5	6	5	5	5	44 = T_{C7}
Case 8	3	4	5	6	5	5	4	5	4	41 = T_{C8}
Case 9	4	4	3	4	3	3	4	5	4	34 = T_{C9}
Case 10	3	3	2	3	3	3	3	4	3	27 = T_{C10}
T_R = Total Overall Raters	52 = T_{R1}	57 = T_{R2}	53 = T_{R3}	63 = T_{R4}	54 = T_{R5}	55 = T_{R6}	53 = T_{R7}	58 = T_{R8}	53 = T_{R9}	498 = GT

morale problem may exist rather than a simple measurement problem. Chapters 16 through 18 describe these management issues and suggest ways of dealing with them.

Computing a Reliability Coefficient

You now need to be able to compute your own reliability coefficient. In Table 1, we have reproduced an example taken from Carter and Newman (1976). It shows the 17 steps needed to compute a reliability coefficient. The example involves nine raters (R = 9) making judgments on ten cases (C = 10). When following this example through, be sure to note where you would need to make adjustments if you wish to compute reliability coefficients for situations involving other than 9 raters and 10 cases. In Table 2, we give an analysis of variance, briefly showing how to obtain a reliability coefficient.

At the bottom of the table are the totals for each *staff member,* abbreviated as T_R.

At the right hand of the table are the totals for each *case,* abbreviated as T_C.

The sum of either the 9 totals for raters (T_R) or the 10 totals for cases (T_C) is the Grand Total (GT), or 498.

Note that:

The letter r = number of raters (r = 9)*

The letter n = number of cases (n = 10)*

---

* To compute a reliability coefficient for values other than 9 raters and 10 cases, simply substitute the appropriate values for "r" and "n" throughout.

Table 2. Analysis of Variance

	Sources of Variance	Degrees of Freedom (df)	Sums of Squares (SS)	Mean Square (MS)
A. COMPUTE SOURCES OF VARIANCE				
STEPS 1–6	Cases (C)	$(n-1)$	$SS_C = \frac{\sum_{C=1}^{n} (T_C)^2}{r} - \frac{(GT)^2}{r \times n}$	$MS_C = \frac{SS_C}{(n-1)}$
STEPS 7–10	Raters (R)	$(r-1)$	$SS_R = \frac{\sum_{R=1}^{r} (T_R)^2}{n} - \frac{(GT)^2}{r \times n}$	$MS_R = \frac{SS_R}{(r-1)}$
STEPS 11–14	Error Term (R) (Rater × Cases)	$(n-1)(r-1)$	$SS_e = \sum_{R=1}^{r} \sum_{C=1}^{n} (X_{RC})^2 - \frac{(GT)^2}{r \times n} - SS_C - SS_R$	$MS_e = \frac{SS_e}{(n-1)(r-1)}$
B. COMPUTE RELIABILITY COEFFICIENT*				
STEP 15	Case Variance Alone	$\frac{MS_C - MS_e}{r} = \hat{\sigma}_c^2$		
STEP 16	Total Variance	$\hat{\sigma}_c^2 + MS_e$		
STEP 17	Reliability Coefficient*	$\frac{\hat{\sigma}^2_C}{\hat{\sigma}^2_c + MS_e}$ = Reliability Coefficient	0.00 if low reliability 1.00 if high reliability	

**A Note of Caution:* Reliability as measured by this procedure only tells you the degree of judgment consistency among the staff. One or more staff members could be rating consistently *high* or *low*, and the reliability coefficient would be insensitive to consistent differences. In order to analyze statistically such factors as the influence of professional training on the rating of different types of cases, use the procedures described in Subsection 3.

Step 1

Square the Grand Total.

$$GT \times GT = (GT)^2$$
$$498 \times 498 = 248{,}004$$

Step 2

Divide the squared Grand Total by the number of cases × number of raters.

$$\frac{248{,}004}{10 \times 9} = \frac{248{,}004}{90} = 2755.6$$

$$\frac{(GT)^2}{rn} = \text{Correction Term}$$

The results of these calculations is called the *correction term* and is usually given by the notation $\frac{(GT)^2}{r(n)}$ where "n" is the number of cases and "r" is the number of raters or staff members.

Step 3

Square the totals for each case and add these squared values.

	T_C (Case Totals)^2	=	Square of Case Total
Case 1:	69^2	=	4961
Case 2:	68^2	=	4624
Case 3:	43^2	=	1849
Case 4:	63^2	=	3969
Case 5:	41^2	=	1681
Case 6:	68^2	=	4624
Case 7:	44^2	=	1936
Case 8:	41^2	=	1681
Case 9:	34^2	=	1156
Case 10:	27^2	=	729
Sum of Squared Case Totals		=	27,010

$$(T_{C1})^2 + (T_{C2})^2 + \ldots + (T_{C10})^2 = \sum_{C=1}^{10} (T_C)^2$$

Step 4

Divide the sum of the squared case totals (from Step 3, above) by the number of raters (9).

$$\frac{27{,}010}{9} = 3001.11$$

$$\frac{\sum_{C=1}^{10} (T_C)^2}{r} = 3001.11$$

Step 5

Subtract the "correction term" (from Step 2) from the result obtained in Step 4.

$$3001.11 - 2755.60 = 245.51$$

$$\frac{\sum_{C=1}^{10} (T_C)^2}{r} - \frac{(GT)^2}{r \times n} = SS_C$$

The result 245.51 is called the *Sum Square for Cases* (SS_C), where T_C = total for each case, r = number of raters, n = number of cases, and GT = grand total.

Step 6

Divide the Sum Square for cases by the number of cases minus 1. (Number of cases minus 1 [or n − 1] is called the *degrees of freedom* for cases.)

$$\frac{245.51}{10 - 1} = \frac{245.51}{9} = 27.279$$

$$\frac{SS_C}{n - 1} = \frac{SS_C}{df_C} = MS_C$$

The result is called the *Mean Square* for cases and is given by the notation MS_C. $n - 1 = df_C$ or degrees of freedom for cases.

Step 7

Square the totals for each rater and add these squared values.

Totals for Rater^2		Square of Rater Total
Rater 1:	52^2 =	2704
Rater 2:	57^2 =	3249
Rater 3:	53^2 =	2809
Rater 4:	63^2 =	3969
Rater 5:	54^2 =	2916
Rater 6:	55^2 =	3025
Rater 7:	53^2 =	2809
Rater 8:	58^2 =	3364
Rater 9:	53^2 =	2809
Sum of Squared Rater Totals	=	27,654

$$(T_{R1})^2 + (T_{R2})^2 + \ldots + (T_{R9})^2 = \sum_{R=1}^{9} (T_R)^2$$

Step 8

Divide the sum of the squared rater totals (from Step 7) by the *number of cases* (10).

$$\frac{27{,}654}{10} = 2765.40$$

$$\frac{\sum_{R=1}^{10} (T_R)^2}{n} = 2765.40$$

Step 9

Subtract the "correction term" (from Step 2) from the result obtained in Step 8.

$$2765.40 - 2755.60 = 9.80$$

$$\frac{\sum_{R=1}^{9} (T_R)^2}{n} - \frac{(GT)^2}{r \times n} = SS_R$$

The result is called the sum of squares for raters and is often denoted by SS_R; T_R = total for each case, n = number of cases, r = number of raters, and GT = Grand Total.

Step 10

Divide the Sum Square for staff members by the number of staff members minus 1. (Number of staff members minus 1 is called the degrees of freedom for staff members.)

$$\frac{9.80}{9 - 1} = \frac{9.80}{8} = 1.225$$

$$\frac{SS_R}{9 - 1} = \frac{SS_R}{df_R} = MS_R$$

The result is called the mean square for raters—staff members—and is often represented as MS_R. $r - 1 = df_R$ = degrees of freedom for raters.

Step 11

Square *each entry* in Table 1 and add these squared values.

sum of the squares = 3050

$$7^2 + 8^2 + \ldots + 3^2 = \Sigma(X_{RC})^2$$

(where X_{RC} = the rating of the "Rth" rater on the "Cth" case)

Step 12

Subtract the correction term from the total obtained in Step 11.

$$3050 - 2755.6 = 294.40$$

$$\Sigma(X_{RC})^2 - \frac{(GT)^2}{r \times n} = SS_T$$

The result is called the total sum square or SS_T.

Step 13

Subtract sum square cases (Step 5) and sum square raters or staff members (Step 9) from total sum square (Step 12).

$$294.40 - 245.51 - 9.80 = 39.09$$

$$SS_T - SS_C - SS_R = SS_e$$

The result is Sum Square error or SS_e.

Step 14

Divide the Sum Square for error by the degrees of freedom for error (degrees of freedom for error = number of cases minus 1 [n − 1] × number of staff members minus 1 [r − 1]).

$$\frac{39.09}{(10 - 1) \times (9 - 1)} = \frac{39.09}{9 \times 8} = \frac{39.09}{72} = 0.543$$

$$\frac{SS_e}{(n - 1)(r - 1)} = \frac{SS_e}{df_e} = MS_e$$

The result is called the Mean Square for error or MS_e. $(n - 1) \times (r - 1) = df_e$ = degrees of freedom for error.

Step 15

Subtract the Mean Square for error (Step 14) from the mean square for cases (Step 6). Divide the difference by the number of staff members (9).

$$\frac{27.279 - .543}{9} = \frac{26.736}{9} = 2.971$$

$$\frac{MS_C - MS_e}{r} = \sigma_C$$

The result is the estimate of variance due to *cases* alone: σ_C.

Step 16

Add the estimate of variance due to cases (Step 15) to the Mean Square for error (Step 14).

$$2.971 + 0.543 = 3.514$$

$$\sigma_C + MS_e = \sigma_{Tot}$$

The result is the variance contributed by cases *plus* variance of staff members across cases, sometimes denoted σ_{Tot}.

Step 17

Divide the estimate of variance for cases (Step 15) by the variance for cases plus staff members across cases (Step 16).

$$\frac{2.971}{3.514} = .845$$

$$\frac{\sigma_C}{\sigma_{Tot}} = \text{Reliability Coefficient}$$

3. IDENTIFYING FACETS INFLUENCING SCALE AND COMMUNICATION DEPENDABILITY AND GENERALIZABILITY WITHIN A SERVICE PROGRAM[2]

The emphasis of this chapter has been on the management applications of measures of a scale's reliability and validity. For quantitative estimates to be useful, they need to provide direction as to which facets may be influencing or limiting the degree of data dependability or limiting the generalizability of the clinical data. Because a scale is at one level of reliability or another is not sufficient to address the clinical and management concerns about facets influencing reliability. Identifying facets is necessary if clinical supervisors or program managers are to take useful administrative steps to change "decreases" to "increases" in scale (and communication) reliability. Procedures are outlined for testing whether certain facets are influencing clinical judgments activities. Followup steps for a clinical supervisor or administrator are outlined to stimulate needed changes and improvement.

Some Basic Assumptions

For the procedures to be useful, certain components of a client-oriented system should be operating. When these procedures are used, a global scale and/or a multifactored behavioral checklist (scale) should be in use for at least 3 to 6 months. Other elements assumed are treatment planning, a review process, and clinical record documentation similar to those outlined earlier. Behavioral scale data (e.g., client level of functioning) should be available with partitions by categories of major client category or service modality. Moreover, the staff-development sessions should be clearly identified and used as part of the clinical supervision process and not as a witch-hunting technique to uncover "bad" clinical staff. In summary, the reliability procedures described will only be useful for the ongoing clinical supervision and management of your program if they can be related to both client impact analysis (e.g., cost-outcome data) and the clinical process.[3]

Two Kinds of Research Questions and Designs

Clinical management applications move in two directions:

---

[2] We are using the word *facet* to indicate a variable which may be influencing data dependability. The meaning of facet is the same as *variable* or *factor* in the general sense, but not necessarily as *factor* is used in the statistical technique called *Factor Analysis*.

[3] As an aside, our experience has shown that unless these assumptions are met, calculations of staff communication reliability can represent a threat to staff and could severely weaken staff morale and productivity.

(1) *Within Therapist Facets*—Do one or more particular client characteristics (e.g., age, sex, symptom, prior history, social and economic situation) have differential effects on clinical judgments *within* a group of therapists?
(2) *Mixed Between and Within Therapist Facets*—Are there differences *between* different specific subgroups of therapists (e.g., clinical speciality area, service-program area, amount of clinical experience, professional discipline) as to the effects of particular client characteristics within each subgroup of therapists?

The first question, addressing within therapist issues, reflects research questions which are of particular interest to clinical supervisors of a serivce unit where staff communication is imperative for both effective and efficient efforts. Another way of stating the within therapist issue is:

> Does the clinical staff *within* our service unit communicate consistently for all of the major categories of clients with which we deal?

The extent to which one or more client characteristics differentially affect clinical staff perceptions and communication may, in turn, be influential on client progress and outcome. This would be the case particularly if the client's treatment plan requires two or more staff to work with the client or with each other on the client's behalf. The staff's judgments may be quite consistent with one client group, but there may be greater divergence with another client group. Consider Figure 6. Suppose we asked four therapists to make judgments on three categories of clients in a staff-development session, and the following results were obtained.

A visual inspection of the results suggests:

— A consistent tendency for *prior psychiatric* hospitalization history to be rated lower than no prior mental-health service history.
— Little consistency within this group of therapists when rating clients with prior mental-health service history.

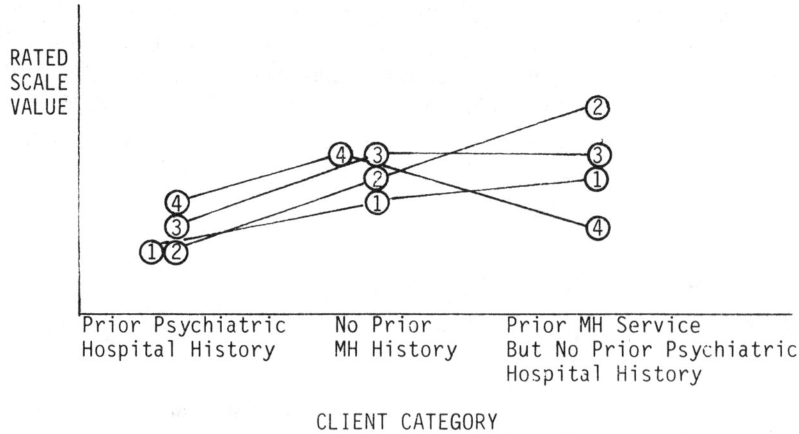

Figure 6. Four Therapists' Judgments of Three Clients

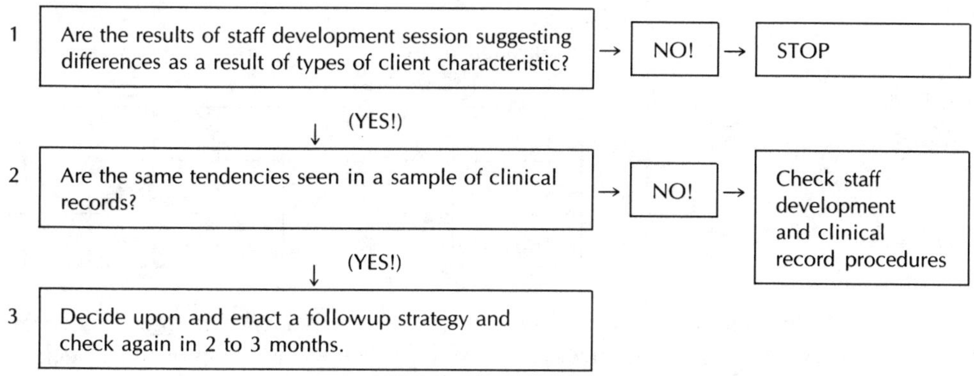

Figure 7. Summary of Management Strategy

Assuming that these trends were statistically significant, you would certainly want to followup the staff-development session with three kinds of activities in sequence:

— First, review a sample of actual client records to determine if these same tendencies exist for actual cases. If these trends appear to hold, you would proceed with the next two steps.
— Second, review the clinical literature and then discuss the results of the staff-development session, the clinical record-sampling results, and the clinical literature review with the staff to decide upon followup strategies which may assure that remediation of the problems can occur. Examples of followup strategies are:
  - Include precautionary questions and checks in the (peer) review procedures which are tailored to signal the problem's repeated occurrence and constructively deal with the problem or issue immediately.
  - Reallocate staff efforts to cover client caseloads which maximize their consistent judgments and minimize their inconsistencies.
  - Provide specialized training or supervision to specific staff on specific types of cases.
— Third, implement the followup strategy and review its impact by another staff development session 2 or 3 months later.

This three-part approach is reasonable only if the tendencies suggested by the results of the staff-development session are both statistically significant and verified (validated) by a cross check with a sample from the clinical records. If the staff-development session results do not correlate with the clinical records review, then you may wish to look at the procedures you employed in the staff development session. Otherwise you may be wasting time, effort and expense, weakening staff morale needlessly. Figure 7 summarizes this management strategy.

Statistical Procedures for Within-Therapist Designs

The statistical procedures will be described by means of an example. Technical notes throughout this section will provide the statistical rationale for the procedures used. These technical notes are set off within boxes and in footnotes. The issues raised in this example concern how a clinical staff of three professionals, working in a partial hospitalization program, are influenced by the presence or absence of prior psychiatric hospitalization in a client's history.

STAFF PERSON (RATERS)	Case Type I: No Prior Hospitalization History ①	②	③	④	⑤	Case Type II: Prior Hospitalization History ⑥	⑦	⑧	⑨	⑩
①	7	7	5	7	6	4	4	3	3	2
②	8	8	6	8	7	5	5	4	4	3
③	9	8	6	8	7	4	5	3	4	3

For this design, there are four facets which can be clearly identified to be influencing the overall variability (sources of variance) among ratings within this group of three raters:

Sources of Variance[4]	Number of Levels	Component of Variance
1. Raters, R	r = 3	σ^2_R
2. Types of Cases, T	t = 2	σ^2_T
3. Raters × Type, RT (Rates × Type Interaction)	rt = 6	σ^2_{RT}
4. (Cases/Types) × Raters, (C/T) × R (Cases within Types interacting across Raters is variance due to error of measurement)	(c/t)r = (5 × 2)3 = 30	$\sigma^2_{(C/T)R} + \sigma^2_{error}$

By partitioning the data into these four sources of variance, we can directly analyze the three critical issues of concern in a staff-development session. The three issues should be addressed in sequence:

(1) Are there sufficient differences among clinical staff in how they rate these types of cases (No Prior vs. Prior Psychiatric Hospitalization History) which might obscure the influence of clinical characteristics of the cases themselves? The following statistical ratio can be used to address this issue:

$$\begin{bmatrix}\text{Coefficient of}\\ \text{Dependability}\end{bmatrix} = \frac{\sigma^2_{Type}}{\sigma^2_{Type} + \sigma^2_{Rater \times Type} + \sigma^2_{(Cases/Type)+Rater} + \sigma^2_{error}}$$

Ideally, the sole consideration in rating clients should be the variability of characteristics peculiar to the type of cases being rated, σ^2_{Type}. As the other influences might increase in value greater than zero, the ratio decreases from a maximum of 1.00. Thus the *Coefficient of Dependability* describes the relative influences of variability among raters with these types of cases, $\sigma^2_{R \times T}$, and the influences of the sample cases used within each type of case ($\sigma^2_{(C/T)R} + \sigma^2_e$). As their influence increases, the ratio decreases. If the ratio decreases from 1.00 to a value below 0.60 or 0.70, a second issue should be addressed.

(2) Are there systematic differences among staff ratings across the types of cases being rated? The statistical ratio used to test this issue is an F-Ratio:

---

[4] In this design, we are concerned with the influence of a facet on a particular group of clinicians. Thus, the facet of *Raters* is treated as a fixed rather than a random effect in this design.

$$F = \frac{\text{(Variance due to R} \times \text{T interaction)}}{\text{(Variance due to random case and error facets)}}$$

$$F = \frac{MS_{R \times T}}{MS_{(C/T)R}} = \frac{\sigma^2_{R \times T} + \sigma^2_{(C/T)R}}{\sigma^2_{(C/T)R} + \sigma^2_e} + \sigma^2_e \geq 1.00$$

Here, the existence of the interaction of $\sigma^2_{\text{Raters} \times \text{Types}}$ is directly tested. Again, the ideal would be that the staff are consistent in their ratings across the types of cases being rated. If they were perfectly consistent, $\sigma^2_{R \times T} \rightarrow 0.00$ and the F–Ratio would approach 1.00. If the F-Ratio is statistically significant, then the nature of the interaction needs to be studied. This leads to the third issue.

(3) What is the comparative consistency of staff ratings within each of the types of cases? Here, there are two steps. First we need to determine if the reliability coefficients of ratings on cases within each of the types of cases will reflect whether the interaction was due to rating variation within or across types of cases. The statistical procedure for estimating the consistency of clinical ratings within each type of case is of the same form as shown in Tables 1 and 2:

$$\begin{bmatrix} \text{Reliability Type 1} \\ \text{Cases} \end{bmatrix} = \frac{\sigma^2_{C/T_1}}{\sigma^2_{C/T_1} + \sigma^2_{(R \times C)T_1} + \sigma^2_e}$$

$$\begin{bmatrix} \text{Reliability Type 2} \\ \text{Cases} \end{bmatrix} = \frac{\sigma^2_{C/T_2}}{\sigma^2_{C/T_2} + \sigma^2_{(R \times C)T_2} + \sigma^2_e}$$

If $(\sigma^2_{R \times C/T_R} + \sigma^2_e) \rightarrow 0.00$, then the Reliability Coefficient $\rightarrow 1.00$. Thus, when you have a significant interaction, $\sigma^2_{R \times T}$, and high within-type reliability, then staff differences are probably a matter of semantics and a group discussion can usually correct the occurrence of a significant interaction. For example, some staff have a consistently different view of how prior hospitalization influences overall functioning.

If $(\sigma^2_{(R \times C)/T_K} + \sigma^2_e)$ is a large value, the reliability ratio would be low and then you need to determine if $\sigma^2_{(R \times C)/T_K}$ within one type of case is significantly greater than the other. Here we can also use an *F*-Ratio (called the *F*-Max Test) to determine if the within-type of cases category variability is approximately equal:

$$F(\text{MAX}) = \frac{\text{Largest } \sigma^2_{(R \times C)T_K}}{\text{Smallest } \sigma^2_{(R \times C)/T_K}}$$

If the *F*(MAX) test suggests that variance of ratings across cases within types of cases differs significantly, then there are three possible lines of followup required:

—Was there one or more of the cases rated contributing to most of the differences? If so, was the case history poorly constructed or was there an additional facet which may have biased ratings, e.g., suicide, incest?

—Was there one or more staff that were responsible for most of the differences? If so, what is their explanation for this? Is individual training and follow-through needed?

—Are there words or phrases in the rating scale which were viewed as having different meanings by different staff? If so, what are the differences and what changes might assist in leveling the differences?

Now let us go through the steps in the computations of the reliability coefficients and the statistical effects test.[5]

Step 1. Set up the data in a fashion which permits you to obtain row and column subtotals and the grand totals. Compute these subtotals and totals.

	Case Type 1						Case Type 2						
	1	2	3	4	5	Subtotal Type 1	6	7	8	9	10	Subtotal Type 2	Rater Totals
RATER ①	7	7	5	7	6	$T_{R_1T_1} = 32$	4	4	3	3	2	$T_{R_1T_2} = 16$	$T_{R_1} = 48$
②	8	8	6	8	7	$T_{R_2T_1} = 37$	5	5	4	4	3	$T_{R_2T_2} = 21$	$T_{R_2} = 58$
③	9	8	6	8	7	$T_{R_3T_1} = 38$	4	5	3	4	3	$T_{R_3T_2} = 19$	$T_{R_3} = 57$
	$T_{C_1} = 24$	$T_{C_2} = 23$	$T_{C_3} = 17$	$T_{C_4} = 23$	$T_{C_5} = 20$	$T_{T_1} = 107$	$T_{C_6} = 13$	$T_{C_7} = 14$	$T_{C_8} = 10$	$T_{C_9} = 11$	$T_{C_{10}} = 8$	$T_{T_2} = 56$	GT = 163

(GRAND TOTAL) ↑

Note that there are five cases within each case type. The notation for subtotals are given by example.

T_{C_1} = Subtotal for Case 1.
$T_{R_1T_1}$ = Subtotal for Rater 1 over the five cases of Type 1 cases.
T_{R_1} = Subtotal for Rater 1 over all 10 cases, disregarding case type and case within case type.
GT = The Grand Total

Step 2. COMPUTE A TABLE OF MEANS

(a) Compute the mean for each rater within each case type, e.g.,

$$M_{R_1T_1} = T_{R_1T_1} \div (C/T_1) = 32 \div 5 = 6.4;$$

$$M_{R_3T_2} = T_{R_3T_2} \div (C/T_2) = 19 \div 5 = 3.8$$

(b) Find the *Rater Means* by dividing the totals for each rater, from Step 1, by the number of cases (c) each rated, e.g.,

$$M_{R_1} = (T_{R_1} \div C) = 48 \div 10 = 4.8$$

---

[5] Technical Note: The design and statistical model employed here uses the procedures for proportionate frequencies in treatment populations. While the example we are using has equal cell frequencies, the procedures allow for the user to vary the number of cases rated within each case type. The number of cases within each case type should be in proportion to the relative numbers of clients with the characteristics distinguishing the case type. If equal cell frequencies in the population are reasonable to assume, then only a few extra computational steps are needlessly expended when using the prescribed procedures. If, however, unequal cell frequencies in the population are expected, then the procedures used here are the safest to employ. For a full rationale of these procedures, see Myers (1979, pages 109–119), and Snedecor and Cochran (1967, pages 475–477).

(c) Find the *Type of Case Means* by dividing the Totals for each case type, from Step 1, by the number of ratings, e.g.,

$$M_{T_1} = (107 \div 15) = 7.13$$

(d) Find the Grand Mean by dividing the Grand Total by the Total Number of ratings, i.e.,

$$GT \div 30 = 163 \div 30 = 5.43$$

Rater	(a) Case Type 1	(a) Case Type 2	(b) Rater Means
①	$M_{R_1T_1} = 6.4$	$M_{R_1T_2} = 3.2$	$M_{R_1} = 4.8$
②	$M_{R_2T_1} = 7.4$	$M_{R_2T_2} = 4.2$	$M_{R_2} = 5.8$
③	$M_{R_3T_1} = 7.6$	$M_{R_3T_2} = 3.8$	$M_{R_3} = 5.7$

(c) TYPE OF CASE MEAN	$M_{T_1} = 7.13$	$M_{T_2} = 3.73$

(d) GRAND MEAN
GM = 5.43

Step 3. Set up a *Sources of Variance* Table (see Table 3) and (a) Compute the "Sum of Squares" by following the five steps cited in Column (3), placing the computed sums of squares in Column (4); and then (b) Compute the Means Square as shown in Column (5).

(3.1) Compute the sums of squares for Raters = SS_R.

$$SS_R = (\text{Total \# Cases}) \sum_{j=1}^{r} (M_{Rj} - GM)^2$$

$$= 10[(4.8 - 5.43)^2 + (5.8 - 5.43)^2 + (5.7 - 5.43)^2]$$
$$10[\quad (0.397) \quad + \quad (0.137) \quad + \quad (0.073) \quad]$$

$$= SS_R = 10(0.6070) = 6.070$$

(3.2) Compute the Sums of Squares for Types of Cases = SS_T.[6]

$$SS_T = r\Sigma C_k(M_{T_R} - GM)^2 = 3[5(7.13 - 5.43)^2 + 5(3.73 - 5.43)^2]$$

$$SS_T = 3[5(2.89) + 5(2.89)] = 86.7$$

6 TECHNICAL NOTE: C_k is equal to five (5) in the present example, i.e., all raters rated an equal number of cases within each case type. If an unequal number of cases were involved, then the value of C_k would vary within each case type as shown.

Table 3. Sources of Variance

(1) Source of Variance	(2) Degrees of Freedom	(3) Steps to Compute Sums of Squares	(4) Sums of Squares* Values	(5) Means Square
RATERS (R)	$(r - 1) = (3 - 1) = 2$	STEP 3.1	$SS_R = \underline{6.070}$	$MS_R = \frac{SS_R}{r - 1} = \underline{3.035}$ $F = 3.640$
TYPES OF CASES (T)	$(t - 1) = (2 - 1) = 1$	STEP 3.2	$SS_T = \underline{86.700}$	$MS_T = \frac{SS_T}{t - 1} = \underline{86.70}$ $F = 104.04$
RATERS BY TYPES (R × T)	$(r - 1)(t - 1) = (2)(1) = 2$	STEP 3.3	$SS_{R \times T} = \underline{0.600}$	$MS_{RT} = \frac{SS_{RT}}{(r - 1)(t - 1)} = \underline{0.300}$ $F = 0.36$
CASES WITHIN TYPES BY RATERS (C/T) × R	Total Number of Ratings minus (r × t) $30 - (3)(2)$ $30 - 6 = 24$	STEP 3.5 (First do Step 3.4, SS Total)	$SS_{(C/T) \times R} = \underline{20.000}$	$MS_{(C/T) \times R} = \frac{SS_{(C/T) \times R}}{T\#r - r \times t} = \underline{0.833}$
TOTAL	(Total Number of Ratings) − 1 = $30 - 1 = 29$	STEP 3.4	$SS_{TOTAL} = \underline{113.367}$	

*Technical Note: The Sums of Squares may be easy to compute if you have a calculator which computes the standard deviation, and the design has an equal number of cases within each case type. If so, try computing the sums of squares values by finding the standard deviations of the means called for in the source of variance term, square the standard deviation value and multiply by the degrees of freedom, and then multiply again by the number of terms required to compute the means.

(3.3) Compute the Sums of Squares for the interaction of Types of Cases by Raters = SS_{RT}.

$$SS_{RT} = \sum_{j} \sum_{r} C_k(M_{R_j}T_k - GM)^2 - SS_R - SS_T$$

$$= [5(6.4 - 5.43)^2 + 5(7.4 - 5.43)^2 + 5(7.6 - 5.43)^2 + 5(3.2 - 5.43)^2$$

$$+ 5(4.2 - 5.43)^2 + 5(3.8 - 5.43)^2] - SS_R - SS_T$$

$$= [5(0.941) + 5(3.881) + 5(4.709) + 5(4.973) + 5(1.513) + 5(2.657)]$$

$$- 6.070 - 86.7 = 0.600$$

(3.4) Compute the total sums of squares, SS_{TOTAL}.

$$SS_{TOTAL} = \left[\begin{matrix}\text{Sum of squared values} \\ \text{of all ratings}\end{matrix}\right] - \left[\frac{(\text{Grand Total})^2}{(\text{Total \# Ratings})}\right]$$

$$= [7^2 + 7^2 + 5^2 + \ldots + 3^2 + 4^2 + 3^2] - \left[\frac{(163)^2}{30}\right]$$

$$= 999. - 885.633 = 113.367$$

(3.5) Compute the Sums of Squares for Cases within Types of Cases by Raters, $SS_{C/TR}$.[7]

$$SS_{C/TR} = SS_{TOTAL} - SS_{RT} - SS_R - SS_T$$

$$SS_{C/TR} = 113.367 - 0.600 - 86.700 - 6.066 = 20.000$$

Step 4. Compute the estimates of the *Components of Variance* needed for the statistical estimates of Dependability, Reliability, and Generalizability using the MS values from STEP 3.

(4.1) $$\hat{\sigma}^2{}_T = \frac{(MS_T - MS_{(C/T)R})}{r(C_{T_1} + C_{T_2})/t} = \frac{86.700 - 0.833}{15} = 5.724$$

(4.2) $$\hat{\sigma}^2{}_{R\times T} = \frac{MS_{R\times T} - MS_{(C/T)R}}{(C_{T_1} + C_{T_2})} = \frac{0.300 - 0.833}{10} = -0.053 \simeq 0.000$$

In theory, it is not possible to obtain a variance, σ^2, or any squared term, less than zero (i.e., having a negative value). In practice, it can occur when MS_{RT} is very small and by chance alone

---

[7] Technical Note: For the present example, the computation of the $MS_{C/TR}$ proceeds directly from the computation of $SS_{C/TR}$, i.e., $MS_{C/TR} = SS_{C/TR} \div df(C/TR)$, where df(C/TR) = the degrees of freedom. For unequal, but proportional, cell frequencies, the degrees of freedom are most easily computed by summing the degrees of freedom within each case type ($C_k - 1$) for all case type by rater combinations. For unequal, disproportional cell frequencies, however, the computations require additional steps. The reader is referred to either Myers (1979, pages 116–119) or Snedecor and Cochran (1967, pages 475–477) to see the required steps described.

MS_{RT} and $MS_{(C/T)R}$ are approximately equal. Thus, if a negative variance does occur, set it equal to 0.000.

(4.3) $\hat{\sigma}^2_{(C/T)R} + \sigma^2_e = MS_{(C/T)R} = 0.833$

Step 5. Estimate the dependability and generalizability of ratings by type of case.

(5.1) $$\text{Coefficient of Dependability} = \frac{\hat{\sigma}^2_T}{\hat{\sigma}^2_T + \hat{\sigma}^2_{RT} + \hat{\sigma}^2_{(C/T)R} + \hat{\sigma}^2_e}$$

$$= \frac{5.724}{5.724 + 0 + 0.833} = 0.873$$

Interpretation: For the three clinicians in this example, 87.3% of the total variance was due to type of cases, Raters × Types, and Error of measurement, and is probably accounted for by the characteristics of the type of case alone, $\hat{\sigma}^2_T$.

(5.2) *Computing a Coefficient of Generalizability.* A second but related issue is the extent to which you can generalize the clinician ratings to other cases with the characteristics of these two types of cases. Here we can use the coefficient of generalizability:

$$\text{Coefficient of Generalizability} = \frac{\hat{\sigma}^2_T}{\hat{\sigma}^2_T + (\hat{\sigma}^2_{RT/t}) + (\hat{\sigma}^2_{(C/R)T} + \hat{\sigma}^2 e/(C_{K_1} + C_{K_2})}$$

$$= \frac{5.724}{5.724 + 0/2 + 0.833/10} = \frac{5.724}{5.807} = \underline{\underline{0.986}}$$

Thus, you may generalize these results to another study, like this one, with the same clinicians and have a 98.6% chance of replicating these same results.

If either of the two coefficients are low, then either $\sigma^2_{R \times T}$, or $(\sigma^2_{(C/T)R} + \sigma^2_e)$, or both, are high. (See Step 6).

Step 6. To test for the significance of $\sigma^2_{R \times T}$.

(6.1) *Compute:*

Technical Note

$$F(\text{obtained}) = \frac{MS_{R \times T}}{MS_{(C/T)R}} = \frac{(C/t\hat{\sigma}^2_{RT} + \hat{\sigma}^2_{(C/T)R} + \hat{\sigma}^2_e}{\hat{\sigma}^2_{(C/T)R} + \hat{\sigma}^2_e} = \frac{0.300}{0.833} = 0.360$$

(6.2) Contrast F(obtained) with the F value in an F-table from a standard statistics text, where in our example:
—degrees of freedom (numerator) = 2

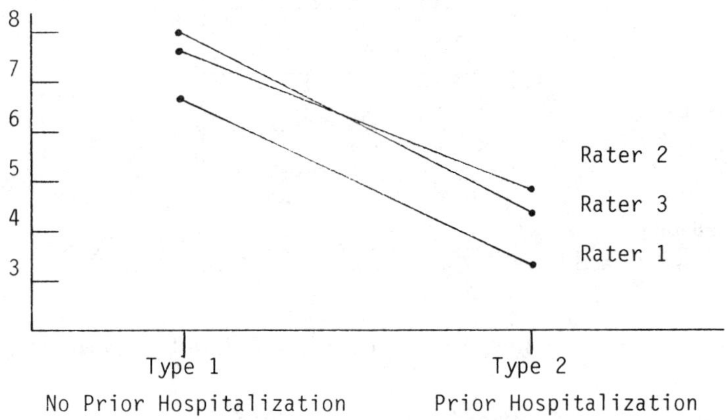

Figure 8. Graph of a Table of Means

—degrees of freedom (denominator) = 24
—probability of F(obtained) $\geq F$(Tabled with 2 and 24 df) > .05.[8]

$F(2, 24, p < .05) = 3.40$

If the obtained value of F is equal to, or greater than, the tabled F–value, then reject the possibility that there is no interaction and start to look carefully at how the case types studied differentially affect clinicians' judgments; e.g., in our example:

$[F(\text{Observed}) = 0.300] < [F(2, 24, p < .05) = 3.40]$

Thus, we would not wish to conclude that the raters were differentially affected by types of cases. That no statistically significant effect occurred can be shown graphically by drawing a graph which plots the means obtained in Step 2, as illustrated in Figure 8. Note that the three rater functions are nearly parallel, which would be the case when no significant interaction, Rater-by-Type, is obtained.

If a statistically significant interaction is obtained, i.e., F(Observed) $\geq F$(From the statistical text table), then you would need to conclude that the types of cases do differentially affect your clinical group. Drawing the figure of Rater-by-Type means will show the nature of the interaction.

Step 7. Computing and comparing the consistency of ratings within each type of case.

(7.1) Using the procedures from Subsection 2, find:

---

[8] If you wish to be more conservative, set p < .10, where "conservative" implies that it would be unwise to falsely accept the null hypothesis that no $\sigma^2_{R \times T}$ exists.

Technical Note

$$\left\{\begin{matrix}\text{Reliability} \\ \text{Within Type 1 Cases}\end{matrix}\right\} = \boxed{\frac{\hat{\sigma}^2_{C/T_1}}{\hat{\sigma}^2_{C/T_1} + \hat{\sigma}^2_{(RC)T_1} + \hat{\sigma}^2_{e}}} = \underline{0.XXX}$$

$$\left\{\begin{matrix}\text{Reliability} \\ \text{Within Type 2 Cases}\end{matrix}\right\} = \frac{\hat{\sigma}^2_{C/T_2}}{\hat{\sigma}^2_{C/T_2} + \hat{\sigma}^2_{(RC)T_2} + \hat{\sigma}^2_{e}} = \underline{0.XXX}$$

(7.2) If either of the values are low, e.g., much below 0.60 or 0.70, then compute $F(\text{MAX})$.

$$\text{OBTAINED–}F(\text{MAX}) = \frac{\text{Largest } MS_{RC/T_K}}{\text{Smallest } MS_{RC/T_{K'}}} = \frac{X.XXX}{X.XXX} = \underline{X.XXX}$$

If OBTAINED–F(MAX) $\geq$ TABLE–F(MAX), $p < .05$, the $(\sigma^2_{CR/T} + \sigma^2_e)$ for within each type of case are probably sufficiently different to review in followup.

Statistical Procedures for the Mixed Between- and Within-Therapist Groups Design

Again, we will use an example to describe the statistical procedures. The issues in this section focus on how two or more groups of clinicians might have different perceptions of the same sets of clients. To demonstrate the procedures we will build upon the example for the within-therapist design by contrasting the ratings of the three partial hospitalization staff from that example with ratings by four staff from the outpatient service on the same 10 cases, five cases within each of the two types of cases. Thus, the overall data for this design is:

		Case Type 1 No Prior Hospital History					Case Type 2 Prior Hospital History				
		①	②	③	④	⑤	⑥	⑦	⑧	⑨	⑩
PARTIAL HOSPITAL	①	7	7	5	7	6	4	4	3	3	2
STAFF	②	8	8	6	8	7	5	5	4	4	3
	③	9	8	6	8	7	4	5	3	4	3
OUTPATIENT	④	7	6	4	6	5	5	5	3	3	2
STAFF	⑤	7	7	5	7	6	4	5	3	4	3
	⑥	6	7	5	7	6	4	4	4	3	2
	⑦	6	6	4	6	5	4	5	4	4	3

For this design, there are six facets which can be clearly identified to be influential toward the overall variability (sources of variance) between and among groups:

Sources of Variance	No. of Levels	Component of Variance
Between Therapist Groups:		
1. GROUPS (G) (Programs)	$g = 2$	σ^2_G
2. Raters Within Groups (R/G)*	$(r_{g_1} + r_{g_2}) = (3 + 4) = 7$	$\sigma^2_{R/G}$
Within Therapists		
3. Types of Cases (T)	$t = 2$	σ^2_T
4. GROUPS × Types of Cases, (G × T)	$(g)(t) = (2 \times 2) = 4$	$\sigma^2_{G \times T}$
5. Raters by Types of Cases Within Groups (R × T/G)	$(r_{g_1})t + (r_{g_2})t = (3)2 + (4)2 = 14$	$\sigma^2_{(R \times T)/G}$
6. (Cases/Types) × Raters/Groups (C/TR/G)	$C(r_{g_1})t + C(r_{g_2})t = 5(3)2 + 5(4)2 = 70$	$[\sigma^2_{C/TR/G} + \sigma^2_{error}]$

The six-part partitioning of the total sources of variance permits you to look at three important issues. The issues focus on the differences in judgments among two or more groups of clinical staff. The design also permits you to pursue the three issues described under the within-therapist design.

(1) Are there sufficient differences among subgroups of clinical staff (e.g., outpatient *vs.* partial hospitalization staff) to obscure the clinical characteristics of the cases being judged? The statistical ratio given below will highlight the degree to which between-therapist group facets, in combination with other facets, influence the judgments due to the type of clients being rated.

$$\text{Coefficient of Dependability} = \frac{\sigma^2_{Type}}{\sigma^2_{Type} + \sigma^2_{G \times T} + \sigma^2_{(RT)/G} + \sigma^2_{C/TR/G} + \sigma^2_{error}}$$

As was true of the within-therapist design, one would hope that the sole consideration in rating a client would be the types of characteristics of the clients themselves, i.e., σ^2_{Types}. But, the degree to which between- and within-therapist facets, ($\sigma^2_{G \times T}$, $\sigma^2_{(RT)/G}$, $\sigma^2_{C/TR/G}$, σ^2_{error}), influence and obscure the judgments is of critical concern. As the ratio approaches 1.00, then these other facets are of little influence. As these other facets take on a greater influence and their respective variance terms become larger, the coefficient will become smaller; approaching 0.00 if they become very large. Thus, the coefficient describes the relative influence of facets related to both between- and within-group difference on the judgment of the types of cases being studied, σ^2_T. Again, if this ratio falls approximately below 0.60 or 0.70, you need to address other issues.

(2) Are there systematic differences among the therapist groups involved in the study? The statistical ratio used to address this issue is the *F*–Test:

$$F = \frac{\text{(Variance due to G} \times \text{T Interaction)}}{\text{(Variance due to rater by case and random error)}}$$

* TECHNICAL NOTE: This design, like the earlier designs, is concerned with the facets influencing a particular group of clinicians. Thus raters within groups becomes a fixed rather than a random effect in this design.

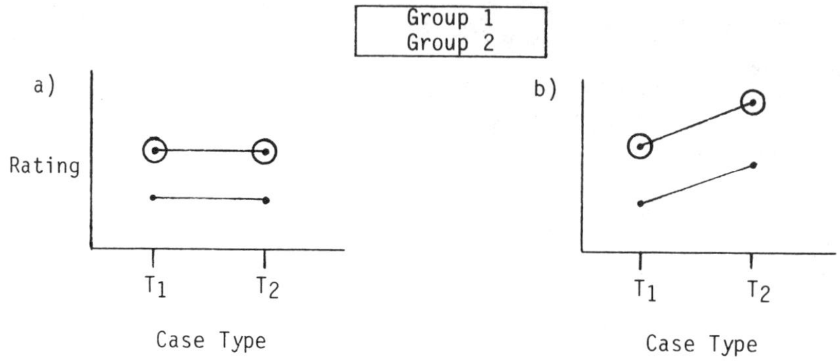

Figure 9. No Interaction Effect

$$F = \frac{MS_{G\times T}}{MS_{C/TR/G}} = \frac{rc\sigma^2_{G\times T} + \sigma^2_{C/TR/G} + \sigma^2_e}{\sigma^2_{C/TR/G} + \sigma^2_e} \geq 1.00$$

Specifically, this F–Ratio will describe whether the interaction of therapist groups and types of cases, $\sigma^2_{G\times T}$, is significantly greater than chance variation in case ratings within types of cases across raters and groups, $(\sigma^2_{C/TR/G} + \sigma^2_e)$. As the ratio becomes significantly larger than 1.00, then we may wish to assume that $\sigma^2_{G\times T}$ exists to a noticeable degree. If the groups of therapists were perfectly consistent in their ratings across the types of cases rated, then $\sigma^2_{G\times T} \rightarrow 0.00$ and the F–Ratio would approach 1.00. Thus, if the F–Ratio is statistically significant, then the nature of the interaction needs to be studied.

(3) What is the nature of the differences in the ways in which the therapist groups differed in their ratings of the types of cases? To address the third issue a sequential-step strategy is required. First, you need to draw a graph of the interaction by plotting the mean rating of each group for each type of case. This should show the general nature of the interaction. Two example figures for no interaction effects (Figure 9(a) and (b)) are contrasted with three examples of significant interaction effects (Figure 10(a–c)).

From the figure you draw you should be able to design followup tests of significance as well as followup estimates of dependability and generalizability. Suppose, for example, we obtained the results given in Figure 10(b). The appropriate followup test would be to determine whether for Type-2 cases the means of groups 1 and 2 are significantly different. Here a t-test or F-test could estimate whether the means are significantly different from each other.[9] The t-test would be:

$$\left(t = \frac{(M_{G_1T_1} - M_{G_2T_1})}{\sqrt{(MS_{R/G}/RC_{K_1}}}\right) \geq t \quad \text{Expected by chance with } p < .01$$

If the followup t-test(s) is/are statistically significant, then the ensuing followup actions would take two paths. One path is to perform further statistical analysis on the therapist ratings *within* each of the therapist groups, using the within-therapist group design procedures described earlier in this unit. This really means that you would be performing two parallel statistical analyses, one analysis on the ratings within each of the groups.

---

[9] TECHNICAL NOTE: If there are two means, the t and F distributions ar edirectly related, $t^2 = F$. With more than two groups an F-test is appropriate. You should also note that the level of significance suggested here is .01 since statistical tests performed after the fact need to be more conservative.

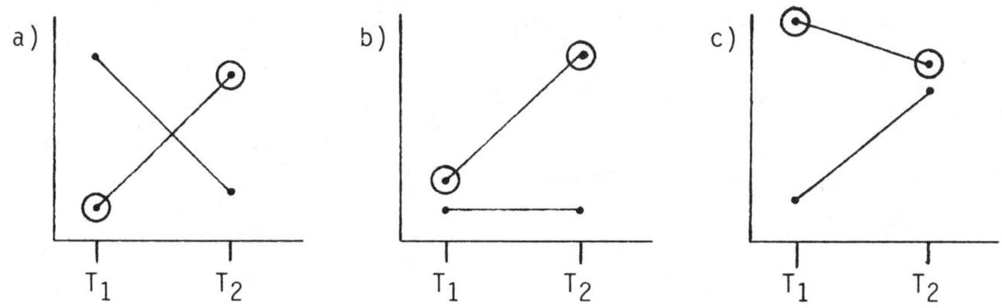

Figure 10. Interaction Effects

The second followup path is more managerial. As we discussed earlier, group discussions, studying samples of actual cases, and tailoring the review processes to attend to these differences are particularly useful approaches to uncover underlying influences and possibly rectify problems which may have resulted.

To demonstrate the actual statistical procedures required to address the three issues, we will go through a step-by-step process using the data described earlier and replicated in Step 1, below.

Step 1. Set up the data in a fashion which makes it easy to compute subtotals for groups, raters/groups, types of cases, as well as a grand total. The detailed steps for computation of group 1 totals are demonstrated for the within-therapist design in Step 1 for that design of cases. Thus, the overall data for this design are as follows:

		CASE TYPE 1						CASE TYPE 2						
		1	2	3	4	5	$T_{R_jT_1G_1}$	6	7	8	9	10	$T_{R_jT_2G_1}$	T_{R_j/G_1}
PARTIAL HOSP. STAFF	①	7	7	5	7	6	32	4	4	3	3	2	16	48
	②	8	8	6	8	7	37	5	5	4	4	3	21	58
	③	9	8	6	8	7	38	4	5	3	4	3	19	57
$T_{C_KG_1}$		24	23	17	23	20	$T_{T_1G_1}$ = 107	13	14	10	11	8	$T_{T_2G_1}$ = 56	T_{G_1} = 163
							$T_{R_jT_1G_2}$						$T_{R_jT_2G_2}$	T_{R_j/G_2}
OUTPATIENT STAFF	④	7	6	4	6	5	28	5	5	3	3	2	18	46
	⑤	7	7	5	7	6	32	4	5	3	4	3	19	51
	⑥	6	7	5	7	6	31	4	4	4	3	2	17	48
	⑦	6	6	4	6	5	27	4	5	4	4	3	20	47
$T_{C_KG_2}$		26	26	18	26	22	$T_{T_1G_2}$ = 118	17	19	14	14	10	$T_{T_2G_2}$ = 74	T_{G_2} = 192
T_{C_K}		50	49	35	49	42	T_{T_1} = 225	30	33	24	25	18	T_{T_2} = 130	Grnd. Tot. GT = 355

Step 2. Compute a Table of Means from Step 1 Totals.

(a) Compute the means for each rater, by type of case, M_{RGT}; e.g.,

$$M_{R_1G_1T_1} = T_{R_1G_1T_1} \div C_K = \frac{32}{5} = 6.4$$

$$M_{R_6G_2T_2} = T_{R_6G_2T_2} \div C_K = \frac{17}{5} = 3.4$$

(b) Compute the Rater means within each group, $M_{R/G}$, e.g.,

$$M_{R_1/G_1} = T_{R_1/G_1} \div (C_{K/T_1} + C_{K/T_2}) = \frac{48}{10} = 4.8$$

$$M_{R_5/G_2} = T_{R_5/G_2} \div (C_{K/T_1} + C_{K/T_2}) = \frac{51}{10} = 5.1$$

(c) Compute the Type of Case means within each group, M_{TG}, e.g.,

$$M_{T_1G_1} = T_{T_1G_1} \div (r \times C \text{ for } G_1T_1) = 107 \div 15 = 7.13$$

$$M_{T_2G_2} = T_{T_2G_2} \div (r \times C \text{ for } G_2T_2) = 74 \div 20 = 3.70$$

(d) Compute the means for each Type of Case, M_T, e.g.,

$$M_{T_1} = T_{T_1} \div (C_{T_1} \times [r_{G_1} + r_{G_2}]) = \frac{225}{5(7)} = 6.43$$

(e) Compute the Grand Mean, $GM = \dfrac{GT}{\text{Total \# Ratings}}$

$$GM = 355 \div 70 = 5.07$$

Step 3. Set up the Sources of Variance Table and

(a) Compute the "Sums of Squares" by following the steps indicated, and
(b) Compute the Mean Squares

(1)

Sources of Variance	Degrees of Freedom	Steps to Compute Sum of Squares	Sums of Squares SS	Mean Squares SS/df
BETWEEN THERAPIST GROUPS				
Groups (G)	$(g - 1)$ $(2 - 1) = 1$	3.1	$SS_G = 6.808$	6.808 $F = 4.55$
Raters within Groups (R/G)	$(r_{G_1} - 1) + (r_{G_2} - 1)$ $(3 - 1) + (4 - 1) = 5$	3.2	$SS_{R/G} = 7.470$	1.494
WITHIN THERAPISTS				
Types of Cases (T)	$t - 1 = 2 - 1 = 1$	3.3	$SS_T = 129.472$	129.472
Groups × Types (G × T)	$(g - 1)(t - 1) =$ $(2 - 1)(2 - 1) = 1$	3.4	$SS_{GT} = 5.624$	5.624
Raters × Types within Group (RT)G	$[(r_{G_1} - 1) + (r_{G_2} - 1)](t - 1)$ $[(3 - 1) + (4 - 1)] \times (2 - 1) = 5$	3.5	$SS_{RT/G} = 4.86$	0.972
Cases within Types, by Raters within Group (C/TR/G)	df_{TOT} − Sum of df listed above = $69 - 13 = 56$	3.7	$SS_{C/TR/G} = 48.409$	0.864
TOTALS	Total Number of ratings = $70 - 1 = 69$	3.6	$SS_{TOT} = 202.643$	

			CASE TYPE MEANS 1	CASE TYPE MEANS 2	RATER MEANS
PARTIAL	STAFF	①	$M_{R_1T_1G_1}$ = 6.4	3.2	$M_{R_1G_1}$ = 4.8
		②	7.4	4.2	5.8
		③	7.6	3.8	5.7
	M_{T_K/G_1}		M_{T_1/G_1} = 7.13	M_{T_2/G_1} = 3.73	M_{G_1} = 5.43
OUTPATIENT	STAFF	④	5.6	3.6	4.6
		⑤	6.4	3.8	M_{R_5/G_2} = 5.1
		⑥	6.2	$M_{R_6G_2T_2}$ = 3.4	4.8
		⑦	5.4	4.0	4.7
	M_{T_K/G_2}		M_{T_1/G_2} = 5.9	M_{T_2/G_2} = 3.70	M_{G_2} = 4.8
	M_{T_K}		M_{T_1} = 6.43	M_{T_2} = 3.71	G.M. = 5.07

(3.1) Compute the Sums of Squares for Groups, SS_G.

$$SS_G = \sum^{g} [(\text{\# of ratings made by all therapists in the Group})(M_G - GM)^2]$$

$$= 30(5.43 - 5.07)^2 + 40(4.80 - 5.07)^2$$

$$= 30(0.1296) + 40(0.073) = 6.808$$

(3.2) Compute the Sums of Squares for Raters/Groups, $SS_{R/G}$.

$$SS_{R/G} = \sum_{j=1}^{r} \sum_{p=1}^{p} (C_{KT_1} + C_{KT_2})(M_{R_jG_p} - M_{G_p})^2$$

$$= (5 + 5)[(4.8 - 5.43)^2 + (5.8 - 5.43)^2 + (5.7 - 5.43)^2]$$

$$+ (5 + 5)[4.6 - 4.8)^2 + (5.1 - 4.8)^2 + (4.8 - 4.8)^2 + (4.7 - 4.8)^2]$$

$$= 10[0.607] + 10[0.140] = 10[0.747] = 7.470$$

(3.3) Compute the Sums of Squares for types of cases, SS_T.

$$SS_{Types} = \sum^{t} [(\# \text{ of ratings in each level of T})(M_{T_K} - GM)^2]$$

$$= 35(6.43 - 5.07)^2 + 35(3.71 - 5.07)^2 = 35(3.6992)$$

$$SS_{Types} = 129.472$$

(3.4) Compute the Sums of Squares for Groups by Types, SS_{GT}.

$$SS_{GT} = \left[r_{G_1} \sum_{j=1}^{t} (\# \text{ cases at each level of T})(M_{G_1T} - GM)^2 \right.$$

$$\left. + r_{G_2} \sum_{j=1}^{t} (\# \text{ cases at each level of T})(M_{G_2T} - GM)^2 \right] - SS_G - SS_T$$

$$= [3[5(7.13 - 5.07)^2 + 5(3.73 - 5.07)^2]$$

$$+ 4[5(5.9 - 5.07)^2 + 5(3.70 - 5.07)^2] - 6.808 - 129.472$$

$$= [(3)(5)(6.0392) + (4)(5)(2.5658)] - 136.280$$

$$= (90.5880 + 51.3160) - 136.280 = 141.904 - 136.280 = 5.624$$

$$SS_{GT} = 5.624$$

(3.5) Compute the Sums of Squares for the Interaction of Raters by Types of cases within groups, $SS_{RT/G}$.

$$SS_{(RT)/G} = (SS_{RTG_1} + SS_{RTG_2} = \sum^{g} [SS_{RTG_1} + SS_{RTG_2}]$$

$$SS_{RT/G_1} = \left\{ \left[\sum^{r} \sum^{t} C_K(M_{RTG_1} - M_{G_1})^2 \right] - r_1 \left[\sum^{t} C_K(M_{TG_1} - M_{G_1})^2 \right] \right.$$

$$\left. - (C_{K_1} + C_{K_2}) \left[\sum^{r} (M_{RG_1} - M_{G_1})^2 \right] \right\}$$

$$SS_{RT/G_2} = \left\{ \left[\sum^{r} \sum^{t} C_K(M_{RTG_2} - M_{G_2})^2 \right] - r_2 \left[\sum^{t} C_K(M_{TG_2} - M_{G_2})^2 \right] \right.$$

$$\left. - (C_{K_1} + C_{K_2}) \left[\sum^{r} (M_{RG_2} - M_{G_2})^2 \right] \right\}$$

Computing SS_{RT/G_1}:

$$SS_{RT/G_1} = \{[5(6.4 - 5.43)^2 + 5(3.2 - 5.43)^2 + \ldots + 5(3.8 - 5.43)^2]$$

$$- 3[5(7.13 - 5.43)^2 + 5(3.73 - 5.43)^2]$$

$$- (5 + 5)[(4.8 - 5.43)^2 + (5.8 - 5.43)^2 + (5.7 - 5.43)^2]\}$$

$$= [5(18.673) - 3(28.9) - 10(0.6067)]$$

$$SS_{RTG_1} = 93.3665 - 86.70 - 6.607 = 0.600$$

Computing SS_{RT/G_2}:

$$SS_{RT/G_2} = \{[5(5.6 - 4.8)^2 + 5(3.6 - 4.8)^2 + \ldots + 5(4.0 - 4.8)^2]$$

$$- 4[5(5.9 - 4.8)^2 + 5(3.7 - 4.8)^2]$$

$$- (5 + 5)[(4.6 - 4.8)^2 + (5.1 - 4.8)^2 + (4.8 - 4.8)^2 + (4.7 - 4.8)^2]\}$$

$$= [5(10.56) - 4(12.1) - 10(0.14)]$$

$$SS_{RT/G_2} = 52.8 - 48.400 - 0.14 = 4.26$$

$$SS_{RT/G} = SS_{RT/G_1} + SS_{RTG/_2} = 0.600 + 4.26 = 4.86$$

(3.6) Compute Sums of Squares Total, SS_{TOT}.

$$SS_{TOT} = \text{Sum of Squares of } all \text{ ratings} - \left[\frac{(\text{Grand Total})^2}{(\text{Total \# ratings})}\right]$$

$$= [7^2 + 7^2 + 5^2 + \ldots + 4^2 + 3^2] - \frac{(355)^2}{70} = 202.6428$$

(3.7) Compute Sums of Squares for Cases within Types By Raters within Groups, $SS_{C/TR/G}$.[10]

$$SS_{C/TR/G} = SS_{Total} - [\text{Sum of all other Sums of Squares}]$$

$$= SS_{Total} - [SS_G + SS_{RG} + SS_T + SS_{GT} + SS_{RT/G}]$$

$$= 202.643 - [6.808 + 7.470 + 129.472 + 5.624 + 4.86]$$

$$SS_{C/TR/G} = 202.643 - 154.243 = 48.409$$

Step 4. Compute the estimates of the *Components of Variance* needed for the statistical estimates of Dependability, Reliability, and Generalizability.

(4.1) $$\hat{\sigma}^2_T = (MS_T - MS_{C/TR/G}) \div [(r_1C_K + r_2C_K) \div t)]$$

$$= (129.472 - 0.864) \div [[3(5) + 4(5)] \div 2]$$

$$\hat{\sigma}^2_T = 128.608 \div 17.5 = 7.349$$

[10] *Technical Note:* For the present example, the $MS_{C/TR/G}$ is computed in the regular fashion, i.e., $MS_{C/TR/G} = SS_{C/TR/G} \div df_{C/TR/G}$. For the general case of how to compute the degrees of freedom, footnote 7.

(4.2) $$\hat{\sigma}^2_{GT} = (MS_{GT} - MS_{C/TR/G}) \div \frac{\text{Total \# Ratings}}{gt}$$

$$= \frac{(5.624 - 0.864)}{70/(2)(2)} = \frac{4.76}{17.5} = 0.272$$

(4.3) $$\hat{\sigma}^2_{RT/G} = (MS_{TR/G} - MS_{C/TR/G}) \div \left[\frac{(\text{Total \# ratings})}{(C_{K_1} + C_{K_2})/t}\right]$$

$$\hat{\sigma}^2_{RT/G} = \frac{0.972 - 0.864}{70/[(5 + 5)/2]} = \frac{0.108}{14} = 0.008$$

(4.4) $$(\hat{\sigma}^2_{C/TR/G} + \hat{\sigma}^2_e) = SS_{C/TR/G} \div df_{C/TR/G} = MS_{C/TR/G} = \frac{48.409}{56} = 0.864$$

Step 5. Estimate the Dependability and Generalizability of Ratings by Type of Case.

(5.1) $$\left\{\begin{matrix}\text{Coefficient}\\ \text{of Dependability}\end{matrix}\right\} = \frac{\hat{\sigma}^2_{Type}}{\hat{\sigma}^2_T + \hat{\sigma}^2_{GT} + \hat{\sigma}^2_{RT/G} + (\hat{\sigma}^2_{C/TR/G} + \hat{\sigma}^2_e)}$$

$$= \frac{7.349}{7.349 + 0.272 + 0.008 + 0.864} = \frac{7.349}{8.493} = 0.865$$

Interpretation: Across the two groups of clinicians, ratings of cases were 86.5% influenced by the characteristics of the case types relative to the other influences in interactive combination with groups.

(5.2) $$\left\{\begin{matrix}\text{Coefficient}\\ \text{of Generalizability}\end{matrix}\right\} = \frac{\hat{\sigma}^2_{Type}}{\hat{\sigma}^2_{Type} + (\hat{\sigma}^2_{GT})/t + (\hat{\sigma}^2_{RT/G})/tg + \dfrac{(\hat{\sigma}^2_{C/TR/G} + \hat{\sigma}^2_e)}{(C_{K_1} + C_{K_2})g}}$$

$$= \frac{7.349}{7.349 + \dfrac{0.272}{2} + \dfrac{0.008}{4} + \dfrac{0.864}{20}} = \frac{7.349}{7.5302} = \underline{0.976}$$

Thus, you may generalize these results to another study, like this one, with the same clinicians, and have a 97.6% chance of replicating the results.

If either of the two coefficients is low, then $\sigma^2_{G\times T}$, $\sigma^2_{RT/G}$, or $(\sigma^2_{C/RT/G} + \sigma^2_e)$ singly or in some combination are sufficiently high to warrant continued analysis (see Step 6).

Step 6. Test for the significance of σ^2_{GT}.

(6.1) Compute

TECHNICAL NOTE:
$\dfrac{r_{(C/T)}\sigma^2_{GT} + \sigma^2_{C/TR/G} + \sigma^2_e}{\sigma^2_{C/TR/G} + \sigma^2_e}$

$$F(\text{Obtained}) = \frac{MS_{GT}}{MS_{C/TR/G}} = \frac{r_{(C/T)}\sigma^2_{GT} + \sigma^2_{C/TR/G} + \sigma^2_e}{\sigma^2_{C/TR/G} + \sigma^2_e} = \frac{5.624}{0.864} = 6.509$$

(6.2) Contrast F(Obtained) with F-value in an F-Table from a standard statistical text, where for our example:
—degrees of freedom numerator, $df_{GT} = 1$
—degrees of freedom denominator, $df_{C/TR/G} = 56$
—Probability of F(Obtained) $\geq F$(Tabled with 1 and 56 df) > 0.5.[11]

Reject the possibility that there was no G × T interaction ($\sigma^2_{GT} \rightarrow 0.00$) if F(Obtained) $\rightarrow F$ (Tabled with 1 and 56 df).

For our example, then:

$$[F(\text{Obtained}) = 6.509] > [F(1{,}56,\ p < .05) = 4.02]$$

the contrast table tells us that there is a statistically significant variation among the groups in their average (mean) ratings of the types of cases. This statistically significant result would lead us to the next steps to determine the nature of the differences (i.e., issue (3) discussed earlier).

Step 7. Describe the nature of the G × T Interaction.

(7.1) Draw a figure to describe the interaction

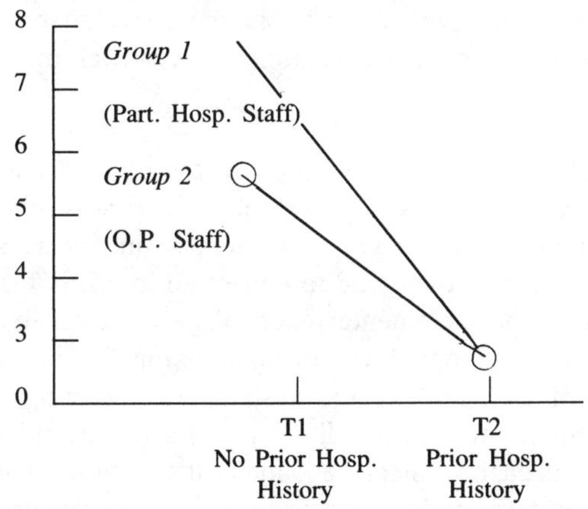

It would appear that the two groups of therapists differed primarily on their ratings of Type 1 cases, i.e., those with no prior hospitalization. Therefore, we would wish to test for this difference.

(7.2) Test for the "Simple Effect" within the G × T Interaction.[12]

$$\left[t(\text{Observed}) = \frac{(M_{G_1T_1} - M_{G_2T_2})}{\sqrt{(MS_{R/G})/rC_{K_1}}} \right] \geq [t(df_{R/G} = 5,\ p < .01) = 4.032]$$

$$t(\text{Observed}) = \frac{(7.13 - 3.73)}{\sqrt{(1.494)/15}} = \frac{+3.400}{0.0996} = \frac{+3.400}{0.315} = 10.794$$

---

[11] If you wish to be more conservative, set $p < .10$. In this case, it may be unwise to falsely accept the null hypothesis that no σ^2GT exists.

[12] Note that the more conservative value of ($p \leq .01$) is used. This is because this sort of statistical test is performed after we have inspected the data. Such comparisons must be done cautiously (see Myers, 1979, 292–4).

Since [t(Observed) = 10.794] > [t(5, p < .01) = 4.032], we conclude that the two groups of therapists differ in their ratings of Type 1 cases. Specifically, the outpatient staff tend to view cases with no prior hospitalization history less favorably than do the partial hospitalization staff. The statistical and managerial followup steps are described at the end of the earlier discussion of the third issue for this type of design.

4. GENERALIZING RESULTS ACROSS SERVICES AND ACROSS PROGRAMS

Two questions which frequently are raised have a negative answer but a positive solution which is relatively simple to implement. The two questions are:

— "Will two or more clinical services using the same scales use them in exactly the same manner?"

No, but, if the scales refer to similar types of clients, the data can be easily transformed to permit aggregating data and making generalizations across services on that same set of clients.

— "Will two or more catchment area programs using either the same scales or different scales on similar types of clients use the scales in the same manner?"

Again, the simple answer is "No," but we suggest that the data can be easily transformed to permit aggregating data and making generalizations across programs on that same set of clients.

The basis for asserting that a relatively simple transformation of the clinical data will permit intra- and interprogram generalizations rests on two suppositions. The first is that if the measures are taken on a similar set of clients (e.g., clients of roughly similar ages, socioeconomic, and problem-area characteristics), then they tend to be related to each other in a predictable fashion. A specific example might be "elementary schoolage children in urban settings entering service at the lower to middle range level of functioning." The second supposition is that the major components of a client-oriented system are operating in the programs generating the data; e.g., both a global and a multidimensional scale are used routinely. Global scale observations are made at each clinical encounter; the multidimensional observations are made at intake, in review, at termination, and in followup. Moreover, there should be two or more people routinely involved in the review process on at least a sampling basis (see Chapters 5 and 6), and there should be regular staff-development sessions similar to those described in Chapters 13 and 14. Thus, if all services within each program are operating within a client-oriented system, and the data are taken on similar clients, then data aggregation and generalization should be possible.

When data are collected on similar objects (clients in our case), and under similar conditions (as in client-oriented systems), then a simple linear transformation of the data ought to allow the data to be aggregated across programs. The procedures for you to test whether this is possible in your own situation are relatively straightforward. There are three steps. These are described in Table 4, and a numerical example shows how to apply these steps.

Table 5 gives an example of a linear transformation procedure.

Once the transformation coefficients ($b_{A.B}$ and k) have been obtained, then average ratings across programs can be aggregated and/or compared in statistical analysis of process or outcome data for cost outcome, cost effectiveness, and evaluation research studies. The major cautions to be aware of in the use of these data are:

Table 4. Steps for Testing Where Between-program Clinical Data Can Be Aggregated

STEP 1: Have each of the program's clinical staff independently rate the same case histories in their respective staff-development sessions. Try to insure that the procedures for conducting the staff-development sessions are as comparable as possible and have at least 10 case histories rated, more if possible and convenient.

STEP 2: Compute the mean ratings within each program.

	PROGRAM		
CASE	*A*	*B*	*C*
1	$\bar{X}_{1A}$	$\bar{X}_{1B}$	$\bar{X}_{1C}$
2	$\bar{X}_{2A}$	$\bar{X}_{2B}$	$\bar{X}_{2C}$
.	.	.	.
.	.	.	.
.	.	.	.
20	$\bar{X}_{20A}$	$\bar{X}_{20B}$	$\bar{X}_{20C}$

$\bar{X}_{ij}$ is the mean rating for the ith case by the staff in the jth program.

STEP 3: Select one program as the standard* (we will use Program A for our example) and do a linear transformation on each of the other program's data to the standard (A) by finding:

3.1 The linear correlation coefficient between each program's average (mean) ratings and the standard program's mean ratings on the same cases.

$$r_{jA} = \frac{N[\Sigma(\bar{X}_{ij})(\bar{X}_{iA})] - (\Sigma\bar{X}_{ij})(\Sigma\bar{X}_{iA})}{\sqrt{[N\Sigma(\bar{X}_{ij})^2 - (\Sigma\bar{X}_{ij})^2][N\Sigma(\bar{X}_{iA})^2 - (\Sigma\bar{X}_{1A})^2]}}$$

3.2 Test to determine if a sufficiently high proportion of the variance is shared between the two programs.

Proportion of Total Variance Described by Linear Transformation = r^2, or
Percent Total Variance = $r^2 \times 100$

As r^2 approaches 1.00 (or 100%), then the linear transformation will be a near perfect method of aggregating data across programs, provided that interpretative generalizations using the transformed data are kept to inferences about average clinical ratings on clients similar to those covered in the sample case histories.

3.3 If r^2 is sufficiently high (e.g., accounting for more than 75% or 80% of the total variance), then perform the linear transformation of all the data in the other programs to that of the standard program scale as follows:

Transformed Value in the jth Program = $(\bar{X}_{ij}) = b_{A.j}\bar{X}_{ij} + k$

where

$$b_{A.j} = \frac{N(\Sigma\bar{X}_{ij}\bar{X}_{iA}) - [(\Sigma\bar{X}_{ij})(\Sigma\bar{X}_{iA})]}{N(\Sigma\bar{X}_{ij})^2 - (\Sigma\bar{X}_{ij})^2}$$

$$k = \frac{\Sigma(\bar{X}_{ij})^2(\Sigma\bar{X}_{iA}) - [\Sigma(\bar{X}_{ij}\bar{X}_{iA})(\Sigma\bar{X}_{ij})]}{N\Sigma(\bar{X}_{ij})^2 - (\Sigma\bar{X}_{ij})^2}$$

*The standard program selected should be the one with the highest within-program reliability coefficient.

Table 5. Example of Linear Transformation Procedure

CASES N = 10	RAW PROGRAM MEANS A	RAW PROGRAM MEANS B	CALCULATIONS $(\bar{X}_{iA})^2$	CALCULATIONS $(\bar{X}_{iB})^2$	CALCULATIONS $(\bar{X}_{iA})(\bar{X}_{iB})$
1	$\bar{X}_{1A} = 2$	$\bar{X}_{1B} = 3$	4	9	6
2	$\bar{X}_{2A} = 3$	$\bar{X}_{2B} = 4$	9	16	12
3	2	2	4	4	4
4	4	5	16	25	20
5	5	6	25	36	30
6	7	8	49	64	56
7	5	6	25	36	30
8	3	4	9	16	12
9	6	6	36	36	36
10	$\bar{X}_{10A} = 6$	$\bar{X}_{10B} = 7$	36	49	42
SUMS =	43 $\Sigma\bar{X}_{iA}$	51 $\Sigma\bar{X}_{iB}$	213 $\Sigma(\bar{X}_{iA})^2$	291 $\Sigma(\bar{X}_{iB})^2$	248 $\Sigma(\bar{X}_{iA})(\bar{X}_{iB})$

$$r = \frac{N\Sigma(\bar{X}_{iA})(\bar{X}_{iB}) - (\Sigma\bar{X}_{iA})(\Sigma\bar{X}_{iB})}{\sqrt{[N\Sigma(\bar{X}_{iA})^2 - (\Sigma\bar{X}_{iA})^2][N\Sigma(\bar{X}_{iB})^2 - (\Sigma\bar{X}_{iB})^2]}} = \frac{[10(248)] - [(43)(51)]}{\sqrt{[10(213) - (43)^2][10(291) - (51)^2]}}$$

$$r = \frac{287.00}{(281)(309)} = \frac{287.00}{294.6676} = .974$$

$r^2 \times 100 = 94.86\%$ of the total variance accounted for by the linear relationship between $\bar{X}_{iA}$ and $\bar{X}_{iB}$. Since the proportion of the total variance accounted for by a linear transformation is so high, .974, we shall proceed with the linear transformation.

The Linear Transformation Coefficients $b_{A.B}$ and k for $\bar{X}'_{iB} = b_{A.B}\bar{X}_{iB} + k$.

$$b_{A.B} = \frac{N\Sigma(\bar{X}_{iA})(\bar{X}_{iB}) - (\Sigma\bar{X}_{iA})(\Sigma\bar{X}_{iB})}{N\Sigma(\bar{X}_{iB})^2 - (\Sigma\bar{X}_{iB})^2} = \frac{[10(248)] - [(43)(51)]}{10(291) - (51)^2} = \frac{287}{309}$$

$$b_{A.B} = 0.9288$$

$$k = \frac{\Sigma(\bar{X}_{iB})^2(\Sigma\bar{X}_{iA}) - \Sigma(\bar{X}_{iB})(\bar{X}_{iA})(\Sigma\bar{X}_{iB})}{N\Sigma(\bar{X}_{iB})^2 - (\Sigma\bar{X}_{iB})^2}$$

$$k = \frac{(291)(43) - (248)(51) = -135}{[10(291)] - (51)^2 \quad = \quad 309}$$

$$k = -0.4369$$

THE TRANSFORMATION TABLE

$\bar{X}_{iA}$	$\bar{X}_{iB} = (0.9288\bar{X}_{iB} - 0.4369)$
1	0.49
2	1.42
3	2.35
4	3.28
5	4.21
6	5.14
7	6.06
8	6.99
9	7.92

— Use means in the statistical analysis collected on similar groups of clients in clinical settings which have the major components of a client-oriented system operating.[13]
— Insure that the percentage of the total variance accounted for by the linear transformation ($r^2_{Aj} \times 100$) is reasonably high (more than 75% or 80%).
— Insure that the annual (sample) studies on scale validity are performed. Some examples of validity studies are described in the last part of this chapter (Subsection 5).

5. COMPLETING THE PICTURE: VALIDITY STUDIES

Recall that in a client-oriented system, many of the routine clinical activities in treatment planning and review assure routine validity checks on individual clients. Specifically, a standard part of a client-oriented system involves two or more people (experienced staff or significant others), in addition to the client, independently assessing the client's multiple problems, strengths, and supports, as well as the client's global level of functioning. These routine clinical procedures on individual clients, however, only increase the probability that the scales you are using are valid across clients over time. The routine procedures do not, by themselves, provide measures of content, predictive, or construct validity. These issues require specifically designed studies.

Obtaining measures of validity are ordinarily time consuming and expensive. The procedures outlined here are designed to be as simple as possible, but they are still sufficiently time consuming to be scheduled as studies performed once a year or once every 2 years. In general, validity studies should be performed on small but representative samples of clients in 1- or 2-year cycles.

The procedures for conducting validity studies have ten general steps:

(1) Divide your client population into the same target groups your clinical staff identified when establishing the scales (Chapter 2).
(2) For each target group identify subgroups of clients by their respective categories of concern (Chapter 5).
(3) For each of the subsets of client groups, identify observable behavioral and/or life-situation patterns which would be expected for clients performing at the low, middle, and high levels of functioning (Chapters 5 and 6).
(4) Select a means for observing (measuring) the behaviors and life-situation patterns described in the preceding step.
(5) Design a sampling strategy, i.e., a means of sampling a small group of clients which is representative of each of the subgroups of clients of clinical concern.
(6) Have two or more knowledgeable colleagues review the five preceding steps and revise accordingly.
(7) Set a schedule of which client subgroups will be sampled and observed first, second, etc. Here is where you need to consider the two practical matters of time and urgency; e.g., validity studies on serious problem and expensive clients ought to rank high in the scheduled order.
(8) Obtain the client sample and corresponding measures.

---

[13] *Technical Note:* By using means, you are permitting the Central Limit Theorem to work for you. Moreover, you will be meeting more of the assumptions of standard statistical practices.

(9) Test the degree to which the obtained measures on sampled clients correspond to the predicted levels described in Step 3, above.

(10) Since the correspondence between predicted and obtained is never perfect, decide whether the deviations are sufficiently important to require further study via either a more microscopic study of the clients' behaviors, the clinical procedures, and the scales' construction, or a repeated sample of another set of clients to determine if the questionable results recur. We would suggest, for practical reasons, to consider a replication first. If the results are replicated, then the more microscopic studies of process and scales will be needed.

Most people who have had one graduate level statistics and research methods course should be able to follow the 10-step outline to design their own validity studies. There are, however, some additional hints which can be helpful. Below we have outlined these hints in line with the corresponding steps in the 10-step outline.

Steps 1–3: Try to help staff identify target groups and categories of clients with unique (mutually exclusive behavioral and/or life-situation patterns.

Step 4: Select means of observing (measuring) client behaviors which are:

4.1 Observable to an impartial observer, or

4.2 Obtained with a psychometrically established measuring instrument, e.g.,
- —Psychiatric Status Schedule (Spitzer, Endicott, Fleiss, & Cohen, 1970)
- —PARS (Ellsworth, 1979)
- —Denver Community Mental Health Questionnaire (Ciarlo and Reihman, 1977)
- —Oregon Quality of Life Scale (Bigalow, 1979)

4.3 Capable of differentiating levels of behavioral patterns (low, middle, and high)

4.4 Practical to use.

There are several cautions you need to exercise when using established psychometric instruments. First, these instruments were (typically) not tested in your service area with the unique set of clients in your sample. Thus, the best that they can offer are some correlated measures which should be sufficiently sensitive to differences among low, medium, and high levels of behavioral patterns (performance). Moreover, you need to be cautious in using these established measures in the fashion for which they were designed. For example, a global level of functioning measure describes a person's ability to function in his/her ordinary community setting within a particular (current) timeframe, and not necessarily as a predictor of future functioning. Thus, be careful not to use a set of followup measures (e.g., PARS, the Denver Scale, or the Oregon Quality of Life Scale) as the yardstick for estimating the validity of a level of functioning measure obtained at termination. If you did obtain these measures at termination, instead of at 3-, 6-, or 12-month followup periods, then they may serve as measures of construct validity. An additional caution in using established scales is that their multifactored structured may not be the same as those you are assuming to underlie your measures of client behavior patterns and/or life situations. In summary, in selecting your means of estimating both content and construct validity, check to insure the correspondence of the established psychometric scales' client norm groups and the underlying multifactor structures to your behavioral and life situation criteria for low, medium, and high levels of client performance.

Steps 5, 8, 9, 10: The sampling strategy ought to combine both stratification and matching of clients by the characteristics uniquely identified with the mutually exclusive client groups. Once these qualifying client characteristics are identified by group (low, middle, high), then selection should be as random as possible (using the usual random number table, slips of numbered paper drawn from an urn, and so forth). While 30 or more sample clients within each major group is ideal, you can often get away with a sequential sampling procedure which starts with smaller samples. That is, start with a sample of 12 clients within each major group. If this small sample provides adequate indiction of predicted results, then stop sampling. If the results are not adequate, then repeat the sampling until more than 30 clients are included in each major group. If questionable validity estimates are still indicated, then more microscopic analyses are required. An example, adapted from Jones and Newman (1971), is described in Table 6.

Step 9: Analyses of correspondence between obtained and expected or predicted results should be kept as simple as possible for these validity studies. Simple correlation coefficients and χ^2tests will often suffice. The simplest example of applying a χ^2test of ''poorness-of-fit'' would be to sort clients as follows:

	CLIENTS RATED AS:			
	Low	Mid–Low	Middle	Mid–High
OBSERVED Your Rating Scales	X_{10}	X_{20}	X_{30}	X_{40}
EXPECTED: Measured by Independent Observer or External Rating Scale	X_{1E}	X_{2E}	X_{3E}	X_{4E}

where X_{ij} is the frequency of clients in category.

$$\chi^2 = \frac{(X_{observed} - X_{expected})^2}{X_{expected}} =$$

$$\chi^2 = \frac{(X_{10} - X_{1E})^2}{X_{1E}} + \frac{(X_{20} - X_{2E})^2}{X_{2E}} + \frac{(X_{30} - X_{3E})^2}{X_{3E}} + \frac{(X_{40} - X_{4E})^2}{X_{4E}}$$

If $\chi^2_{(obtained)}$ is greater than the value in a χ^2 table under degrees of freedom equal to the number of pairs of $(X_{observed} - X_{expected})^2$ contrasts and there is an error probability of .80 or greater, then worry about problems of validity.

If your program does not have a staff member who is particularly adept with statistics, you may wish to use the procedures suggested in the Carter and Newman (1976) monograph. These procedures are reproduced for your convenience in Tables 7 and 8.

Table 6. Sequential Sampling and Testing: Hypothetical Example of a Bayesian Approach*

The Problem

A counselor is faced with a decision regarding the use of a behavioral scale as an aid in placement of clients in community-support programs. The test will be used only if it has correlation equal to or greater than .50 with the criterion (independent assessment by two trained professionals). From past experience with behavior scales in other circumstances, the counselor's data suggest that the correlation between scale and performance will be .60, and furthermore, that the interval between .50 and .70 would approximately constitute a plus or minus one standard deviation interval for the coefficient. To make the assumption of a normal prior distribution more tenable, all coefficients are transformed into Fisher's z functions. Thus, the prior distribution has a mean of .69 ($r = .60$, $z = .69$) and a standard deviation of .16 ($[z_{.70} - z_{.50}]/2 = .16$). The criterion, the z transform of .50, is .55.

The counselor then takes a sample of 50 randomly selected clients and finds a correlation between the scale and performance of .71 (expressed as a Z transform) with a standard error of $\sqrt{1/(50 - 3)} = .15$. The question then is whether a classical inferential process serves the counselor better than a Bayesian inferential process in aiding the counselor's decision as to whether to use the behavioral scale.

The Classical Approach

Here the counselor simply contrasts the two Z values (.71 and .55) to test the null hypothesis that there is "no difference" with p (Type I error) .05:

$$\frac{z - z_0}{\sqrt{1/(N - 3)}} = \frac{.71 - .55}{.15} = 1.061$$

The conclusion would be: "Do not reject the null hypothesis." Further, by computing a confidence interval and transforming the z functions back to correlation coefficients, the counselor may expand his nonrejection statement to say that the interval .40 to .76 has a .95 probability of covering the true predictive value. This is, however, the limit of inference allowed with this problem.

The Bayesian Approach

There are a number of inferential developments possible under a heading Bayesian inference. The one that seems most appropriate for this problem would be to first establish a posterior distribution based on the prior distribution and the sample, and to contrast it with the criterion of .55. From this procedure, a definite probability statement can be made regarding the criterion and the efficiency of the behavioral scale.

In accordance with the formulation suggested by Schlaifer (1961), the mean (M_2) and standard deviation (sd_2) of the posterior distribution are:

$$M_2 = \frac{M_1(h_1) + M_2(h_2)}{h_1 + h_2} \qquad (sd_2)^2 = \frac{1}{h_1 + h_2}$$

where

M_1 = prior mean (.69)
M_2 = sample mean (.71)
h_1 = reciprocal of prior variance ($1/.16^2$)
h_2 = reciprocal of sample variance ($1/.15^2$)

In this example, the values are M_2 of 0.70 and sd_2 of 0.11. The posterior distribution and criterion can then be used to establish an explicit probability statement such as:

$$p\left[Z < \frac{.70 - .55}{.11} = 1.36\right] = 0.087$$

The verbiage of inference here takes a different tack than the classical procedure. Given the posterior distribution, the probability of obtaining a value Z less than .55 is .087 or less than one in 10. Thus, the chances are better than

* Adapted from Jones and Newman (1972). The original example dealt with the issue of adopting a new aptitude test. Thus, the initial sample size is large (N = 50).

Table 6. (*Continued*)

nine out of 10 that the new scale will have a predictive value equal to or greater than the criterion. The criterion value, .55, becomes the lower limit of prediction for the counselor's probability statement, rather than the pivotal quantity of an interval. The counselor is not accepting or rejecting the sample data, but rather incorporating the data in a probability statement. The choice of the behavioral scale would be justified by the probability statement, and not simply because the test is "no different" from the criterion.

According to a Bayesian view, the sample data should now be incorporated into the counselor's information for further decision making. For example, if the counselor wishes to draw another sample of 50 and run the correlation again, information from the first sample can be used in evaluating results of future samples. Specifically, the critical value (C_v) can be determined below which the behavioral scale's correlation with performance would be suspect. Before collecting data on a second sample, the C_v could be estimated (Schlaifer, 1961) as follows:

$$C_v = \frac{\text{criterion } (h_2 + h_3) - M_2(h_2)}{h_3}$$

$$= \frac{.55\frac{1}{.11^2} + \frac{1}{.15^2} - .70\frac{1}{.11^2}}{\frac{1}{.15^2}} = .27$$

Thus, given the posterior distribution (based on prior distribution and first sample), the counselor should not reject the scale unless the second sample correlation is less than a *Z* of .27.

Table 7. A Procedure for Relating Behavioral Data to Levels of Functioning*

Step 1

A secretary, student, or volunteer draws a sample of 60 cases from each of your program's target groups. The person drawing the sample should be instructed in the procedures governing client confidentiality. Usually supervision by a professional would be required. Each case should have had at least three clinical service encounters at which time behavioral data (on a checklist or in case notes) were recorded along with level of functioning. Thirty of these should be cases that were rated at "functional" levels (e.g. 5–9 on the Montgomery County scale) at intake or at time of last service contact. Within the bounds of these restrictions, the selection of cases should be random.

Step 2

Sort the 60 cases from each target group by level of functioning.

Step 3

For the cases within each level of functioning, sort in three categories:

—*Improved* level of functioning since intake or review
—*Maintained* same level of functioning
—*Regressed* to a lower level

Step 4

A panel of at least two direct service (clinical) staff persons reviews the behavioral checklist and level-of-functioning data recorded for cases in the three categories: "improved," "maintained," and "regressed." (You may want to assign different staff persons to different target groups and even to different levels of functioning. Reviewing over 30 case histories can be arduous.)

Step 5

After reviewing (independently) the data for "improved," "maintained," and "regressed" cases at each level of functioning, each panel member develops a "model" or summary of behavioral characteristics and/or behavioral changes that represents a typical profile of clients who improved, were maintained, or regressed. *The model should depict the recorded data and not what the clinician feels ought to be the case.*

Step 6

A secretary assembles the panel members' "model" profiles and each member reviews the other members' profiles.

(*continued*)

Table 7 *(Continued)*

Step 7

The panel must then form a consensus about the behaviors exhibited by clients in each target group, at each level of functioning, that justifies their status as "improved," "maintained," or "regressed."

Step 8

The "model" profiles what the staff agrees will constitute the "external criteria" against which assigned levels of functioning are checked. The panel discusses the fit of the "model" behavioral profiles to the level of functioning data and judges the appropriateness of the ratings. It is useful to invent and use an "appropriateness of fit" scale for this exercise, like the following:

Suggested Scale Format
for Judging Appropriateness of Fit

0 1 2 3 4 5 6 7 8 9 10

▼ ▼

Totally Inappropriate ⟶ Perfect Fit

Step 9

A secretary selects two more cases from each level of functioning within each target population and the panel rechecks the judgments made above. By rating the "appropriateness of fit" between behavioral data and assigned levels of functioning, you will be ascertaining validity by reference to external (behavioral) criteria.

*Adapted from Carter & Newman (1976).

Table 8. Procedures for Relating Behavioral and "Life Situation" Data to Behavioral and Level of Functioning Records*

Step 1

Select a representative sample of cases from the group of cases analyzed as described in Table 7. The sample should include 4–8 clients from each target group, half of whom are "functional," half "dysfunctional."

Step 2

A direct-service person (other than the staff member or members responsible for the client's therapy) conducts interviews with both the client and his/her immediate family. The interviews should be structured to check the presence or absence of the behaviors found in the case records or checklists and to ascertain facts about the client's "life situation" (residence, marital status, employment, or school attendance) that could be used to verify assigned level of functioning.

Step 3

The panel and the interviewer rate independently the degree of correspondence between the "facts" of the interview and of those appearing in the case records

Step 3 *(continued)*

(behaviors, life situation, and level of functioning). Again, the use of a 0–10 scale to rate "degree of correspondence" between interview findings and case record information (see following chart) is helpful.

Suggested Scale Format
for Rating "Degree of Correspondence"

0 1 2 3 4 5 6 7 8 9 10

▼ ▼

No Correspondence ⟶ Perfect Correspondence

If the panel agrees that an acceptable number of cases show high correspondence, no more research is necessary. If there are serious contradictions between interview "facts" and case records, you should take 4–8 more sample cases from each target group and repeat the process. If discrepancies persist, your client record system (behavioral records and/or level of functioning scale) may not be valid.

*Adapted from Carter & Newman (1976).

Chapter 15

Technical Chapter
Creating Your Own Clinical Evaluation Scales*

> We Are Not Reinventing the Wheel!
> We Are Just Building One Suitable to Our Terrain.

Some programs wish to develop their own clinical-evaluation scales, or wish to extensively modify existing scales. This chapter will help you identify and outline the major steps in such scale development. The chapter is designed primarily for use by a committee comprised of clinical supervisors, program managers and research and evaluation staff. The outline of the chapter is:

— EXAMPLE OF AN OVERALL OUTLINE FOR ADAPTATION AND IMPLEMENTATION (Table 1) (with references to where in this text you can find the detailed procedures)
— EXAMPLE OF A DETAILED OUTLINE IN SEQUENTIAL STEPS: The details of each of the steps described in the overall outline are provided.
— EXAMPLE OF A 3-STEP PROCESS FOR CREATING A MENTAL HEALTH FUNCTIONING SCALE WITH SUBSCALES
— PROGRAM IMPLEMENTATION

1. EXAMPLE OF A DETAILED OUTLINE

Sequential Steps for Developing and Implementing a Mental-Health Functioning Scale

The outline provided below gives the major steps for performing the tasks shown in Table 1. We have also referenced other sections of the book (where possible) which discuss the necessary details of how to accomplish these tasks.

(1.0) Specification of the needs for mental-health functioning measures (Chapter 2).
(2.0) Assessment of the feasibility of development and implementation of a measure (to include but not limited to the following):

* The procedures described in this chapter were first conceived by Gordon Gibson, South Bloomington (IN) CMHC.

Table 1. Example of an Overall Outline for Planning and Developing of Scales

Illustration of a timeline of development and implementation of the mental-health functioning scales with references to other sections of text

YEAR 1

	APR.–JUL.	JUL.–OCT.	OCT.–JAN.	JAN.–APR.	APR.–JUL.	JUL.–OCT.	OCT.–JAN.	JAN.–APR.	APR.–JUL.	JUL.–OCT.
ACTIVITY	Identify Measures Assess Feasibility Specify Needs	Strategy Development	Organization Sanction Colleague Feedback	Identify Entry Points			Clinician Development of Scale	Assess Reliability Clinician Training Case Histories	Collect Data	Simulate Studies Validate w/Other Measures Reassess Reliability
TEXT REFERENCE	Chap. 2 System Design Chap. 3 Clinical Process Chapters 9, 10, and 12 Records Chap. 12	Chapters 1, 2, 12, and 13	Chapters 18 and 19 Organizational Structure Chap. 20 Management Questions				Chapters 2, 12, and 13	Chapters 12 and 13 Chap. 13 Chap. 14		Chap. 14 Chap. 14 Chap. 13

(2.1) Clinical records system with problem orientation (Chapters 9–11).
(2.2) Cooperation of CMHC constituent interests (internal and external political aspects).
(2.3) Workable mental-health information system, preferably automated (Chapters 25–28).
(2.4) Quality assurance program in operation
(2.4.1) Utilization/peer review functions (Section II).
(2.4.2) Clinical records audit review functions (Section III).
(2.4.3) Clinical care evaluation review functions (Chapter 6 and Chapters 20–24).
(2.5) Evaluation research resources (Chapters 20–24).
(2.6) Environmental setting stability (Chapters 18 and 19).
(3.0) Development of an overall strategy.
(3.1) Design around a Community Mental Health Center (CMHC) service where other evaluation is in progress.
(3.2) Design into a CMHC service where inquiries are precipitating a proposed evaluation.
(4.0) Identification of potential mental-health functioning measures (Chapter 2 and this chapter).
(5.0) External feedback on the strategy and measure from colleagues (Chapter 12).
(6.0) Determine level of organization support and sanction for implementation (Chapters 18 and 19).
(7.0) Identification of the potential entry points for development and implementation (Chapter 18).
(8.0) Clinician modification/development of the scale.
(8.1) Review of the need for developing and utilizing the scale.
(8.2) Request clinician statements of client behaviors representing each behavioral domain with multiple levels of severity.
(8.3) Clinicians judge the behavioral statements with the scale levels (Chapters 12–15).
(8.4) Aggregate ratings to develop the new scale (this chapter).
(9.0) Develop case histories to be used in the staff training for interclinician consistency in judgment (Chapter 13).
(10.0) Training sessions for clinicians using the mental-health functioning scale (Chapters 12–14).
(10.1) Train clinicians for making consistent judgments controlling for reactivity factors and definitional drift.
(10.2) Assess reliability of the judgment process with the scale.
(11.0) Conduct periodic review of the assessment of reliability utilizing subsequent training sessions (Chapters 12–14).
(12.0) Validate the measure with other data from evaluation measures assessing client behavior (Chapter 14).
(13.0) Simulate clinical judgments studies: for program planning, development, evaluation, and cost effectiveness inquiries (Chapters 20–22).

2. EXAMPLE OF THREE STEPS TO CREATING A MENTAL-HEALTH FUNCTIONING SCALE

The procedure involves three major steps. First, a small committee should identify the major subscale factors, and then create 20 sentences which may represent the range of behaviors which possibly cover the range of each subscale. Second, have a group of clinical staff members rate

Table 2. Major Subscale Factors

Subscale 1 Personal Self-Care Behavior	Subscale 2 Interpersonal Social Behavior	Subscale 3 Vocational Educational Behavior	Subscale 4 Stress Tolerance Behavior	Subscale 5 Special Interest Behavior	Global Scale Client's Overall Functioning
behavioral statement no. 1.1	behavioral statement no. 2.1	behavioral statement no. 3.1	behavioral statement no. 4.1	behavioral statement no. 5.1	global level no. 1
↓	↓	↓	↓	↓	↓
behavioral statement no. 1.20	behavioral statement no. 2.20	behavioral statement no. 3.20	behavioral statement no. 4.20	behavioral statement no. 5.20	global level no. 20

each statement (presented in random order on a 0–100 scale) from lowest to highest. Select the nine or ten behavioral statements with the lowest variability and which are spread out approximately evenly over the range of the scale. Third, combine the subscales and the global scales for an overall assessment instrument to be used in treatment planning and review.

Let's examine each step in detail. In the first step, a small committee identifies major factors underlying the global scale and then creates 20 overall statements representing the range for each subscale from Lowest (Level 1) to Highest (Level 20), as illustrated in Table 2. Note that subscale number 5 is a special-interest scale, to cover behavioral measures on a specific set of clients (alcohol abusers).

Second, for each subscale obtain the clinician judgments of behavioral statements reflecting self-care functioning domain. Use a 0–100 scale, with 0 = the Lowest Level of the behavioral dimension. An example is shown in Table 3.

Third, assemble the 9 or 10 behavioral anchors for each subscale, and combine as your clinical assessment instrument (see Table 4).

Table 3. Chart for Recording Clinicians Judgments of Behavioral Statements

Subscale Behavior Statements	Clinicians														Average* Judged Level
	01	02	03	04	05	06	07	08	09	10	11	12	13	14	
behavioral statement no. 1.1															
behavioral statement no. 1.20															

*Select the 9 or 10 behavioral statements which have minimal variability and which represent approximately equal distances from each other in the order of low to high. Remember, a scale should have 9 or more points to be useful for communicating behavioral changes.

Table 4. Clinical Assessment Instrument

Subscale 1 Personal Self-Care Behavior	Subscale 2 Interpersonal Social Behavior	Subscale 3 Vocational Educational Behavior	Subscale 4 Stress Tolerance Behavior	Subscale 5 Special Interest Behavior	Global Scale Client's Overall Functioning
behavioral anchor 1.1	behavioral anchor 2.1	behavioral anchor 3.1	behavioral anchor 4.1	behavioral anchor 5.1	global level 1.0
behavioral anchor 1.2					global level 2.0
behavioral anchor 1.8	↓	↓	↓	↓	global level 8.0
behavioral anchor 1.9	behavioral anchor 2.9	behavioral anchor 3.9	behavioral anchor 4.9	behavioral anchor 5.9	global level 9.0

3. PROGRAM IMPLEMENTATION

Appoint a small committee to plan the implementation of the scale. Be sure the clinical leadership is represented on the committee. The three initial steps are:

(1) Go through the outline given in this chapter and rate the feasibility of your program staff performing each step. Let
  0 = Total impossibility
  1 = Done with a great deal of difficulty
  2 = Done with some difficulty
  3 = Done easily

(2) Draft a revision of the list of steps to meet difficulties envisioned.

(3) Draft the necessary timelines given your responses to (1) and (2) above.

For overall program implementation, turn this chapter over to a small committee to plan the implementation of the scales.

SECTION V
THE FISCAL SYSTEM

DESIGNING THE COSTING SYSTEM—AN OVERVIEW

The costing system addresses two questions:

(1) As costs are related to clinical efforts, what are the key fiscal, yet client-oriented questions?
(2) If program costs are analyzed, what are the fundamentals of cost-finding and rate-setting?

Each question is analyzed in depth in Chapters 16 and 17.*

Chapter 16: Relating Costs to Clinical Effort outlines the need to know costs and how good cost-finding can help find the answers. The kinds of cost questions good managers should be asking are reviewed along with applications of costing to programs and target groups.

Chapter 17: Analyzing Program Costs is a thorough review of program-cost analysis. The fundamentals of cost-finding are outlined and applied in an extended exercise. Chapter 17 concludes with managerial illustrations of how the results of cost-finding can be used. Finally, a brief checklist can help evaluate someone else's cost-finding through a list of good and incisive questions to ask.

---

* Parts of both chapters are adapted from Sorensen, J. E., & Hanbery, G. W. (1979). *Using financial management in mental health organizations*. Rockville, MD: NIMH.

Chapter 16

Relating Costs to Clinical Efforts

How Much Did It Cost to Run the Outpatient Service?
What Is the Cost Per Hour of Service?
How Much Did It Cost to Treat Kids in the Children's Program?
What Is the Average Cost Per Treated Case This Year?

OBJECTIVES

All four questions are good cost-accounting questions. The first one asks about a *total* cost of a *service,* the second about a *unit* cost of *service,* the third about the cost of a *program* (a target group), and the fourth about an *episode* of care cost. Responding to these and related questions can be tough, especially if timely and accurate data are wanted. The objectives are:

To identify what proper cost-finding can do;
To illustrate the linkage of cost data to management questions.

There are four sections:

(1) THE NEED TO KNOW COSTS
(2) WHAT COST-FINDING CAN DO
(3) LINKING COST DATA TO QUESTIONS
(4) COSTING PROGRAMS AND TARGET GROUPS

While this chapter may sound like it is for an accountant, the chief executive, program managers, and evaluators in a mental-health facility are likely to benefit the most. While accountants or business managers may perform the underlying analyses, *users* of cost-finding need to understand why it is needed and to see how costs can be linked to clinical efforts.

1. THE NEED TO KNOW COSTS

A good human-services manager needs to know how current resources are being consumed. In the Broadway stage play *The Music Man,* a salesman ". . . had to know his territory," and in human services, a good manager has to know his or her costs. In most mental-health organizations, 60–80% of the costs are personnel. Clinicians comprise a large segment of mental-health organization costs and the first step in costing is a statistical description of the clinician: In what service did the clinician spend his/her time? How was time spent? With what type of and how many clients? At what location? Inadequate statistical data on staff activity and services provided lead naturally to inadequate costing. And poor costing means poor answers to cost questions. Linking accounting data to operating statistics is called *cost-finding* and is one of the major systems needed to perform good cost analyses.

2. WHAT COST-FINDING CAN DO[1]

Information as to the amount of money spent on an activity is not particularly useful unless the expense is related to a stated volume of activity. Knowing Mental-Health Organization A had a total outpatient expense of $500,000 and that Organization B had an outpatient expense of $900,000 is not useful unless one also knows the quantity of effort and type of patients the expense represents. The relationship between dollars and units of service gives meaning to the two separate parts.The subsystems designed to capture the statistical data must be using the same organizational unit specification as that used for accounting. If not, statistical data and accounting cannot be matched for assessing the cost for various types of services provided.

The term *cost-finding* may be defined as "a system of allocating and reallocating costs from a point of data collection into different sets or subsets of costs." Simply stated, cost-finding is any method that attempts to charge all relevant costs—both direct and indirect—to final producing functions or activities, or what accountants have traditionally called "revenue producing functions." (Since accountants trace expenses to the cost centers that produce the final product or service, the term "final producing cost center" has been coined for human-service organizations.) Unlike production organizations with easily identified products, human-service organizations often have difficulty in identifying the appropriate final production (or revenue producing) activities.

The evolution of the *type of service* concept suggests that one natural way to collect and allocate expenses is by the basic types of service or programs that are provided. In mental-health organizations, for example, inpatient, outpatient, emergency service, partial hospitalization, and consultation and education represent one possible description of varied services. One could also choose type of patients, such as children, adolescents, adults, and geriatrics as being final (or revenue) producing centers. These types or units of service can be accumulated to describe the costs of effort allocated to an individual or a group of clients' treatment episode, or to a community oriented consultation/education activity.

No matter which of the several possible ways is selected, some rational and systematic method of charging all expenses, both direct and indirect, must be utilized to assign those expenses to the final (or revenue producing) activities. Full-cost allocation is appropriate even

---

[1] Adapted from J. E. Sorensen and David W. Phipps. (1975). *Cost-Finding and Rate-Setting for Community Mental Health Centers,* DHEW Publication No. ADM 76–291, Washington, DC: U.S. Government Printing Office.

though some of the defined activities may be subsidized in part or entirely by some level of governmental funding; knowing the total expense of a program can be useful in evaluating cost-efficiency or cost-effectiveness, or in planning of alternative sources of financial support if government funding ceases.

Determination of Rates for Services

The degree of emphasis placed on collection for services varies widely among mental-health organizations. In some organizations, intensive efforts are made to collect a very high percentage of the expenses incurred for client services. In others, very little effort is expended to make such collections, despite requirements to recover costs such as those in Public Law 94–63. As the expense of services increases and the availability of general public funds decreases, the need to recover a higher proportion of the expenses from clients, patients, and third-party payors becomes increasingly important. These developments require the determination of rates for services offered by human-service organizations.

Because of the diversity of services rendered in mental-health organizations, the statistical base for the rate can be problematic; in mental-health organizations, for example, using frequency of visits, patient contacts, or duration and intensity of treatment for determining patient charges based on averages for most patients (e.g., average cost per patient day or visit) may lead to unsatisfactory rates. Some types of service, such as inpatient and partial hospitalization, might rely heavily on average cost for the portion of service cost accruing from the usual hospital facilities including room occupancy, meals, housekeeping items, and nursing care because these may be relatively uniform for all patients. On the other hand, because the amount of professional staff services used in outpatient services may be highly varied, a cost per hour or quarter hour may be a more appropriate rate. Expenses such as the direct professional service would probably vary considerably and therefore could be misleading if based on averages tied to "patient visit." A self-study exercise illuminates this problem.

Self-Study Exercise. Calculate the cost per visit and hour for an outpatient service and then contrast the precision of the two rates. Suggested solutions are at the end of the exercise.

DEFINITIONS

A *visit* is defined as an encounter greater than 10 minutes but less than 3 hours.
An *hour of service* is based on client time (quarter hours) in the service (and does not include chart time).

1. Cost and Statistical Data

A. Total cost of outpatient service	$900,000
B. Total client visits	30,000
C. Total hours of direct client service	20,000
D. Cost per visit	$_____
E. Cost per hour	$_____
F. Cost per quarter hour	$_____

2. Analysis of Precision

	System Using Visits	System Using Hours
A. How much would be charged for a 15-minute medication check?	$___	$___
B. How much would be charged for a 2.5 hour testing session?	$___	$___

3. What is your conclusion about these two measures? Which one does the best job of linking resources and client services? If you were linking resources to client outcomes, which one would you prefer?

ANSWERS:

1. (D) \$30; (E) \$45; (F) \$45 ÷ 4 = \$11.25
2. (A) \$30, \$11.25; (B) \$30, 2.5 × \$45 = \$112.50
3. Hours, since visits averages so heavily.

Negotiation with Third-party Payors

As the expense of mental-health services has increased, many third-party payors have made revisions in their contracts to increase the coverage of services and, at the same time, have refused to pay for certain client or patient charges not covered by their contracts. They have also increased their auditing procedures to determine costs being buried within the overall or average rates being charged patients, especially those expenses that are not—in their judgment—properly charged. Universities, for example, have discovered federal agencies disallow certain costs in developing overhead rates for contracts. Costs dealing with student-health and counseling services are systematically disallowed in determining the reimbursable costs because these costs have little or no relevance to the governmental contracts. In a similar way, costs of newborn services are disallowed in hospital rates for geriatric patients covered by Medicare.

As this trend continues, the individual mental-health organization will need to have accurate records to prove the validity of charges made to each client or patient. Direct services can offer little problem if adequate records are maintained, but the organization must also be able to recover the cost of indirect service as well. A systematic and logical cost-finding methodology becomes imperative if the organization expects to recover charges. The cost-finding system must be designed to eliminate duplications or omissions and to distribute all costs fairly. Although there is no absolutely accurate way to distribute indirect costs, methods do distribute such costs fairly. For example, the costs of administration can be allocated to all of the services (or products) created by a human-service organization, using as the ratio the total direct costs of a program to the total direct costs of all programs. While other bases for such calculations could be used, a consistent application of an equitable cost allocation method should raise few arguments with third-party payors.

Information for Funding Agencies and Other External Groups

If a significant portion of a mental-health organization's total revenue comes from public sources—federal, state, or local sources—there will be a need to provide fiscal reports to the funding agencies about expenses within established accounting methodologies. Such reports frequently focus on the cost and outcome of various service programs and/or service modalities. Funding agencies are usually not unreasonable when they ask for valid information about the costs of various programs; the request, however, often appears unreasonable because the organization has a poor or undeveloped management information system (MIS).

Some mental health care program costs, for example, have been called into question because the information furnished to funding agencies has been based on crude averages. In one mental hospital, for example, as the type of treatment changed from purely custodial care to intensive therapy, the expense information furnished led to a misleading interpretation—while the daily population had decreased by nearly 80%, the total expense of treatment had more than tripled. The error occurred in the way the treatment population characteristics were related to the type of care, cost of treatment rendered, and outcome. As another example, treatment modalities vary widely from one mental-health center to another because some centers favor the use of high-cost intensive therapy with a rapid turnover in the patient population, whereas others use a longer-term approach with lower cost per patient for a given time period and a smaller patient roster. These two examples highlight why comparisons of cost per patient can be a meaningless exercise. Only if the costs per episode for comparable problems are accompanied with measures of outcome can meaningful analysis proceed.

Because there is not any unanimity of opinion about the most effective types of programs in mental-health organizations, programs will differ and so will their costs. Perhaps from the vantage point of several years' experience and good records both as to costs, on the one hand, and the outcomes or benefits obtained by the individuals and communities served on the other, some determination of the most effective programs will be possible. But unless good records are kept about both costs and outcomes, the answer may never be identified.

Information for Managerial Analysis

Although the need to furnish accurate and meaningful cost information to patients, clients, third-party payors, and funding agencies is becoming increasingly important, usually there is minimal direct opportunity for consumers or funders to change the expenditure patterns of mental-health organizations. The specifics of this challenge are usually left to the management of the individual organization (although some funding sources may think they can and should influence expenditure patterns). This specific responsibility highlights the information needs of management.

One especially useful managerial application of cost-finding flows from a comparison of the revenue generated by the target population, service, or program to the total cost of operating the service or program. Management can identify whether or not the service is producing a net income or requiring a subsidy. From this type of analysis, meaningful adjustments to the rate structure may be achieved as well as evaluating the overall financial desirability of the specific service or program.

Cost finding is useful in rate setting, negotiation, and evaluating the overall financial aspects of a specific service, but it is not a substitute for a budgetary control system that provides financial control over, and administrative evaluation of, specific individuals responsible for these services.

3. LINKING COST DATA TO MANAGERIAL QUESTIONS

In general, cost accounting will identify how resources were consumed. Specifically you may find out how staff spent their time, how many units of service they generated, the cost per unit of that service, and the cost of treating a particular client or group of clients. What would a manager do if the outpatient service received the following report?

(1) Percent of total staff time purchased (excluding vacation, holiday, and sick day) spent in direct client contact 28%
(2) Cost per delivered *hour* of mental health outpatient service $122.00

Sound efficient? Probably not. If service time were increased to 50% in the setting the unit cost would fall to about $42 an hour (a reasonable cost per hour of a service for adult clients within the middle ranges of level of functioning). Clearly production was too low. Through these two measures, great insight into the use of resources is revealed. Overstaffing, underproduction, and poor client recruiting may be the culprits. But in days of rising inflation and shrinking resources, such measures can highlight poor use of resources and stimulate corrective managerial action.

Often mental-health managers are unsure of what a unit cost should be. In one southern state, for example, cost per child in residential treatment facilities varied by over 200% between providers! In an urban setting of the same state, costs of the program varied by 50%. Managers at the state level were fretting over these wide variations and wondering why they existed (and how they could explain them if they became known). A partial answer was variation in the resource used, the size of operation, and the geographic and environmental circumstances. Another source was the variation in financial and cost-accounting practices. Just to find out what *is* the cost per unit is a major task besides the additional burden of deciding what *range* of costs is acceptable performance.

Unit costs focus managerial attention on input and process at the same time. The manager must now simultaneously keep a watchful eye on cost of staff, client volume, and staff activity. Better management of resources is likely to follow. In a large mental-health/mental-retardation center in Texas, for example, unit cost reports stimulated productivity, reduced unit costs, and, best of all, increased the number of clients served and the level of service per client with almost no change in the budget. (Effects on client outcomes are important and will be discussed in Chapter 21.) Forty percent increases in productivity have occurred with no change in total budget. The movement to managing and/or funding on a unit-cost-of-service basis appears to be both logically and empirically sound when coupled with data on client characteristics, problems, and problem severity.

Self-Study Exercise. Assume you are the Executive Director of a community mental-health center. Your information system has provided the following selected information on last year's operation:

		Service	
Line #	Variable	Partial Care	Outpatient
1.	Active Unduplicated Client Count (end of fiscal year)	100	250
2.	Actual Units of Service	3,600 days 14,400 hours of service	12,500 hours of client contact
3.	Average Daily Attendance: actual	4.5 individuals per group	625 individuals per day
4.	Number of Fulltime Equivalent (FTE) Treatment Staff	20	40
5.	Number of Days a FTE Is Available for Treatment Service (excluding annual leave, holidays, etc.)	200	200
6.	Number of Planned Hours Per Day Available for Treatment Services	5	3.2
7.	Number of Treatment Teams	4	8
8.	Total Cost of Service	$500,000	$1,000,000
9.	Statewide Average Unit Cost of Comparable Centers	$70	$45

(A) Based on the foregoing information, is the center doing a good job with its resources? Yes? No? Can't Tell? Why? ______________________________

____

____

____

Hints: (1) Calculate the cost per unit of service and compare it to the statewide average, viz., (line #8 ÷ line #2) vs. line #9.

(2) Calculate the percentage of planned time for service actually spent in the service, line #2 ÷ (line #4 × line #5 × line #6).

(3) How many clients are seen per staff member per day? (line #3 ÷ line #4).

(B) How much harder will each service have to work to bring their costs in line with the statewide average?

Partial Care: ____

____

Outpatient: ____

____

Hint: Divide the statewide rate into the total cost to see how many units of service are required given existing costs. Then relate the units to individual daily workload.

(1) (line #8 ÷ line #9) − (line 2a) = Extra workload

(2) (Extra workload ÷ line #5) ÷ line 20 = extra workload

(C) Prepare a graph to communicate the results of your analysis in question B, above: (Hint: Prepare a before and after bar chart for each service.)

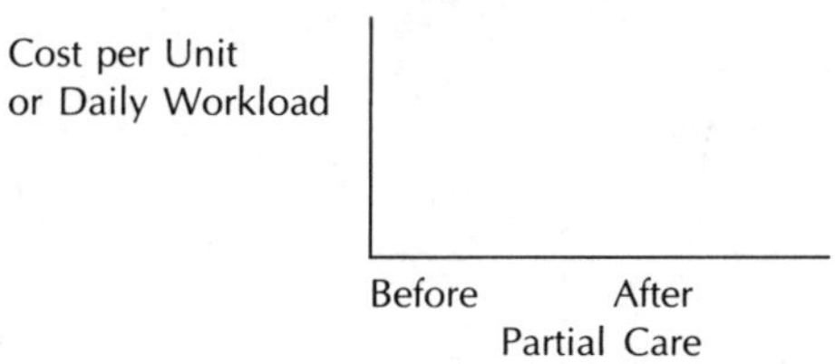

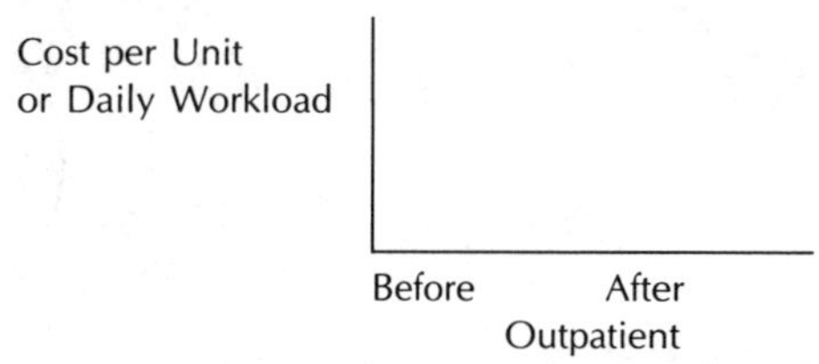

The graphs may be helpful in explaining the change needed to bring the centers' rates into line.

4. COSTING PROGRAMS AND TARGET GROUPS

Once services have been costed, a number of other interesting questions can be probed. How much does the elderly program cost? If the unit cost of various services is known, and if the services received by the elderly can be identified, then the cost of the program can be estimated (viz., multiply the units of service by the unit cost and sum all costs for the target group). Unit costs by service give answers to many critical questions about the resource use in a mental-health agency.

Self-Study Exercise. Assume the following cost and activity schedule based on last year's operations:

	Rates	Units	Total Cost of Service
Inpatient Day	$150	200	$ 30,000
Partial Hospitalization	70	4,500	315,000
Outpatient Hour	40	20,000	800,000
Consultation/Education Hour	30	2,500	75,000
		TOTAL	$1,220,000

You have been requested to explain how much of the last year's dollar resources were consumed by the following target groups:

Target Group	Services Received			
	Inpatient Days	Partial Days	Outpatient Days	Consultation/Education (C/E) Hours
Children and Adolescents	50	400	1,500	100
Adults	100	4,000	18,000	1,800
Elderly	50	100	500	100
Not identified	—	—	—	500
TOTAL	200	4,500	20,000	2,500

(A) Prepare a "pie" graph indicating the amount of dollars devoted to each target group. (Hint: For each target group multiply the units of service times the unit-cost rates. Sum over the services and then calculate the percentage each group is to the total. Include both dollars and percentages in the "pie" graph. Be careful that the proportions of the pie and the percentages look reasonable.)

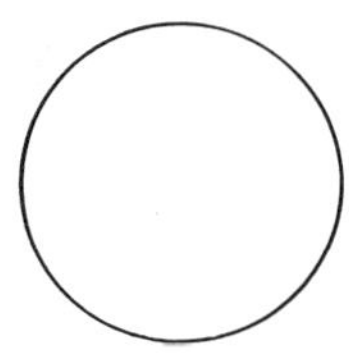

(B) Now assume you find out from research and evaluation that the population and needs of your catchment area are as follows:

	(1) Population	(2) Percent in Need	(3) Index (1 × 2)	(4) Percent Distribution of ( )
Children and Adolescents	10%	20%	.02%	20%
Adults	60%	8.33%	.05%	50%
Elderly	30%	10%	.08%	30%
	100%	—	.10%	100%

What program (or policy) questions arise?
(Hint: Compare column 4 to your pie graph.)

Chapter 17
Analyzing Program Costs

How Do I Go About Costing My Services?
How Can I Use Cost-Finding to Analyze and Manage My Clinical Services?
What Are the Best Ways to Present Cost-Finding Results?
How Do I Use Cost-Finding to Improve My Fee Revenue?
What Question Should I Ask About Cost Reports?

The objectives of Chapter 17 are to reveal how cost-finding procedures relate costs to clinical efforts and eventually to client outcomes. Specific techniques develop a manager's ability to:

Analyze how staff time is used and at what cost;
Search for alternative uses of staff efforts;
Calculate cost-based rate schedules for services;
Present cost analyses in an understandable form.

Knowledge of fiscal issues is explored through six sections:

(1) FUNDAMENTAL CONCEPTS needed to understand and do costing.
(2) MANAGERIAL APPLICATIONS OF COST FINDING to illustrate how
— Costs are related to continuity and quality of care
— Staff resources can be better managed
— Cost reports can identify management options
(3) EXPANDING COST-FINDING TO MULTIPLE SERVICES to see applications in complex multiservice settings.
(4) PRESENTING THE RESULTS OF COST-FINDING in an understandable way to insure comprehension and use.
(5) COST-FINDING IMPLEMENTATION develops a general approach to working cost analysis into an organization.
(6) REFERENCES for further reading.

1. FUNDAMENTAL CONCEPTS OF COST-FINDING

Relating clinical effort to costs requires combining accounting and clinical statistical information to form the total and per-unit costs of service. These cost calculations are useful for rate setting, negotiations with third-party payors, presentations to funding agencies and other external groups, and managerial analyses. Properly formulated, good costing procedures can provide useful data for *cost-outcome studies* (namely, cost per unit of change in some behavioral index) and *cost-effectiveness analyses* (namely, cost comparisons between different treatment outcomes). Cost accounting, then, becomes a vital element of the information system and management decision process, starting with the simple costing of programs through sophisticated cost-effectiveness studies.

Managers can use time analyses and unit costs to assess the productivity and efficiency of clinical-service programs. Patterns of staff time utilization can aid in reallocating staff effort to improve overall fiscal viability and survival. Treatment personnel can see the steps required to do a competent job of costing and managing the valuable resource of clinical staff effort. Others can gain an overview of the role of the fiscal system and develop a model against which varying mental-health settings can be compared.

The basics of cost-finding will be simplified and illustrated so they can be put to immediate use. The practical graphic presentations can be adapted to any type of mental-health organization.

Basic Cost-Finding

Cost-finding may focus on a number of cost objectives. The object of interest may be the total cost of a specific service (e.g., outpatient), the total cost of a support function (e.g., administration), or the cost per unit of service (e.g., cost for outpatient visit or cost per hour of delivered outpatient service). Figure 1 portrays a simplified six-step cost-finding method on a step-by-step approach. In Step 1, organizational units are classified as to:

- Client service
- Community service
- Administrative support service

In Step 2, each type of expense (e.g., salary, fringe benefits, telephone, rent, depreciation) is classified by ease of traceability (e.g., directly or indirectly) to the three general types of service. In Step 3, total direct and indirect administrative support-service costs are allocated to client and community services. In Step 4, direct, indirect, and allocated administrative costs are combined on a service-by-service basis so the *total* cost of each service can be computed. Step 5 accumulates the units of service delivered and by dividing total costs of a service by the units of service (e.g., total visits, hours, days), a *cost per unit of service* results (Step 6).

Self-study Exercise. The beginning exercise leads you through the steps of cost-finding and rate-setting for a small outpatient clinic involving five professional staff.[1] The exercise addresses the following issues for the hypothetical clinic:

---

[1] For ease of learning, we are using this simple example of an outpatient unit with five professional staff. The principles of cost-finding used here parallel those of a larger multiservice program. If it will aid your conceptualization, consider this example a large mental-health program with five service components instead of five professional staff.

			SERVICES			
Step 1: ALLOCATE ORGANIZATIONAL UNITS TO SERVICES				CLIENT		
		TOTAL	ADMINISTRATIVE SUPPORT	A	B	COMMUNITY
Step 2: TRACE EXPENSES TO SERVICES	*DIRECT*					
	Salaries	$630*	$ 50	$200	$300	$ 80
	Fringe Benefits	120	10	40	60	10
	Other Direct Costs	50	15	10	20	5
	INDIRECT					
	Depreciation, etc.	80	5	50	20	5
		$880	$ 80	$300	$400	$100
Step 3: ALLOCATE ADMINISTRATIVE COSTS			$(80)‡	+30	+40	+10
Step 4: DETERMINE TOTAL COST OF EACH CLIENT AND COMMUNITY SERVICE			——	$330	$440	$110
Step 5: ACCUMULATE UNITS OF SERVICE				10	10	5
Step 6: CALCULATE UNIT OF SERVICE COST				$ 33	$ 44	$ 22

*All dollars and units are in thousands.

‡Allocation based on total cost of service before allocation of administration; viz., $300 + $400 + $100 = $800; $80,000 ÷ $800 = 10%; $300,000 × .10 = $30,000.

Figure 1. Simplified Cost-Finding

(1) How are staff allocating their time across the array of client and client-related services, or the consultation and education services, and at what costs?
(2) Are there alternative arrangements for the allocation of staff effort and corresponding costs across the array of services?
(3) What are reasonable fee schedules for each of the units of service?

Table 1 presents a comprehensive breakdown of time accounted for by the hypothetical outpatient clinic staff of five people. Two people, Dr. Able and Ms. Capable, also have administrative responsibilities. Dr. Able is medical director and supervises staff development. Ms. Capable supervises administrative/clerical staff, takes primary responsibility for interagency coordination, and directs research and evaluation.

Table 2 starts the step-by-step exercise where you will:

(1.1) Determine the overhead costs for staff efforts expended on nonchargeable activity (or what we call "staff time overhead costs").
(1.2) Compute the total overhead costs per chargeable hour by combining administrative and facility overhead with staff time overhead.
(1.3) Compute actual staff costs per hour for each staff person.
(1.4) Demonstrate that multiplying the cost per hour times the total chargeable hours accounts for total costs.
(1.5) Compute service costs per *hour* and per *unit* of service basis.

Finally, a short set of brief questions are provided to illustrate:

(1) How rates for services can be established, and
(2) How cost-finding may be related to program analysis.

Table 1. Accounting of Staff Time—3-Month Period

	Client Services						Client Related Services						Nonclient Services							
	a. Psychiatric Eval. b. Testing c. Individ. Therapy d. Group Therapy e. Family Therapy					Total Client Serv.	f. Phone Contact g. Staff Conf. 1 h. Intra-Agency Conf. 1 i. Chart Time & Corresp. 1 j. Travel					Total Client Relat. Serv.	k. Inter-Agency Conf. l. Staff Devel. m. Speaking Engage. 2 n. Research & Eval.				Total Nonclient Serv.	Total Acc't Time	Contract Time	Unacc't Time (P-O)
	a.	b.	c.	d.	e.	a–e	f.	g.	h.	i.	j.	f–j	k.	l.	m.	n.	k–n	O	P	Q
Dr. A. (MD)	120	—	120	20	40	300	10	50	10	30	—	100	5	25	10	—	40	440	480	40
Dr. B. (MD)	100	—	120	30	70	320	20	60	10	30	—	120	—	20	—	—	20	460	480	20
Ms. C. (MA Psych.)	—	120	40	40	—	200	40	60	50	40	10	200	30	20	10	20	80	480	480	0
Mr. D. (MSW)	—	100	40	20	—	160	50	60	40	90	20	260	10	10	—	20	40	460	480	20
Ms. E. (Caseworker)	—	—	90	30	—	120	60	60	40	120	20	300	10	10	—	40	60	480	480	0
TOTALS (HOURS)	220	220	410	140	110	1100	180	290	150	310	50	980	55	85	20	80	240	2320	2400	80

1. The state funding agency will reimburse all costs related to a client's quality assurance process, provided that both staff effort and individual clients can be identified in an audit.
2. The clinic requests a donation or fee for all speaking engagements and limits staff to 10 hours per quarter.

(1.1) *Compute the staff time overhead cost:* complete Table 2, using the appropriate data from Table 1. Insert correct information where blanks are marked by a (☐ ?)

Table 2. Computing Staff Time Overhead Cost

	Ten Steps	Dr. A.	Dr. B.	Ms. C.	Mr. D.	Ms. E.	Total
1.	Total Chargeable Client Hours	300	320	200	☐ ?	120	1100
2.	Total Client-Related Service Hours	100	☐ ?	☐ ?	260	300	980
3.	Total Chargeable Client-Related Service Hours (see Table 1, note 1; sum of Cols. g, h, and i)	☐ ?	100	☐ ?	190	220	750
4.	Total Nonclient Service Hours	40	20	☐ ?	40	☐ ?	240
5.	Total Chargeable Nonclient Service Hours (see Table 1, Note 2 and Col. m).	10	—	10	—	—	20
6.	Total Chargeable Hours: Sum Rows (1), (3), and (5) from above; cross add the totals for Dr. A. through Ms. E. for Grand Total.	400	☐ ?	☐ ?	350	340	☐ ? (TOTAL CHARGEABLE HOURS)
7.	Total # Contracted Hours	480	480	480	480	480	2400
8.	Nonchargeable Hours Row (7) less (6)	80	60	120	☐ ?	☐ ?	530
9.	Hourly Salary Rate including Fringe	25	15	15	10	5	—
10.	Staff Overhead Costs Row (8) × (9), then sum across Row (10)	$2000	☐ ?	1800	☐ ?	700	☐ ? (STAFF OVERHEAD COSTS)

Who contributed the most to staff time overhead costs ________________?;
The least ________________________________?

Answers to 1.1: Total Chargeable Hours, 1870; Staff Overhead Costs, $6700; Most, Dr. A.; Least, Ms. E.

(1.2) *Compute the total overhead costs per chargeable hour:* Combine staff time overhead with administrative staff and facilities overhead and divide by the total chargeable hours.

(1) Staff Time Overhead Costs (Table 2, Row 10) = $ _____ ?

(2) Administrative & Facility Overhead (given) = $ 30,700

TOTAL OVERHEAD COSTS [(1) + (2)] = $ _____ ?

(3) Compute Overhead Costs per Chargeable Hour:
[Divide Total Overhead Costs, (1) + (2) Totals, above, by the Total # Chargeable Hours, Table 2, Row (6)]

$ _____ ? / Hours _____ ? = $ ☐ ? per hour

Answers to 1.2: Staff Time Overhead Costs, $6700; Total Overhead Costs, $37,400; Cost per Hour: $37,400/1870 = $20

(1.3) *Compute the total cost per hour for each staff person:* Combine the hourly salary (including fringe) with the overhead rate per chargeable hour:

Table 3. Total Cost per Chargeable Hour

	Variable	Dr. A.	Dr. B.	Ms. C.	Mr. D.	Ms. E.
		1	2	3	4	5
1.	Hourly Salary, including fringe	$25	$15	$15	$10	$5
2.	Overhead costs per chargeable hour	□ ?	□ ?	□ ?	□ ?	□ ?
3.	Total cost per hour	□ ?	□ ?	□ ?	□ ?	□ ?

(Note overhead is allocated equally to each staff person.)

(1) This method of cost finding computes overhead costs per ________ hour? [See Item 1.2, (3) above.]

(2) The staff nonchargeable time overhead costs per hour were then allocated *equally* to all staff's hourly rate even though each staff person contributed different amounts to the overhead costs. (See Item 1.1, Row 10.) Does this seem proper? Offer reasons why you think it is proper. ________________________________

____

____

Answers to 1.3:
Table 3, Row 2, Columns (1) to (5) are all $20;
Table 3, Row 3, Columns (1) to (5) are $45, $35, $35, $30, $25 respectively;
(1) Chargeable
(2) Several reasons are plausible; first, the method is simple; second, since all non-chargeable time costs must be carried by chargeable time, averaging these costs *within* a service is a reasonable way to distribute these costs.

(1.4) Any cost finding system must demonstrate the system accounts for all of the costs.
Computing Total Expenses Paid for During the Period:
(1) Compute the clinical staff salary expense for the period:

Table 4. Total Treatment Staff Salary Costs

		Dr. A.	Dr. B.	MA Psych.	MSW	Caseworker	Total
		1	2	3	4	5	6
A	Salary & fringe	$25	$15	$15	$10	$5	—
B	Contracted hours	480	480	480	480	480	—
C	Salary Paid	$12,000	□ ?	$7,200	$4,800	$2,400	□ ?

(2) Add period general overhead [Item 1.2, (2)] to total salaries paid +30,700
(3) TOTAL PERIOD EXPENSES [Combine (1) + (2)] = $ ______ ?
Computing Total Costs Based on Total Chargeable Hours:
(4) Compute cost of the chargeable hours for each staff person:

Table 5. Total Costs Based on Chargeable Hours

		Staff					
		Dr. A.	Dr. B.	MA Psych	MSW	Caseworker	Total
ID	Variable	1	2	3	4	5	6
D	Client hours	300	☐ ?	200	160	120	1100
E	Chargeable client-related hours	☐ ?	100	150	190	220	750
F	Chargeable nonclient hours	10	—	☐ ?	—	—	20
G	Total chargeable hours Row 6, Table 2	400	420	360	☐ ?	340	1870
H	Staff cost per hour	$45	$35	$35	$30	$25	—
I	Total Cost (cross-add Columns 1–5)	18,000	☐ ?	12,600	10,500	8,500	☐ ?

The sum in (3) (which represents the period expenses) should equal the sum found in I–6 (total costs of chargeable hours). If they are not equal, there are errors in the costing or reconciliation calculations.

Answers to 1.4: (C-2) $7,200; (C-6) $33,600; (3) $64,300; (D-2) 90; (E-1) 320; (F-3) 10; (G-4) 350; (I-6) $64,300; (I-2) $14,700

(1.5) Compute service costs in either cost per hour *or* cost per unit of service.
—Simple Average Costs, e.g.,
Psychiatric Evaluation: Done by psychiatrist only.
(A) Average MD cost per hour = $_____ ? Rate Per Hour
Unit of Service Cost: If one unit of psychiatric evaluation service takes an average of 1.5 hours;
(B) Unit of Service Cost = (1.5) × Rate Per Hour = $_____ ? Per Unit
Family Therapy: Done by psychiatrist only.
(C) With one Unit of Service at 1.0 hours = $_____ ?
—Weighted Average Costs, e.g.,
Individual Therapy:
Take Sum of the Products:
(120 hrs.) × (MD, Dr. A, Cost/Hour) = $ 5,400
(120 hrs.) × (MD, Dr. B, Cost/Hour) = 4,200
(40 hrs.) × (MA Psych., Cost/Hour) = 1,400
(40 hrs.) × (MSW, Cost/Hour) = 1,200
(90 hrs.) × (Caseworker, Cost/Hour) = 2,250
TOTAL 410 hrs. $14,450
Total Costs/Total Hours = Cost Per Hour
($14,450)/(410) = ($35.24 Per Hour)
Since one Unit of Service equals one Hour, a Unit of Service costs $35.24.
Group Therapy: To be computed by using the Weighted Average Method, where one Unit of Service equals 1.5 Hours.

Take Sum of the Products:

	(20 hrs.) × (MD, Dr. A, Cost/Hour)	= $ 900
	(30 hrs.) × (MD, Dr. B, Cost/Hour)	= 1,050
(D)	(40 hrs.) × (MA Psych., Cost/Hour)	= $_____ ?
(E)	(□ ? hrs.) × (MSW, Cost/Hour)	= $_____ ?
	(30 hrs.) × (Caseworker, Cost/Hour)	= 750
(F)	TOTAL 140 Hours	= $_____ ?
	One Unit of Service × Cost Per Hour	= Cost Per Unit of Service
(G)	(1.5 Hours) × ($ □ ? Per Hour)	= $_____ ? Per Unit

Testing: Using the Weighted Average Method for Ms. Capable and Mr. Dream to perform psychological testing, find costs per hour and cost per unit of psychological testing service, when one unit of testing service equals 2.0 Hours.

One Unit Hour of Service × Cost Per Hour = Cost Per Unit of Service

(H) (2.0 Hours) × ($ □ ? Per Hour) = ($ □ ? Per Unit)

Note the difference between simple and weighted average costs.

Compute the average costs per hour of clinical effort by averaging over all five clinical staff:

(I) Simple Average = ___________? Per Hour

Suppose you were to charge this amount for individual therapy instead of the weighted average of $35.24. How much money would you lose for rendering 410 hours of individual therapy over a 3-month period?

(J) Loss = ___________?

(K) Explain why the weighted average for individual therapy is greater than the simple average. ______________________________

____

____

____

(L) Explain what you might do to reduce the costs of individual therapy. ______

____

____

Answers to 1.5:

(A) (45 + 35) ÷ 2 = $40; (B) 1.5 × $40 = $60

(C) 1.0 × 40 = $40; (D) 40 hours × $35 = $1,400

(E) 20 hours × $30 = $600 (F) Total $4,700

(G) 1.5 × ($4,700 ÷ 140 or $33.57) = $50.355

(H) 120 × $35 + 100 × $30 = $7,200
$7,200 ÷ (120 + 100 hours) = $32.73
2.0 × $32.73 = $65.46

(I) ($45 + 35 + 35 + 30 + 25) ÷ 5 = 170 ÷ 5 + $34.00

(J) ($35.24 − $34.00) × 410 = $508.40

(K) The weighted average takes into account *both* the rate and the number of hours by each clinician. The overall rate is influenced by the relative cost contribution of each clinician. The simple average only examines the rate and assumes each individual contributes an equal amount of time to the service, which isn't true in our example.

(L) Shift the mix of treatment staff, for example, by having fewer MD hours (Dr. A) and more MSW hours.

2. MANAGERIAL APPLICATIONS OF COST FINDING

Costs Incurred by Coordinating Continuity and Quality of Care

There is a greater potential for continuity and quality of care when staff devote time helping another agency understand each other's clinical record and service tracking system. The following Self-study Exercise is an example of estimating the costs of such staff efforts.

Self-Study Exercise

(2.1) Mr. Dream and Ms. Elpsome spend four hours with the Child Welfare Agency discussing what client information is available to staff from the respective agencies. Assume these four hours represent a reimbursable activity. What are the costs of this meeting to the clinic?

Answer: $\$30 \times 4 + \$25 \times 4 = 120 + 100 = \$220$

(2.2) If you were to consider the impact of this investment on continuity of care with children, what kinds of observations and outcomes about child clients would you hope to make over the next three to six months? In the following Table, list two or more sets of objectives (left side), and the sources and resources needed for data collection and analysis (right side).

Objectives	Sources and Resources for Data Collection
Less duplication of efforts by MH and Child Welfare Agency.	*Source:* Monthly billing (client ledger) card. Contrast of services rendered reports of each agency for child clients before and after the meetings with child welfare. *Resources:* Secretarial staff sample 20 child clients who are receiving services from both agencies and contrast services rendered.

Note: This example also demonstrates how most consultation and education activities and their related cost effectiveness could be reviewed.

Analyzing the Costs of an Individual Staff Person's Activities

One of the most important assets is staff time. The staff member's mix of chargeable and nonchargeable time becomes important to the financial viability of the organization. The following Self-study Exercise focuses on the individual and the mix of hours.

Self-Study Exercise

(1) Dr. Brut spent 4.5 hours on the phone talking to one patient's family last quarter. If these hours were reimbursable, how much cost would be allocated for this service? $__________?

Answer: $\$35 \times 4.5 = \$157.50$

Allocation of Staff Time and Costs: The Management Resources

There are a number of issues which both the clinical staff and management have to address in deciding upon the allocation of professional staff time. Consider the following issues:

— What are the present allocations of staff time and concomitant costs by:
  - Direct services (which are chargeable)?
  - Indirect client-related services (only some of which are chargeable)?
  - Nonclient related services, Consultation and Education (only some of which are chargeable)?

— How are the staff-time allocations and unit of service costs *relatively* distributed?

— How do unit-of-service costs *and* third-party reimbursement fee schedules compare?

All of these issues can be analyzed by a number of different means. The following Self-study Exercise will help you develop an approach to address these tough issues.

Self-Study Exercise. Table 6 summarizes the hours, percentage of time, and total costs by type of chargeable service. Client Services ($39,500), Client-Related Services ($24,000), and Nonclient Services ($800) total the cost for the period ($64,300). Table 7 summarizes the hours, percent time, and direct salary costs in nonchargeable and unaccounted time. The total cost is $6,700 ($2,400 + 2,800 + 1,500) and represents the staff time allocated to overhead. The $6,700 is already distributed to each type of service in Table 7 as part of the overhead rate addition of $20 to each chargeable hour. Four questions are explored:

1. Who does what?
2. Who costs what?
3. Who produces revenue?
4. How do I avoid bankruptcy?

(1) WHO DOES WHAT (using Tables 6 and 7)?
The total number of hours the clinic has contracted with staff:
(Client Hours) + (Chargeable Client-Related) + (Chargeable Nonclient Related) + (Nonchargeable Client-Related) + (Nonchargeable Nonclient-Related) =
(A) 1,100 + 750 + 20 + 230 + 220 + 80 = ______ ?
Percent of total contracted hours:
(B) Percent time on client services = ______ ?
(C) Most of the client services were provided by psychiatrists who spent ______ ? hours or ______ ? percent of the total clinic's contracted hours?
(D) Most of the chargeable, client *related* services were provided by ______________ (name the staff person)?
(E) Most of the nonchargeable, nonclient related services were provided by ________ ________ (name the staff person)?
(F) Do the issues raised in (A) through (E) above address what kind of clients were served with what outcomes? YES ____ NO ____

(2) WHO COSTS WHAT (using Table 6)?
The total costs for the two MDs rendering 620 hours of client services can be calculated by multiplying, for each MD, (# hours) × (total cost per hour);

Dr. A.	300 × $45 =	$13,500
Dr. B.	320 × $35 =	11,200
	TOTAL	$24,700

What were the costs of the MA Psychologist rendering client services?

Table 7. Summary of Percent Time by Categories of Nonchargeable Service Activity and Unaccounted Time*

Staff	Client-Rel. Services		Nonclient Related		Unaccounted Time	
	%	Hrs.	%	Hrs.	% Hrs.	Hrs.
MD Totals	1.2	30	2.0	50	2.5%	60
MA Psych.	2.1	50	2.9	70	0.0%	0
MSW	2.9	70	1.7	40	0.8%	20
Caseworker	3.3	80	2.5	60	0.0%	0
TOTALS	9.5	230	9.3	220	3.3%	80

*These direct salary costs already have been allocated to chargeable service activity. Once a nonchargeable hour becomes chargeable, then the costs of the units of service have to be recalculated. Percentages are figured on percent of total time.

Table 6. Summary of Percent Time and Cost Allocated by Chargeable Service Activity*

Staff†	Client Services			Client-Related Services			Nonclient Services		
	% Hrs.	Hrs.	Cost	% Hrs.	Hrs.	Cost	Hrs.	Hrs.	Cost
MD	25.8%	620	$24,700	8.0%	190	$ 7,550	.4%	10	$450
MA Psych.	8.3%	200	7,000	6.2%	150	5,250	.4%	10	350
MSW	6.7%	160	4,800	7.9%	190	5,700	—	—	—
Caseworker	5.0%	120	3,000	9.2%	220	5,500	—	—	—
TOTALS	45.8%	1100	$39,500	31.3%	750	$24,000	.8%	20	$800

*Note the total costs for the period under review are $64,300 ($39,500 + $24,000 + $800). This total is consistent with earlier analyses where staff salaries, and administrative staff and facility costs were totaled ($33,600 + $30,700 + $64,300).

†The MD totals are combined. Once individual cost figures have been established, costs and time may be summarized by classification of clinician and simplifies reports without altering costs by averaging.

(G) ______ ? hours × $ ______ ? = $ ______ ?

What were the costs of the Caseworker to render chargeable client-related services?

(H) ______ ? hours × $ ______ ? = $ ______ ?

(I) Do service costs always reflect caseload and the impact of the service activities? YES ____ NO ____

(3) WHO PRODUCES WHAT REVENUE?

Since each staff person was contracted to render 480 hours, the two psychiatrists were contracted for 960 hours. Suppose only direct client services were reimbursed. What percent of the psychiatrists' contracted hours were spent in income producing services (chargeable)?

(J) ______ ? : 960 = ______ ? percent

(K) Is income necessarily related to kinds of clients served and impact of service? YES ____ NO ____

Answers to Questions 1, 2, and 3:
(A) 2400 (B) 45.8 (C) 620 hours, 25.8% (D) Caseworker
(E) Ms. C, the psychologist (F) No (G) 200 hours × $35 = $7,000
(H) 220 hours × $25 = $5,500 (I) No (J) 620 : 960 = 64.58%
(K) No

(4) PERFORMING AN ANALYSIS OF CLINICAL-RESOURCE MANAGEMENT. ("WHERE THERE IS LOSS, THERE CAN BE BANKRUPTCY")

The MSW, Mr. Dream, has provided 100 hours of testing for the clinic (see Table 1). It costs the clinic $30 per hour for Mr. Dream's services (see Table 3); however, the established fee schedule is $25 per hour.

(A) What is the net loss to the clinic for Mr. Dream's 100 hours of testing ______ ?
Ms. Capable is a psychologist trained in testing. She has done
(B) ______ ? hours of testing. Considering her costs per hour,
(C) what were the net losses for Ms. Capable's testing ______ ?
(D) What were the total losses to the clinic for testing ______ ?
(E) Describe ways the clinic could lose less, or no, money on testing by reallocation of staff time, and still provide 220 hours of testing ______________________

____

____

____

____

(F) Suppose that Ms. Capable, the psychologist, supervises the caseworker Ms. E in testing and the caseworker receives 60 hours of supervision from the psychologist under the title of Staff Conference. (Recall staff conferences are reimbursable at cost.) Calculate the change in potential gain in revenue from testing and staff conferences by reallocating clinical staff time. ______ ?
Staff conference: 60 hrs. × (sum of Ms. C's and Ms. E's costs) = ______ ?
Using the strategy described above, assume the MSW, Mr. Dream, will have 50 hours free to allocate elsewhere. Likewise, Ms. Capable would have 20 hours available for reallocation. Where might you assign them to maximize income and clinical impact?
(G) ____

____

____

(H) Identify potential negative outcomes on clients. For each one describe what precaution needs to be taken to insure that if problems arise, they are dealt with immediately. ______________________________________

____

____

____

____

Answers for Question #4:
(A) ($30 − 25) × 100 = $500 (B) 120 (C) ($35 − 25) × 120 = $1,200
(D) $500 + $1,200 = $1,700
(E) Use the caseworker under the supervision of the psychologist.

(F) Additional revenue 60 hours × ($25 + $35) = $3,600.
(G) Allocate the hours to services where the fee is in excess of the cost, e.g., Group or Family Therapy, or to replace high-priced MDs in Individual Therapy to reduce the costs of the service.

Cautions in Reallocating Staff: An Optional Exercise

While reallocating staff efforts can turn losses into profits, the profit motive may lead to reallocation decisions harmful to clients. The effects on client outcome must be monitored as well. One exercise you may try here is to reallocate staff to more profitable activities and then list all of the potentially good and bad clinical outcomes which may result. For example, suppose you moved the social worker out of testing and into family therapy under the supervision of a psychiatrist. (a) List the clinical outcomes which are potentially good; (b) potentially bad; (c) identify review and supervision procedures to promote (a) and diminish (b).

3. EXPANDING COST-FINDING TO MULTIPLE SERVICES

The cost-accounting system must have access to units of service at the same level of detail desired for cost-finding. Examples include:

(1) Inpatient care: Days received (which enables cost per day and per episode).
(2) Intermediate or partial care: Hours or days of received service (or some standard number of hours, such as 4 hours = 1 unit of partial day; this permits a cost per episode or month computation).
(3) Outpatient and ambulatory services, such as
    (a) Hours of rendered service
    (b) Clients enrolled/attending
    (c) Visits
    (d) Treatment types (e.g., number of units of individual vs. group therapy)
    (e) Ancillary services, (e.g., testing) associated with primary services received (e.g., counts or relative value units)

Minimum information requirements to measure the cost elements for client-oriented costing would require direct (or traceable) costs sorted by program (e.g., mental health), organizational unit (see Chapter 2), service (e.g., outpatient), and object of expenditures (e.g., salary). A fairly sophisticated accounting system is required and implies the existence of a set of procedures for allocating overhead costs to the final producing cost centers.

The Basics of Multiservice Cost-Finding

Cost-finding (and rate setting) involves six basic procedures:

(1) Identify various types of service
    — Client (e.g., inpatient, outpatient)

— Community (e.g., Consultation and Education)
— Support (e.g., administration)

(2) Describe salary, wages, and fringe benefits based on the time staff spend in each service.
(3) Allocate other direct and indirect expenses (e.g., travel, depreciation)—sometimes called "overhead"—to each service.
(4) Reallocate support-services costs (e.g., administration) to client and community services.
(5) Total each client and community service cost. This is the *total* cost of the service.
(6) Divide the total cost by the number of units of service (e.g., hours, visits) to produce the unit cost. At this level of sophistication, the cost-accounting system can provide total costs of programs, cost per unit of service, cost per time period, and cost per treatment episode for subsequent cost-efficiency analysis.

To illustrate how one might establish a cost-finding system for a mental-health organization, complete the following Self-study Exercise for a center with all of the essential services, including administration. This example assumes that direct, indirect, allocated costs, and units of service have been accumulated for each type of service.

Self-study Exercise. Assume you are the Director of a center which offers the following five basic services:

— Inpatient (on contract)
— Other 24-hour care
— Partial care (6-hour day program)
— Outpatient
— Consultation and Education

Your accountant has prepared the following analysis using the suggested cost-finding model in Table 8. (Several key numbers have been deleted to enhance learning in this exercise.)
Reviewing the basic steps:

Step 1: (A) How many different services are being costed in Table 8? N = ____
(B) How much is the total cost of the center? $ ____

Step 2: The salary and fringe were allocated based on the proportion of staff time spent in each service. The decimals in parentheses indicate the proportion of the total $1,000,000 salary applicable to that service.
(C) What is the percentage for administration? ____ %
(D) How much salary cost is allocated to administration? $ ____
(E) What is the percentage for outpatient services? ____ %
(F) How much salary cost should be allocated to outpatient services? $ ____

Step 3: Other expenses (e.g., photocopying, travel) and indirect expenses (e.g., depreciation) are traced to each service on the proportion of salary costs allocated to each service. (In all likelihood, a more complex method of tracking costs to services would be used.)
(G) What is the total of other direct cost? $ ____
(H) What is the total indirect cost? $ ____
(I) What percentage of the other direct cost is being allocated to outpatient services? ____ %

Table 8. Cost by Service

Type of Expense	Total Cost	Administration	I/P (Day)	O/24 (Day)	Partial (Encounter)	O/P (Hour)	Community C & E (Hour)	
								Step 1
DIRECT EXPENSES:								
Salary & Fringe:	$1,000,000	$100,000	$50,000	$150,000	$150,000	[ ] ?	$50,000	Step 2
	(100%)	(10%)	(5%)	(15%)	(15%)	(50%)	(5%)	
Other	100,000	10,000	5,000	15,000	[ ] ?	5,000		
INDIRECT	200,000	$ 20,000	10,000	30,000	30,000	100,000	10,000	Step 3
TOTAL COST	$1,300,000	[ ] ?	$65,000	$195,000	$195,000	$650,000	$65,000	
Allocate Administration		130,00	+ [ ] ?	+ 21,671	+ 21,671	+ 72,228	+ 7,215	Step 4
		(100%)	(.0555)	(.1667)	(.1667)	(.5556)	(.0555)	
	-0-							
TOTAL COST	$1,300,000		$72,215	$216,671	$216,671	[ ] ?	$72,215	Step 5
Units of Service			415	3611	5416	20,635	1804	
Cost per Unit (Rounded to nearest dollar)			$ 174	$ 60	$ 40	[ ] ?	$ 40	Step 6

(J) How much of the other direct cost should outpatient services receive? $______

Step 4: Since the cost of administration is to be borne by all the client and community services, the general administrative costs are allocated to all other services.

(K) What is the total cost of administration? $______

One statistical basis for the allocation is salary (and fringe). By totalling all salaries paid to services other than administration, you have the denominator (bottom number) for a ratio which uses the salary (and fringe) of a given service as the numerator (top number) on a service-by-service basis. The ratio is multiplied by the total cost in administration and the derived number is added to that service's cost. Eventually, all of the administration costs will be allocated to other services, and subtracted from administration, thus leaving a zero balance in the administration column.

(L) What is the total salary paid to services other than administration? $______
(M) What is salary paid to inpatient services? $______
(N) What is the relationship of inpatient services' salary percentage to the total salary used as an allocation base? ______%
(O) How much administration was allocated to inpatient services? $______
(P) Is this basis for allocation (salary) fair to the inpatient unit and why? ______

______

______

Step 5: By totalling the columns, the total cost of the service can be computed.

(Q) What is the total cost of the outpatient services? $______
(R) What is the total cost of all of the services? $______

Step 6: By incorporating the units of service, a cost per unit of service can be computed.

(S) How many outpatient hours of service were rendered? ______
(T) What is the cost per unit of service for outpatients? $______

Congratulations! You have just performed a complete cost finding!

ANSWERS TO THE COST-FINDING EXERCISE:

Step 1: (A) 6 (B) $1,300,000

Step 2: (C) 10% (D) $100,000 (E) 50%
(F) .50 × $1,000,000 = $500,000

Step 3: (G) $100,000 (H) $200,000 (I) 50%
(J) .50 × 100,000 = $50,000

Step 4: (K) $100,000 + $10,000 + $20,000 = $130,000
(L) $900,000 = $1,000,000 less administration of $100,000
(M) $50,000 (N) 50,000/90,000 = .0555
(O) .0555 × $130,000 = $7,215
(P) Your opinion for the last item, but another basis could be number of fulltime equivalent service-staff hours.

Step 5: (Q) $500,000 + $50,000 + $100,000 + $72,228 = $722,228
(R) $72,215 + $216,671 + $216,671 + $722,228 + $72,215 = $1,300,000

Step 6: (S) 20,635 (T) $722,228 ÷ 20,635 = $35

(A) If you wanted to spend no more than 10% of your resources on administration, did you succeed? ________

(B) If you wanted to produce outpatient services at less than $38 per hour, did you succeed? ________

(A) Yes; 10% × $1,300,000 = $130,000 which is the total cost of administration.

(B) Yes; outpatient cost per unit was $35.00

4. PRESENTING THE RESULTS OF COST-FINDING

Presenting cost-finding results in an understandable manner can be a challenge. If chargeable time is accumulated, the following method may prove to be useful.

The following four cost components are added to obtain the total cost per hour of a service:

(1) *Salary budgeted rate,* which equals total cost of contracted hours divided by total contracted hours.
(2) *Salary overhead rate,* which equals total cost of nonchargeable and unaccounted for time divided by total chargeable hours.
(3) *Other direct cost rate,* which equals all nonpersonnel costs, clearly or reasonably identified with a program, divided by total chargeable hours.
(4) *Indirect (allocated) cost rate,* which equals allocated indirect overhead divided by total chargeable hours.

Figure 2 presents a sample of the cost indices that result from this approach. The cost components of each team are summarized for an outpatient adult program for a selected period of time. The salary overhead rate is a dynamic measure which monitors the utilization of administrative effort (i.e., amount of nonchargeable and unaccounted for time) as well as the cost of that effort.

Cost per Hour

The hypothetical data presented in Figure 2 indicate that Team 1 is able to deliver an hour of direct service in the adult outpatient program for $34.45. The details of the cost in Figure 2 include:

(1) $8.11 for the professional time to deliver the service.
(2) $14.01 for the administration of the program.
(3) $1.71 for other direct expenses.
(4) $10.62 for facilities and allocated indirect expenses.

The average cost per hour of delivered service in the outpatient adult program across all teams in the center is $33.23.

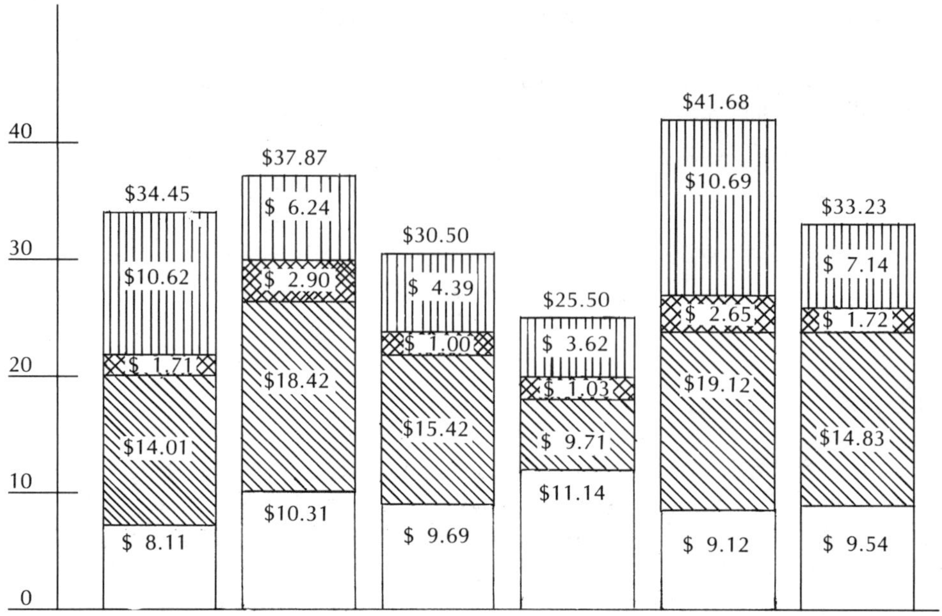

		TEAM 1	TEAM 2	TEAM 3	TEAM 4	TEAM 5	OVERALL
COSTS:		$25,302	8,234	8,044	5,814	10,762	58,156
		4,066	3,822	1,827	1,651	2,640	14,008
		33,394	24,314	28,295	15,649	19,063	120,715
		19,322	13,613	17,756	17,921	9,087	77,699
		$82,086	49,983	55,922	41,035	41,552	270,578
HOURS:	PRI	1,628	1,029	1,398	1,379	652	6,086
	CO	404	190	404	76	89	1,163
	C/E	351	101	31.5	154	256	893.5
		2,383	1,320	1,833.5	1,069	997	8,142.5
STAFF:	FTE	13.7	9.0	10.3	7.0	7.5	47.5
Average TOTAL COST		$34.45	$37.87	$30.50	$25.50	$41.68	$33.23

KEY:

= Indirect (allocated) Cost Rate
= Other Direct Cost Rate
= Salary Overhead Rate
= Budget Rate

FTE = Full Time Equivalent Staff Person
PRI = Primary Therapist
CO = Co-therapist
C/E = Consultation/Education

Figure 2. Comparison of Hypothetical Costs per Delivered Hours in Adult Outpatient Program

Changing Statistical Definitions

Different ways of counting units of service can result in very different conclusions about unit costs. Figure 3 presents cost-finding data from a centralized children's outpatient and evaluation program. Four approaches to accumulating total delivered hours of service lead to four different calculations of cost per hour:

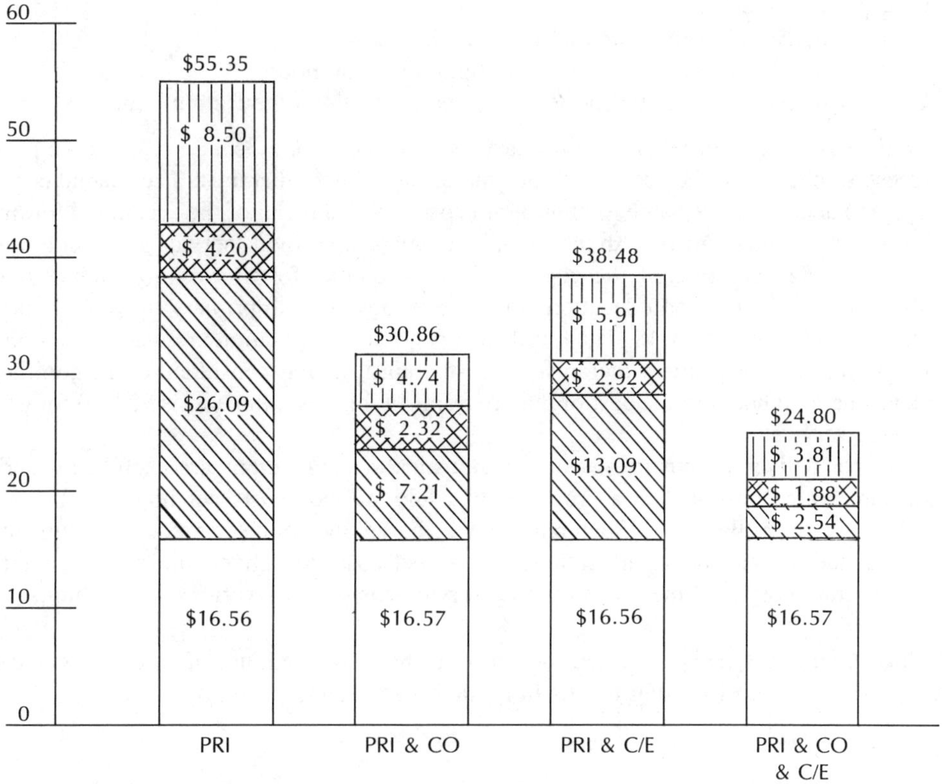

		PRI	PRI & CO	PRI & C/E	PRI & CO & C/E
COSTS:		$ 3,586	3,586	3,586	3,586
		1,772	1,772	1,772	1,772
		11,009	5,458	7,944	2,394
		6,991	12,542	10,056	15,606
		$23,358	23,358	23,358	23,358
HOURS:	PRI	422	422	422	422
	CO	0	355	0	355
	C/E	0	0	185	185
		422	757	607	942
STAFF:	FTE	3.00	3.00	3.00	3.00
Average TOTAL COST		$55.35	$30.86	$38.48	$24.80

KEY:
- = Indirect (allocated) Cost Rate
- = Other Direct Cost Rate
- = Salary Overhead Rate
- = Budget Rate

FTE = Full Time Staff
PRI = Primary Therapist
CO = Co-therapist
C/E = Consultation/Education

Figure 3. Comparison of Costs per Chargeable Hour Children Outpatient and Evaluation

(1) Cost per delivered primary therapist hour.
(2) Cost per delivered primary and co-therapist hours.
(3) Cost per delivered primary and consultation/education hours
(4) Cost per delivered primary, co-therapist, and consultation/education hours.

In the case of cost per delivered primary therapist hour ($55.35), all costs of the program are expressed in terms of the accounted for time of the primary therapist. The second computation ($30.86) deals with the same total program costs divided by all of the accounted for time of both primary and co-therapists. (An individual therapist may provide service as either a primary or co-therapist.) In contrast, if the co-therapists' accounted for time is not included in the analysis, but consultation and education hours are combined with primary therapist hours, the cost per delivered hour is $38.48. The fourth cost per hour computation in Figure 3 combines all accounted for hours (as primary therapist, as co-therapist, and as consultant to the community) and relates the total hours to the cost of the program. In this case, the cost is $24.80 for an hour of delivered service.

Cost per delivered hour using varying statistical accumulations are useful in describing how resources are consumed in a program. In addition, such costs per hour can be used in establishing fees or billing rates. Such rates may be based upon either: unit costs within specific services (including reasonable allocations of indirect costs to delivery units), or centerwide average program costs obtained by summing service costs across various service units.

Self-study Exercise. This exercise is designed to show you the kinds of questions you can ask if you present your cost-finding results in a graph like Figures 2 and 3.

Using 2:

(A) What is the total cost for Team #1? ________

(B) How many hours of primary, co-therapy, and consultation/education hours did Team #1 provide? ________

(C) What is the average cost per hour of service? ________

(D) How much is the cost of nonchargeable and unaccounted for staff time (viz., salary overhead rate)? ________

(E) What percentage of the total average cost is staff-salary overhead (viz., nonchargeable and unaccounted for time) for Team #1? ________

(F) How does this percentage compare to Team #5's percentage? ________________

(G) Does Team #5 appear to be out of line? ________________

(H) What might account for Team #5's higher unit cost? ________________

(I) What if you find out that Team #5 was just recently organized. Which direction would you expect the salary overhead rate to go—up or down—when the cost-finding is done again? Why? ________________

(J) What if you compare the budgeted unit cost for Team #5 ($35) and you found the salary overhead was supposed to be $15. What could you do? ______________________

____

____

Using Figure 3:

(K) How do you interpret the large decrease in unit cost when you combine co-therapist hours with primary hours ($55.35 to $30.86)? ______________________

____

____

(L) How do you interpet the large decrease in unit cost when you combine consultation/education with primary treatment hours ($55.35 to $38.48)? ______________________

____

____

(M) What is the rate you would present to the county board (and newspaper) to indicate the cost of your operation? Why? ______________________

____

____

Answers:

(A) $82,086 (B) 2,383 (C) $34.45 (D) $14.01

(E) $14.01 ÷ $34.45 = 40.6% or slightly over 40%

(F) Team #5 has a higher unit cost, some 20% higher ($41.68 − $35.45 = $7.23; $7.23 ÷ $34.45 = 20.9%). The salary overhead rate of Team #5 is 45.8% of total unit cost ($19.12 ÷ $41.68) and is a higher proportion than for Team #1 (45.8% vs. 40.6%).

(G) Possibly, since Team #5 has a unit cost more than 25% higher than the average ([$41.68 − 33.23] ÷ 33.23 = 25.42%). As an aside, Team #4, which is so much lower, is also of interest.

(H) Team #5 may be a relatively new team and still is building up chargeable hours. Team #5 also may have a more difficult type of client, which might explain why their production is lower. Also, if Team #5 covers a highly dispersed catchment area, there may be a great deal of travel time.

(I) Lower, for two reasons: (a) as chargeable time increases (nonchargeable and unaccounted time decreases), fewer dollars of salary cost will appear in the salary "overhead"; (b) more units of chargeable time will lower the salary overhead per unit of time.

(J) The salary-overhead rate gives you a simple and easy comparative handle on the cost of nonchargeable and unaccounted for time. By comparing the budgeted and actual, you can spot problem areas quickly.

(K) The decrease in unit cost ($55.35 to $30.86) reflects a great deal of teamwork rather than individuals working separately.

(L) The difference between primary and primary combined with consultation/education ($55.35 to $38.48) indicates that the program is providing a considerable amount of service time to the community in working with schools, judges, the police, and others.

(M) $24.80, since this rate represents the average cost per unit of service provided, whether to a client (primary or co-therapist) or community service.

5. QUESTIONS FOR THE FISCAL PERSONNEL

Often managers will be confronted with fiscal reports but will not be sure if the information is OK. Listed below are a series of questions to assess the quality of the fiscal data. While the list isn't exhaustive of every question that could be asked, generally a conclusion can be reached about the quality of the reports. The type of answer is ranked as a ''good'' or a ''not-as-good'' response.

	A GOOD RESPONSE	NOT-AS-GOOD RESPONSE
(1) On what accounting basis is the costing based?	Full accrual accounting basis.	Cash basis accounting (worst) or modified accrual (better as far as expenses are concerned, but not good on revenues).
(2) How are the salaries (and fringe) allocated to services?	Actual time and effort basis.	Budget estimate by fiat (''You're supposed to spend 40% of your time in *X* service'').
(3) How are other direct costs allocated?	To specific services depending on utilization of item.	In proportion to salary expense.
(4) How are indirect costs reallocated?	On specific statistical bases that assure reasonable allocations (e.g., sq. footage for rent or depreciation).	In proportion to salary expense.
(5) Are administrative and other support service costs allocated to client and community service?	Yes.	No.
(6) How are the units of service defined?	Client (or staff) time basis (e.g., per hour or quarter).	Event or encounter basis (e.g., outpatient visit or partial day).
(7) How frequently is the cost-finding performed?	Semi-annually (or yearly).	Every once in a while.
(8) Are current levels of costs divided by current levels of activity to see if actual cost per unit equals budgeted unit cost?	Yes.	No.

	A GOOD RESPONSE	NOT-AS-GOOD RESPONSE
(9) Do current levels of service activity times the existing rates equal or exceed the total budget?	Yes.	No.
(10) Are the bases used for the allocation of costs (direct, indirect or allocated administrative) consistent from time period to time period?	Yes.	No.

6. REFERENCES

Sorensen, James E. & Phipps, David W. (1975). *Cost-Finding and Rate Setting for Community Mental Health Centers,* National Institute of Mental Health, DHEW Publication No. (ADM) 76–291, Washington, D.C.: U.S. Government Printing Office.

SECTION VI

MANAGEMENT SUPPORT—PART I: FOCUSING PERSONNEL ROLES ON THE CLIENT

The measure of program success is how well clients realize a program's goals. Objectively defining program goals using client behaviors was described in Chapter 2. The focus of Section VI is on the management organization (its structure and its climate) and how management can use client process, outcome, and related cost data as one means of supporting the clinical process in meeting program goals. The organization of Section VI follows from this client-oriented focus of a supportive management structure. The three chapters of Section VI describe how management responsibilities and activities can be designed and maintained with client-oriented program goals and outcomes as the measure of management's functional operations.

Chapter 18: Linking Management Roles describes ways to identify service-management and organizational role responsibilities, lines of coordination and authority by how each administrative level relates to, and supports, the program's goals and consumer products.
Chapter 19: Diagnosing and Guiding Organizational Climate describes symptoms indicating the organization is not operating in an appropriate fashion and suggests ways of remedying the underlying problems.
Chapter 20: Formulating Management Questions and Data Summaries relates client characteristics, service efforts and outcomes to program goals. The questions raised and the data analyzed by management establish the management style and climate of your organization.

Products from Section VI along with Section VII (Data Analysis for Management Use) will provide the basis for day-to-day operations, i.e., who is responsible for what? A clear understanding should emerge of who uses what data and for what purposes. Section VI is the basis for the management portion of an information system and aids in:

— Evaluating staff and revising job descriptions.
— Evaluating service efforts, costs, and outcome.
— Planning programs and budgets.
— Analyzing program policies.

Chapter 18

Linking Management Roles: Identifying Service-Management and Organizational Roles

Human Services Do Have a Product—A Functioning Citizen in the Community—And the Organization of These Services Must Be Structured to Focus Efforts on Achieving the Product.

The principal objective of Chapter 18 is to identify how roles functionally support the therapeutic process with or on behalf of the client/consumer. In Section I, a program's clinical processes were designed to focus on assisting clients within program goals (see Chapter 2). Now, in this chapter, organizational components are designed to be client-oriented, i.e., components of the service organization will be linked to how they support the delivery of services to consumers.

Chapter 18 describes how job descriptions can be developed to focus personnel activities on the client.

(1) FEATURES OF CLIENT-ORIENTED JOB RESPONSIBILITIES, COORDINATION, AND AUTHORITY reviews the features of a client-oriented organizational structure relative to more traditional approaches.
(2) AN EXAMPLE AND SELF-STUDY EXERCISE ON CLIENT-ORIENTED ROLE RESPONSIBILITIES reviews the salient features of job responsibilities.
(3) COMPLETING THE DESIGN OF A JOB DESCRIPTION: Provides a step-by-step description of how people in your organization could participate in the development of their own job descriptions.
(4) PRODUCTS AND PITFALLS: Reviews the possible pros and cons of assuming this approach.

Program implementation strategies will be discussed at the end of the chapter.

Through a series of exercise tasks, Chapter 18 will lead to an appreciation of the unique style of a client-oriented organizational structure. The consistent focus on management's responsibility to support the therapeutic process may feel awkward. Management authority is not relinquished. Instead, the client-oriented approach delegates responsibilities to achieve a program's major product of functioning client/consumer.

1. FEATURES OF CLIENT-ORIENTED JOB RESPONSIBILITIES, COORDINATION, AND AUTHORITY

First, the traditional and client-oriented approaches are distinguished, and second, five key features of the client oriented approach are identified.

The Traditional and Client Oriented Approaches

The Traditional Approach emphasizes the lines of authority, responsibility, and coordination. The policy makers and ''upper'' levels of management are at the top of the table of organization; the direct service staff, therapist, and the client are at the bottom of the table of organization.

The Client-Oriented Approach focuses on the questions and decisions made by consumers and direct-service personnel to assist clients to function at their highest level. Personnel at all other organizational levels are required to define their responsibilities by how their decision making supports the therapeutic process. Then, lines of coordination and authority are drawn to support the therapeutic process.

The two approaches are not in conflict. The client-oriented approach includes the key features of the traditional approach since lines of authority and coordination are still clearly defined for all levels of management. But these lines are drawn only after designing, and in support of, a therapeutic-clinical process whose goals are to assist clients to function at their highest level in their ordinary community setting.

The client-oriented approach is a traditional approach. The focus on product, client outcomes, and the processes needed to produce that product, is a classical approach to designing the management structure of an organization by focusing on rules, responsibilities, and goals.

FIVE KEY FEATURES OF THE CLIENT ORIENTED APPROACH

A client-oriented management structure features five salient characteristics

(A) *The Organization of the Therapeutic Process Design* focuses on moving clients toward their treatment goals. All of the components described in the ''Clinical Process Design'' chapters (3–8) are needed before a client-oriented organizational structure can be sensibly designed.
A note of caution: If the clinical process does not focus on clients' moving toward treatment goals—e.g., optimal level of role performance or functioning—then a client-oriented system could become a staff-oriented system.

(B) *Job Responsibilities* at each administrative level start with the client/consumer and are defined by
   (1) Roles and objectives supporting the position(s) closer to the client and direct service staff
   (2) Questions and information to meet roles and objectives
   (3) Possible sources of required information
   (4) Limitations of role or information, e.g., issues of
   —Confidentiality of data sources and means of data transmissions
   —Limitation of inference given the source of data
   —Practical limitation of ease and expense of collecting, processing, and using the data or performing the job roles and objectives

(C) *Lines of Coordination* describe ''Who must interact.'' At each administrative level, lines of coordination are drawn so job responsibilities can be accomplished with a minimum of bureaucratic interference. The guiding principle is, ''Who must interact in support of the therapeutic process?''

(D) *Lines of Authority* describe ''Who assigns and monitors the tasks performed under each job responsibility.''

(E) *Specific Criteria of Role Performance* describe the details of role objectives, performance measures and activities, i.e.,
   (1) Expected products, relative to supporting the clients' therapeutic processes
   (2) Measures of performance achievement
   (3) Program of activities

2. AN EXAMPLE AND SELF-STUDY EXERCISE ON CLIENT-ORIENTED ROLE RESPONSIBILITIES

Self-study Exercise on Client-Oriented Role Responsibilities

The first self-study exercise highlights the identification of role responsibilities and how we can maintain an emphasis on the client products in the development of these responsibilities. Later, we will describe ways to complete the task by identifying lines of coordination, authority, and criteria of role performance. This exercise involves two tasks:

Task 1. Review the example of job responsibilities given in Table 1.
Task 2. Answer the questions below.
(Spend no more than 10 minutes on this task.)

(1) The vertical organization of the Decision Structure places the ____________________ (person) at the top.

(2) The personnel closest to the top are those who have _______________ contact with the client.

(3) Next down the line are those who are involved in the review and supervision of the therapeutic interaction between the _______________ and the _______________.

(4) The columns of the Table describe the role responsibilities of each person in the organization in terms of four characteristics:
   (a) ____________________
   (b) ____________________
   (c) ____________________
   (d) ____________________

(5) Notice that within any one position (row), there is a direct relationship across columns (a), (b), (c), and (d) which describes role responsibilities for each person in the organization. In the space below, use your own words to describe the relationship across the columns, and how it describes the role responsibilities for someone at an administrative level closest to your own.

____

____

____

Table 1. Example of Client-oriented Role Responsibilities*

Administrative Level	a. Roles	b. Questions Raised & Information Needs	c. Possible Information Source	d. Notes & Limitations
Client, Relative, or Legal Guardian	–Describes problems & resources –With staff person, decides upon goals of treatment –Contributes to treatment plan decisions	–What can you do to help me? –What services will I receive? –What do I need to do? –What progress am I making? –Does the treatment plan need change? –Are we approaching my goals?	–Copy of service plan/goals ''contract'' –Progress notes –Review records	–Client has right to information in his/her chart & to determine limitations on its use
Intake Worker	–Assesses client's problems & decides *with client* on possible treatment plan at intake & readmission –Relates service plan to goals –Assigns client to principal therapist (requires approval of Case Coordinator)	–What are client's problems & resources? –Who has referred client & what is the clinical history? –What type client (e.g., short term, long, extended) is he/she to be? –Who would be best principal therapist? –Is this person available for an additional client? –Have I completed the forms as required?	–Interview, referral information, clinical records –Service plan (problems/resources/goals) –Developmental history for child/youth –Monthly report of active caseloads –Descriptive information on therapist's specialties –Statistical report of admissions & readmissions aggregated by target population level of functioning	–May act as principal therapist for some short-term clients (6 or less visits)

Principal Therapist	–Approves or amends & implements treatment plan as authorized by client & 3rd-party payor –Works with client to fulfill treatment plan –Maintains clinical records in accord with quality assurance standards –Reviews progress & goals scheduled *with client* –Amends treatment plan/goals as required –Maintains peer relationship with colleagues regarding clients –Decides with client on closure and followup –Reviews time & caseload with supervisor	–Is the treatment plan proposed by intake worker appropriate? –Does client agree to service plan? –Is client progressing at the expected rate? –Do plans or goals need amending? –What are the costs of service relative to progress? –Is the clinical record complete? –Are fees being collected? –What followup measures are needed? –How am I spending my time with my client & at what costs? –How do my cost outcome results compare with others like me?	–Clinical record & service plan –Service plan & goals for client from clinical record –Clinical record-progress notes & review of record with client –Termination form & summary –Consumer evaluation survey form –Staff activity caseload reports	–Participates in staff development session to assure clinical data dependability
"Appropriate Other" or Peer or Case Manager	–Assumes advocacy role after initial contact through closure & followup –Provides peer review –Consults with principal therapist & Case Coordinator as required	–Are client's needs being met during referral & intake procedures? –Are plans & goals realistic & being followed? –Is the clinical record complete, meeting quality assurance standards? –Is next review date assigned?	–Completed problem/resource/ goal record service plan –Referral information –Other agency information –Review information in clinical record	–Advocacy review is "peer" concept, not supervisory. Appropriately, principal therapist & advocate share information, plans/goals, & work as a team on client's behalf.

(*continued*)

Table 1. (*Continued*)

Administrative Level	a. Roles	b. Questions Raised & Information Needs	c. Possible Information Source	d. Notes & Limitations
Target Group Specialist (A secondary role of all direct service staff)	–Maintains service information file for specified target group –Assesses services provided & service gaps –Is consultant, as required, on individual cases –Assists in program planning for specified group	–What services are available in this area for my target group? –What are the specific needs of this group? –What services does this agency provide? –What is the impact of these services? –How can I better assist individual clients of my group as advocate, principal therapist, or consultant?	–Target group service resources –Catchment area demographic survey –Clinical records –Cost outcome matrices for target group	–Information for specified target group only –Data must involve 5 or more clients in each matrix –No data identifying individual clinicians unless coordinated through & with Case Coordinator
Fiscal Management Staff	–Cost finding by unit of service staff program –Income & expenditures –Rate setting –Billing	–What are staff effort costs & income? –Program effort costs & income? –What are 3rd-party payor requirements? –What is potential & actual income?	–Staff & unit activity reports –Client financial liability & payment records –Accounts receivable & paid from 3rd-party payors –3rd-party payor correspondence	–Data confidentiality should parallel that for client & service staff
Case Coordinator, Clinical Supervisor, Clinical Program Service Director	–General supervision, coordination of case management, & quality assurance procedures –Review intake plans/goals –Evaluates staff for training development –Needs assessment & program planning with Exec. Dir., Prg. Adm., Board, other providers	–How many active cases are clinicians carrying? –How many are case managers reviewing? –What are results of the review process & is support needed? –Can clinic charts be easily audited? –How are clinicians allocating time? Effort? –What is the impact of our services? –What are the cost-outcome results among staff?	–Monthly active caseload report –Weekly review report –Supervisory review of clinical records –Monthly/quarterly time & costing reports –Special statistical reports by request –Cost outcome matrices & analysis	–Data organized by target population & disposition for each client –Sample data for each clinician –May appropriately include individual client/clinician data

Executive Director, Assistant Director, Citizen Board for review & approval of administrative action & policy	–Designs, budgets for, & reviews patterns of service –Coordinates services with other agencies & programs –Designs inservice training & research programs –Designs & maintains Management Information System (MIS) subsystems –Program evaluation	–How much are program costs relative to client outcome by types of service? Target population? Clinician classification? Units of service? –Are our quality assurance & MIS procedures working? –Does our staff need training in special areas? –What new programs are needed? –Have we maximized funding & income sources? –What are the results of our consumer evaluation measures? –Do we maintain continuity of care? –Is staff being utilized properly?	–Monthly income & expenditure report –Monthly summary report on client statistics –Time/activity/costing summaries –Cost outcome matrices & analysis –Annual budget projection –Semi-annual budget reports –Consumer evaluation summary reports	–Reports contain no data on individual clients (Rule of 2 & 5: see Chapter 19), unless legal intervention is required
County Administrators (staff and Citizen Board)	–Designs, budgets, coordinates, reviews patterns of service activities in catchment area –Coordinates & evaluates activities with other services –Assesses catchment area needs –Designs countywide training & research programs –Coordinates county consultation and education activities	–What are the year-to-date cost outcome figures for program agencies? –Does budget projection align with projected services? –What categories of clients (& how many) are the program serving? Failing to serve? –What is the impact of services? The cost? –What new programs are needed? –How do cost-outcome reports assist with future planning? –How do the program agencies complement each other's services? –What are the service gaps & duplication?	–Monthly income & expense reports –Annual budget projection –Monthly service reports –Semi-annual admission statistics & client characteristics report –Catchment-area demographic survey –Aggregated cost-outcome data –Summaries of time/activity/cost records by agency, groups of clinician classification, & client groups	–No data on individual clients or staff unless legal intervention by county program office is required by law, e.g., legal commitment procedures.

*Adapted from a ''Position Responsibilities'' chart developed by Barbara Burwell for the Fayette County (Pennsylvania) MH/MR Clinic in 1975.

(6) Overall, the questions you address reflect your position responsibilities in a client-oriented system, and these questions are supposed to be supportive of the positions closer to the roles of direct service providers. One's position responsibilities will only make sense when interpreted in terms of how they support the position closer to the direct service staff. Review the position of the Program Director (or Clinical Supervisor) and describe two examples of how that role can be supportive of the direct service staff.
   (a) ______________________________
   ____
   (b) ______________________________
   ____

(7) Give two examples of Limitations from Table 1.
   (a) ______________________________
   (b) ______________________________

Answers

(1) Client/consumer (2) Direct (3) Client; Direct service staff

(4) (a) Roles and objectives (b) Questions and information needs
   (c) Information services (d) Limits of influence and confidentiality

(5) A role or position responsibility is defined by the questions you ask and the information you use to make decisions.

(6) (a) Insures that the direct service staff get the information they need to fulfill their roles.
   (b) Insures that the direct service staff caseloads are appropriate.

(7) Confidentiality; Can review aggregated data only

3. COMPLETING THE DESIGN OF A JOB DESCRIPTION

The objective is to link job responsibilities and lines of coordination, authority, and performance criteria to the organizational goal of producing functioning citizens. Completing a job description requires five steps:

Step 1. Read through all five steps entirely, including the example provided in Table 2.

Step 2. Describe the six elements of the job position closer to client given in Tables 3 and 4. The six elements of a position are described by the six column headings of the two tables. The guide for identifying this position is someone whose role supports the therapeutic process, and who would directly depend upon the products or support of your role.

Example: If your role is unit program director, above you (toward the client) is the clinical supervisor, and below you might be the Citizen Board, the county or state authority, or hospital administration.

If your role is Evaluation, above you (toward the client) is clinical supervisor or service-unit director.

If your role is fiscal manager, above you (toward the client) is the service-unit program director.

Table 2—Step 5: Specific Activities and Criteria of Role Performance

Instructions: Read the example below and then follow suit by describing one activity criteria and product within your own position's responsibilities.

Priority ______________________

Product and Its Relationship to Supporting Consumer Products ______________________

Example: Outpatient Unit Director, meeting with clinical supervisors to review caseloads, to insure a good match (therapeutically) of clients and staff, which also maximizes staff time and income.

Activities (Ordered)	Standards of Performance	Required Level of Performance	Data Needs	Data Sources	Authority
EXAMPLE Memo schedule of meeting Set agenda Obtain & distribute data on caseload summaries Hold meeting	Staff/Supervisors assigned all clients by areas of speciality & amount of expected clinical effort	–Monthly review meetings –Staff/Supervisors match clients-staff & maximize time & income	Present caseload LOF × Target Group Present Activities: –Chargeable –Nonchargeable Past standards LOF × Target Group	Staff Activity Records	Job Description Sanction from Executive Director
NOW TRY IT YOURSELF					

Table 3. Your Job Responsibilities

	Admin. Level	Roles & Objectives	Questions Raised and Information Needs	Possible Information Sources (You Trust)
START HERE	Position toward client (above you)			
2nd— FILL THIS IN	Your Position (your support of above)			
LAST— FILL THIS IN	Position below you (support you require)			

Step 3. Describe the six elements of your position as it supports the position toward the client and the therapeutic process. The emphasis is not *control* over the position toward the client, but rather how you support that position in the therapeutic process in helping clients function optimally in their ordinary community setting.

Step 4. Describe the six elements of the position below yours, i.e., away from the client. Again, emphasize the position in terms of the kinds of *support you require* to perform your own support role for those closer to the client.

Step 5. Take one product (output) of your job responsibility and, using the Table 2 format, identify the specific activities and criteria of your role related to that product.

Note that the general outline specifying these criteria has three elements:

(a) Your expected products (*outputs*) defined in terms of the products' support of the clients' service package. These outputs ought to be assigned priorities, e.g., ordering from most to least important.

(b) Measures of performance (*achievement*).

(c) Program of activities for (a) and (b), above.

Four concerns and realizations will emerge in developing client-oriented job descriptions. First, lines of *responsibility* start with the clients and their treatment goals, but lines of *authority* start with the policy and upper management levels who sanction responsibilities. Here is the resolution between the traditional and the client-oriented approaches. Second, possible information sources used as a basis for decisions necessary to perform the job imply a trust in the data and the data sources. The quality assurance of data rests upon simple principles detailed later. Dependability of data will increase

Table 4. Limitations, Lines of Coordination and Authority

		The Lines of	
Admin. Level	Limitations: —Confidentiality —Inference —Practicality	Coordination "Who Interacts"	Authority "Who Assigns & Monitors"
Position toward client (above you)			
Your Position			
Position away from client (toward you)			

— If the data are useful to the persons whose roles are to generate the data
— If procedures for detecting and correcting errors in data generation are educational to the persons who generated the data so the source of the error can be easily corrected

Third, job responsibilities may be described too narrowly or too broadly to adequately support a client-oriented system. Finally, can job demands be matched to available staff skills and resources?

4. PRODUCTS AND PITFALLS

Developing a client-oriented management structure has both positive and negative features. One critical feature of a client-oriented management structure is clearly identifying and protecting the territory of all staff. But the recommendations for protecting territory and identifying how the staff can feed into the decision process in an organization structure promote:

(1) More open but protected organizational structure, i.e., more people will understand the data base for decisions, but the identity of clinical decision making will be protected by the clear lines of responsibility and authority.
(2) More decentralization of decisions.

Table 5. Positive and Negative Features of a Client-oriented Decision Structure

Possible Advantages	Potential Pitfalls
(1) Makes staff less paranoid	(1) Makes management more paranoid
(2) Gives decision-making powers to staff	(2) Powers-that-be assume that decisions will flow from top to bottom, e.g., Feds/State/County/Exec. Director and not vice versa
(3) Data are more reliable	(3) The data are less useful for manipulation
(4) Greater confidentiality	(4) Rule of 2 & 5 is theoretically nice—but will people believe it will be enforced?*
(5) More appropriate model for professional "line" people†	(5) Does correlation between "Who's responsible" and "Who makes decisions" breakdown?†

Source: Paul Sherman, Ph.D., Ravenswood CMHC, Chicago, Illinois.

*The "Rule of 2 and 5" is a means of insuring that lines of confidentiality, responsibility, and authority are not bypassed. It states that "No cost outcome data should be transmitted more than two organizational steps beyond the client/therapist interaction or staff decision-making level unless the data have been aggregated to summarize at least five clients or five staff." This rule cuts down on staff mistrust. A more complete discussion of this concept is provided in chapter 19.

†While items 1–4 have complementary pros and cons, item 5's pro and con are not necessarily related to each other.

There are arguments for and against doing this. An example of arguments for and against such decision structures is given in Table 5 provided by Paul Sherman of the Ravenswood CMHC of Chicago, 1974.

The positive and negative features of the client-oriented organizational structure provide a basis for two things: first, to weigh the assets and liabilities of developing such a system; second, to provide a checklist of performance criteria for the system's development. The negative features should be either avoided in the system's design, or handled by incorporating techniques to identify and process the negative events when they occur.

Chapter 19

Diagnosing and Shaping Organizational Climate

Chapter 19 answers three principal questions. First, is the organization operating as it should? Second, if not, what factors are contributing to the difficulties? Third, what remedies might improve the situation?

(1) DIAGNOSING ORGANIZATIONAL DIFFICULTIES describes the major symptoms indicating difficulties exist and how the current organization might be encouraging such difficulties.
(2) IDENTIFYING POSSIBLE REMEDIES describes useful techniques to correct difficulties.
(3) PROGRAM-IMPLEMENTATION STRATEGIES describes an overall approach for designing a client-oriented organizational structure and maintaining its thrust toward program goals.

1. DIAGNOSING ORGANIZATIONAL DIFFICULTIES

Problem or conflict resolution initially requires the recognition of symptoms of existing organizational difficulties. First, one needs to identify the signs that a problem exists. Next is to identify one's own contributions to these difficulties. Finally, one can identify the contributions of others.

Seven symptoms or indicators suggest the organization is not operating properly.

(a) Staff refusal to submit data or reports.
(b) Inability of staff administrator responsible for reviewing and making decisions with the data to keep up with current reports.
(c) Staff/administrator refusal to read reports before making decisions.
(d) Desire of administrator at one level in the chain of command to deal directly with a much lower level, ignoring intermediate levels.
(e) Direct intervention of administrative personnel on behalf of individual clients.
(f) Intervention in direct service personnel matters by anyone but immediate supervisors and agency personnel officers.
(g) A consistent tendency at any level to suppress data or to produce biased reports in order to conform to what is perceived as "expected" or "desirable."

Figure 1 portrays each of the seven organizational difficulties. The occurrence of these symptoms does not mean the organization is sick. All organizations are likely to exhibit each of

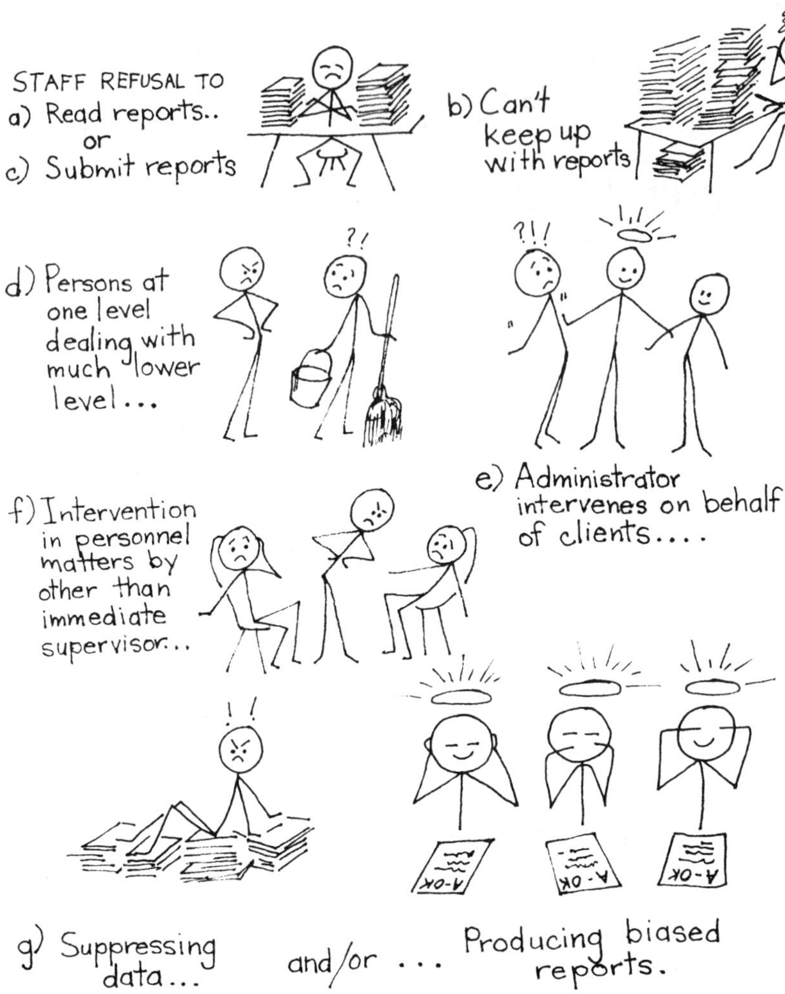
STAFF REFUSAL TO
a) Read reports..
or
c) Submit reports
b) Can't keep up with reports
d) Persons at one level dealing with much lower level...
e) Administrator intervenes on behalf of clients....
f) Intervention in personnel matters by other than immediate supervisor...
A-OK
A-OK
A-OK
g) Suppressing data...
and/or ...
Producing biased reports.

Figure 1. Symptoms of Organizational Difficulties

the symptoms to some degree. The issue is one of degree and to what extent it affects the designated role functions of personnel in the organization and the production of program goals. The objective is to:

— Diagnose the existence of the problem
— Identify possible contributions to the symptoms
— Seek, implement, and test possible remedies

Self-study Exercise on Organizational Difficulties

The following exercise should help you understand how organizational difficulties can arise. After the exercise, some remedies are described. For each symptom given in Table 1, list the possible contributions to the malfunctions

Table 1. Identifying Factors Contributing to Symptoms of Difficulties

First list at least one of *your* contributions to create symptoms. Then list the contributions of others.

Symptoms	Contributing Factors	
	Yours	Others
(a) Staff refusal to submit data or reports		
(b) Inability of staff/administrator responsible for reviewing and making decisions with data to keep up with current reports		
(c) Staff or administrative refusal to read reports before making decisions		
(d) Desire of administrator at one level to deal directly with a much lower level, ignoring intermediate levels		
(e) Intervention of administrative personnel on behalf of individual clients		
(f) Intervention in direct service personnel matters by anyone but their immediate supervisors and agency personnel officers		
(g) A consistent tendency at any level to suppress data or to produce biased reports to conform to what is perceived as "expected" or "desired"		

— you have made (give at least one per symptom)
— others have made (you may do this only after listing the contributions you have made)

Note that you are asked to first identify your contribution to the problem. As Walt Kelly so aptly put it in *Pogo,* "We have met the enemy and they is us." It is important to consider the possibility that your own actions may negatively affect others in the organization.

2. POSSIBLE REMEDIES FOR ORGANIZATIONAL DIFFICULTIES

Possible remedies for reducing organizational difficulties fall into three categories:

(1) A position's roles and objectives are either too broadly or too narrowly defined in terms of questions raised and decisions to be made, and in terms of information needs and availability.

The remedy lies in the development of a more appropriate position description (see Chapter 18).

(2) There may be a mismatching of a staff person's skills to the roles and objectives of the position.

Either staff training and development or reassignment are possible remedies in this case. Again, Chapter 18 can be of assistance for this difficulty.

(3) There may be staff mistrust of:

Who may use what data? and *To what ends?*

Information, Decisions, and Territory

If the symptoms suggest mistrust, consider having staff describe their perceived role around:

— Questions and decisions they feel are primary to their role
— Information they feel would be useful for answering their role questions and decisions
— Which levels of the organizational decision structure would ''You [the staff person] prefer to not know it was you who made a particular decision and what the information base for your decision was?''

As in the parlor game of ''telephone'' where a message, whispered to your neighbor in a circle without feedback, usually breaks down when passed along by two or more people, there appears to be a rule of two in determining: ''They shall not know it was I who made that decision!''

When identification of ''Who was responsible for which decisions'' moves more than two steps away in the organizational decision structure, communication and feedback break down and, as a result, *distrust* appears to increase. Protecting the territory is imperative!

After identifying the general boundaries where staff mistrust may increase, two tactics are available:

— Find the causes for the mistrust, open lines of communication, and perform the necessary education and therapy to maintain a diminished level of mistrust. Usually, improving feedback on decisions will help.
— Assure the protection of someone identifying individual decision makers by *the rule of two and five:*

> No cost-outcome data should be transmitted more than two organizational steps beyond the client-therapist interaction or staff decision level unless the data have been aggregated to summarize at least five clients and/or five staff.

While the staff may grow accustomed to having clinical supervision by other clinicians (peers), nonclinical personnel are not likely to be trusted in reviewing their clinical decisions.

Clearly Identify How Clinical Staff Feed into the Decision Process

The general strategy summarizes cost-outcome data so that:

— Clinical staff as well as management can raise questions, problems, and issues
— Clinical and clinical supervision staff can easily review individual or group data to seek and recommend alternatives
— Management can formulate tests of alternatives and specify boundaries of data outcome as a basis for selecting among alternatives before test data are collected

Table 2. Examples of Possible Remedies*

Symptoms	Possible Remedies
(a) Can't keep up with reports	1. Establish staff committees to outline who gets what information and what are the controls. 2. Provide staff training in utilization techniques. 3. Present advantages of data reports. 4. Use staff input to revise and update reporting system to maximize reliable input.
(b) Refuses to read and submit reports	1. Revise role to concretize time for data input. 2. Prepare question list for goals and objectives. 3. Train for data utilization and staff feedback.
(c) Person at one level dealing with much lower level	1. Reports to decision makers on time. 2. Indicate how decisions relate to data reports. 3. Develop procedure for decisions requiring change-vs.-confrontation. 4. Train for data integration and decision making.
(d) Administrator intervenes on behalf of client	1. Develop organizational chart for lines of responsibility. 2. Specify what each level should be looking for in data reports. 3. Insure communication is total: No one is left out.
(e) Intervention in personnel matters by other than immediate supervisor	1. Clarify real issues and decision to be made. 2. Refer questions and needs to responsible person. 3. Provide feedback and alternatives to clientele "blind spots." 4. Consider staff training and reassessment based on immediate supervisor's report.
(f) Suppressing data	1. Immediate feedback to appropriate supervisors. 2. Tactful redirection. 3. Restricted access to personnel data and reports to provide a buffer.
(g) Producing biased reports	1. Define and clarify data-utilization process: "Who gets what!" 2. Develop review procedure to isolate problems and differences. 3. Provide training and input in assets of accurate data and reports. 4. Clarify goal and objective system. 5. Sprinkle with "M & M's"!
(h) Boredom	Become a consultant

*Remedies recommended by Phillip Grabeau.

— Clinical staff and management get to review the data and understand how the data may affect policy decisions

Another list of remedies developed by Dr. Phillip Grabeau is given in Table 2.

3. PROGRAM-IMPLEMENTATION RECOMMENDATIONS

Chapter 19 focuses heavily on self-study. By themselves, the exercises in Chapter 19 do not provide a means for planning and implementing an entire client-oriented organization structure. Instead, it is a task requiring a coordinated effort by personnel at all levels of the organization.

Some possible steps toward implementing a client-oriented system include:

(1) Forming a small group of 4–8 people who are
  — Easy to work with
  — Represent all the major levels of your organization
(2) Have the group meet for approximately 2–3 hours to go through the self-study exercises in sequence
  — As individuals on one exercise section
  — As a group on that same exercise section

The most important exercise task is Table 3. Here the group identifies performance criteria for the development of a client-oriented organizational structure. If it works for a small, warm-and-friendly group, then proceed.

(3) Next, start pyramiding the process by having all of the clinical and administrative managers attend a workshop covering the exercises in Chapter 19.
(4) Next, have the managers repeat this process with their own staff.

At this point, the process will have moved from upper management levels to line staff. This hardly appears to be a client-oriented approach. But Steps 1–4 are staff development, and Steps 5–7 establish the actual organizational structure. The next step is to reverse the process.

Table 3. Self-study Exercise on Possible Remedies for Organizational Difficulties

For each symptom, describe remedies which best suit your program.

Symptoms	Remedies
(a) Staff refusal to submit data or reports	
(b) Inability of staff/administrator responsible for reviewing and making decisions with data to keep up with current reports	
(c) Staff or administrative refusal to read reports before making decisions	
(d) Desire of administrator at one level to deal directly with a much lower level, ignoring intermediate levels	
(e) Intervention of administrative personnel on behalf of individual clients	
(f) Intervention in direct service personnel matters by anyone but their immediate supervisors and agency personnel officers	
(g) A consistent tendency at any level to suppress data or to produce biased reports to conform to what is perceived as ''expected'' or ''desired''	

(5) Have direct service staff negotiate their job descriptions with their supervisors.
(6) Have the administrative staff negotiate job descriptions with their supervisors.
(7) Have the executive management staff negotiate their job descriptions with the key people from Steps 5 and 6, above.

Repeat Steps 5 through 7 until all dust is settled.

THE FINAL PRODUCTS

After creating the job descriptions of all staff and the design of the clinical service processes, the basis exists for every other component in a program, e.g., clinical records, fiscal, and information systems.

While clinical records, fiscal, and information systems may be developed before completing the design of the clinical service and organizational structure, the first three systems will not be completed successfully until the latter two components are in place.

A RECOMMENDED REFERENCE

Mager, R. F., & Pipe, P. (1970). *Analyzing Performance Problems*. Belmont, CA: Fearon Publishers.

Chapter 20

Formulating Management Questions and Data Summaries

Your Questions Are Your Management Style

The questions you ask represent your management style. But what is implied by the questions you ask? Do your questions focus on your product? Do you ask what happened to the client? Will the questions you ask focus your program's efforts and resources on its principal product: a functioning client? The objective of Chapter 20 is to formulate management questions and data summaries focusing attention on the relationships among client characteristics, services rendered, and outcomes.

Seven major segments are previewed:

(1) MANAGEMENT STYLE AND THE QUESTIONS YOU ASK: Describes how the questions you ask can influence your program.
(2) CLIENT-ORIENTED QUESTIONS: Describes how to formulate questions focusing on client characteristics, service efforts, costs, and outcomes.
(3) INCOMPLETE QUESTIONS: Describes the consequences of incomplete questions, i.e., what can happen when questions fail to focus on the relationships among client characteristics, service efforts, and client outcomes.
(4) UTILITY OF DATA SUMMARIES: Describes how data summaries should and should not be used.
(5) QUESTIONS AND DATA SUMMARIES (A SYSTEMS APPROACH): Describes a technique for designing data summaries to address client-oriented questions.
(6) CONSTRUCTING TABLES AND GRAPHS: Describes some of the technical features of data summaries in a nontechnical fashion.
(7) PROGRAM-IMPLEMENTATION STRATEGIES: Describes how you can help staff start to formulate better questions.

1. MANAGEMENT STYLE AND THE QUESTIONS YOU ASK

The questions you ask reflect your managerial concerns. The questions you ask will shape reports leading either to decisions or to more refined questions. As a result, the questions you ask focus the attention and direction of those who hear the questions and those who feel they are

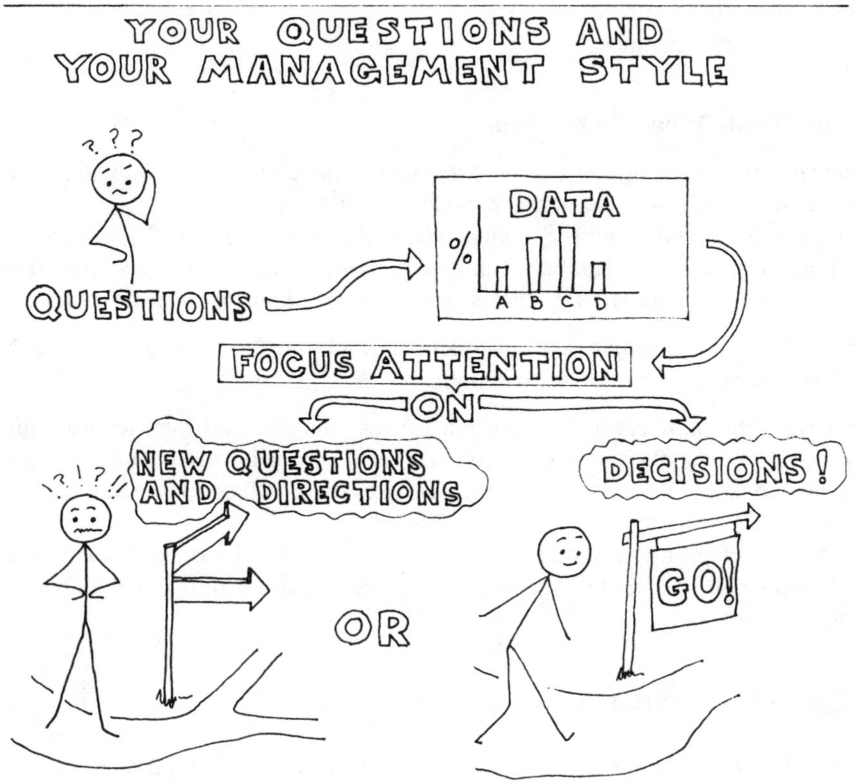

Figure 1. Your Questions and Your Management Style

affected by the answers, including your staff, your Board, and regulatory agencies. Those who hear and are affected by the questions you ask will either meet or resist the perceived expectations of the questions. Seldom will they be neutral, even if there is a pretense of neutrality. The questions you ask and the resulting reports and decisions you make become your style of management.

A Note of Caution on This Unit

Because the concepts in this unit often run counter to time-honored ways of thinking, some may feel an unexpected awkwardness. At issue is whether the standard management questions focus attention on the functioning client/consumer. You may at first find it difficult to reformulate the typical questions you ask into client-oriented questions. You may even feel annoyed at what is being labeled an "incomplete" question. But bear with the process. By the time you finish the exercises, you should have a whole new perspective on the questions you and your staff should ask, and on the management style of your entire organization.

2. CLIENT-ORIENTED QUESTIONS

Management using client-oriented questions will focus on the relationships of three variables:

— Client/consumer characteristics (Diagnostic, problem severity, demographic, supports)

— Services (Resources and activities)
— Client/consumer outcomes

Examples of Client-Oriented Questions

What were the different cost-outcome results for moderate and severely depressed clients for whom group therapy was the primary mode of treatment?

(*Note*: Service costs reflect the amount and value of service effort. An increase in costs comes with an increase in the number of units of service, or when the cost per unit of service increases, e.g., one hour of MD time costs more than one hour of caseworker time.)

What is the relative progress of dysfunctional and mid-functioning clients in the partial hospitalization program over the last 6 months?

What were the numbers and proportion of low, middle, and high level of functioning clients on each staff person's caseload last month? What proportion of direct and indirect service time was rendered by outpatient staff to middle and low level of functioning schoolage children?

In general, a client-oriented question will balance client and service characteristics during the clinical episode and client outcome and revenues afterwards. An incomplete question tends to upset the balance.

3. INCOMPLETE QUESTIONS

Incomplete questions could divert attention away from your principal product: services which reliably help clients to function optimally. A question is considered incomplete if it leads to inquiries and decisions fragmenting the combined concerns of client characteristics, service efforts, and outcomes. The result might be that the incomplete question might focus staff concerns in a biased way. A note of caution is needed here. You need not feel guilty about having asked incomplete questions in the past. Many such questions come from a time when outcome measurement was not considered possible and, therefore, the only questions were incomplete questions.

Let us inspect the characteristics of an incomplete question. Questions which address one or two—but not all three—variables of a client-oriented question are incomplete because they fragment managerial attention and effort. Managerial questions affect the attention, expectation, and behavior of those who hear the questions and feel they are affected by the potential decisions. Fragmented questions will lead to fragmented management. Consider some examples which are purposely designed to overstate the potential negative impact of an incomplete question.

Variable	Problem & Example of Fragmented Question
1. Client/consumer characteristics	*Turnstile Management:* "How many clients with *X* characteristic were served regardless of service cost and outcome?" "If they want us to serve left-handed alcoholics, then let's recruit left-handed alcoholics. Now, what do we *do* for left-handed alcoholics?"
2. Services Resource & Activity	*Sweatshop Management:* "How many hours of direct service were produced regardless of client characteristics and outcome?" "I don't care if it helps the client. If we don't get paid for it, we stop working."
3. Client/consumer outcome	*Ends-Justify-Means Management:* "How many improved, regardless of intake characteristics and service costs?" "Go out and find people who will improve and refer those problem clients elsewhere."

Many managers have fed into these three management styles. Yet, none of us would personally characterize ourselves as being the Grinch with the "turnstile," the "sweatshop" or the "ends-justify-means" style of management. Most managers try to balance their questions and thereby create management concerns which reflect and relate client characteristics, service resources, and efforts to outcomes.

The exercise tasks which follow will ask you to distinguish between client-oriented questions and incomplete ones, and give you practice in restating the incomplete questions to make them better. Then, in the last parts of the chapter, you will be shown how to answer the question with well-formulated data summaries.

Self-study Exercise Tasks

Review each of the three incomplete questions given below. Select at least one of the three questions and:

(1) List three possible negative, nonclient-oriented directions which could be taken because of the question's fragmented focus of attention.

(2) Write one or two client-oriented (or appropriate followup) questions which touch on the same topic, but are expanded to encompass all three variables of:
- — Client characteristics
- — Services
- — Outcomes

Then, repeat this process for each of the other two questions below. If you have difficulty formulating client-oriented questions, review the examples given earlier in the chapter.

Question A: What proportion of clinical staff time is devoted to direct, indirect, client-related, consultation and education, and unaccounted activities?

POSSIBLE NEGATIVE DIRECTIONS ______________________

____

____

A MORE COMPLETE QUESTION ______________________

____

____

Question B: What was the number of active clients in each minority category, e.g., Black, Spanish-speaking, Oriental, Native American?

POSSIBLE NEGATIVE DIRECTIONS ______________________

____

____

A MORE COMPLETE QUESTION ______________________

____

____

Question C: What was the proportion of clients admitted to each outpatient service unit last quarter?

POSSIBLE NEGATIVE DIRECTIONS ______________________

____

____

A MORE COMPLETE QUESTION ______________________

____

____

4. UTILITY OF DATA SUMMARIES: THE DOUBLE-EDGED SWORD

A good client-oriented data summary will clearly address the issue for decision makers at the identified level in the organization, with the bottom line being insight into the program's impact on clients. A corallary criterion could be described as a double-edged sword. Any data summary should raise questions which, if pursued by the responsible person(s), could direct inquiry back to a set of client's clinical records, and be useful for clinical supervision and staff development. Or, the data summary could direct inquiry toward program management and policies and thereby be useful to program directors, citizen boards, and regulatory agencies.

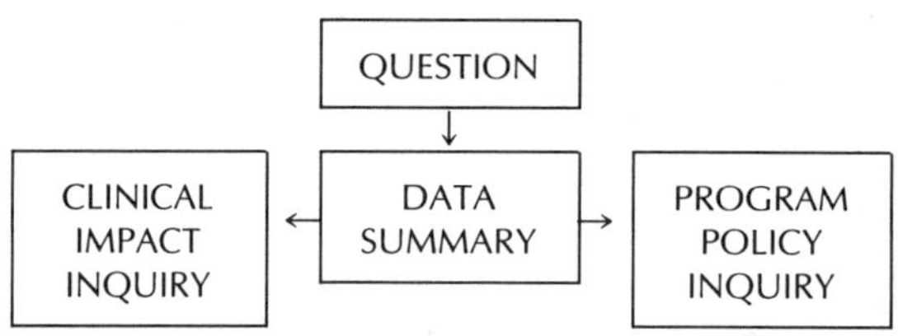

Utility for Clinical Supervisors
(See Chapter 21)

Utility for Program Directors, Citizen Boards, & Regulatory Agencies
(See Chapter 22)

In a hard-nosed fashion, we would recommend that any data summary which does not lead inquiry and utility in both directions is incomplete. You may wish to restrict who is to pursue each avenue of inquiry, e.g., by employing the ''Rule of 2 and 5'' (see Chapter 19). Nevertheless, a good client-oriented data summary functions like a double-edged sword which systematically raises questions.

5. QUESTIONS AND DATA SUMMARIES (A SYSTEMS APPROACH)

A good way to develop data summaries is to follow four systematic steps:

(1) Identify the QUESTION.
(2) Organize a data summary—a TABLE or FIGURE—addressing the question.
(3) Outline the potential UTILITY of the data summary by the kinds of decisions made possible by using the data.
(4) Specify the CAUTIONS and LIMITATIONS of the data summary in terms of
 (a) Practical resources and analysis techniques available
 (b) Limits of what can or cannot be inferred from these kinds of data
 (c) Limitations of decisions given role of the decision maker. (These limitations were discussed in Chapter 19.)

An abbreviated outline of the four steps is:

(1) QUESTION
(2) TABLE OR FIGURE
(3) UTILITY
(4) CAUTIONS & LIMITATIONS

Self-study Exercise

Using the information provided in the example in Table 1, identify:

(1) Client Characteristics ____________________
    Service Area ____________________
    Outcomes ____________________

(2) A utility for
    A Clinician ____________________
    ____
    A Program Director ____________________
    ____

(3) Give one more example for each of the following:
    A Utility ____________________
    ____
    A Caution ____________________
    ____

Answers

(1) Adults with and without prior hospitalization; Outpatient; Level of functioning change, % in each change category, $\$\bar{X}$.

(2) and (3) See "Utility" and "Caution" information at the bottom of Table 1.

Self-study Exercise Tasks

Return to questions A, B, or C that you worked with in the last exercise task. For one of those three questions, consider your revised "better question," and create two one-page presentations of

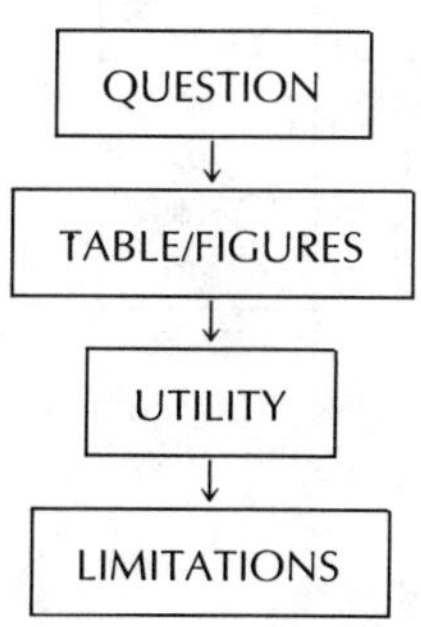

Table 1. Client-oriented Question-data-utility-caution

1) ISSUE: What were the relative cost outcome episode results for the outpatient program when comparing clients with prior or no prior hospitalization history?
2) DATA: For a 5-month period, each cell provides percent of group in row, number, and average costs.*

Prior Hospit. History	Clients Started Dysfunctional				Clients Started Functional			
			Improved		Regressed			
	Regressed	Maintained	Still Dysf.	To Funct.	To Dysf.	Still Funct.	Maintained	Improved
YES $N = 20$		5% 1 $1365.90	10% 2 $374.11	5% 1 $422.79	5% 1 $ 965.46	10% 2 $755.86	35% 7 $1238.76	30% 6 $694.13
NO $N = 57$		5.3% 3 $ 327.38			5.3% 3 $1027.59	12.3% 7 $474.62	42.1% 24 $ 537.54	35% 20 $661.09

(3) UTILITY:

a) *For Clinicians:* How do my results compare with the whole outpatient program?
b) *For the Utilization Review Committee:* Were there differences in resource utilization and outcome for these two groups?
c) *For Quality Assurance and Supervision:* What followup activities took place for discontinued clients who regressed to the dysfunctional level or who were maintained at the dysfunctional level?
d) *For Service Program Managers:* What changes in available resources might improve the cost-outcome picture?
e) *For Policy Levels:* Could policy changes affect differences in resource allocation and outcomes?

4) CAUTIONS:

a) Are these data supported by what is in the clinical records? (Check by inspecting a random sample.)
b) Are these results consistent with other past time periods? (Check by performing a retrospective study.)
c) Would these results also be true in the future? (Check by running a prospective study.)

*Data from Paul Sherman, Ravenswood Hospital CMHC, Chicago, Il.

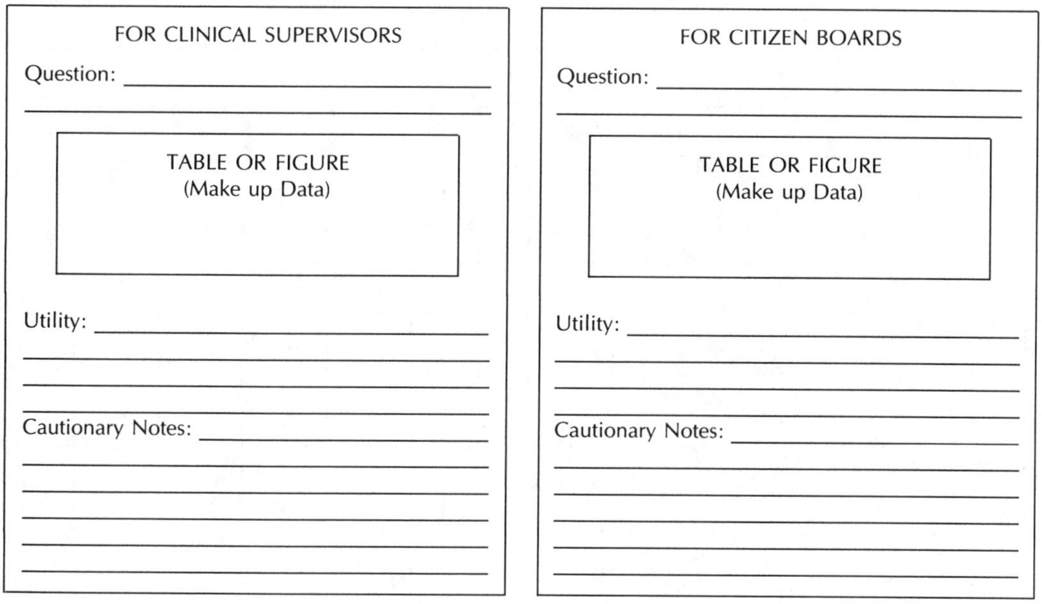

Figure 2. Exercise Format

Figures 2–3 and Table 2 provide examples of a format and figures you should use for this exercise.

In keeping with the concept of the double-edge sword, we are asking you to create two presentations. One presentation will be for use by clinical supervisors and the other for Citizen Board members. While the overall format of your presentation to each group may be the same, you need to ask whether each of these two groups (clinical supervisors and Citizen Boards) should have the data aggregated and presented in the same fashion. Probably not, since their use of the data and direction of decision making differ.

To help you in this task, an example of a client-oriented figure summary is provided in Figure 3. You may also consider using the cost outcome matrix format shown in Table 2.

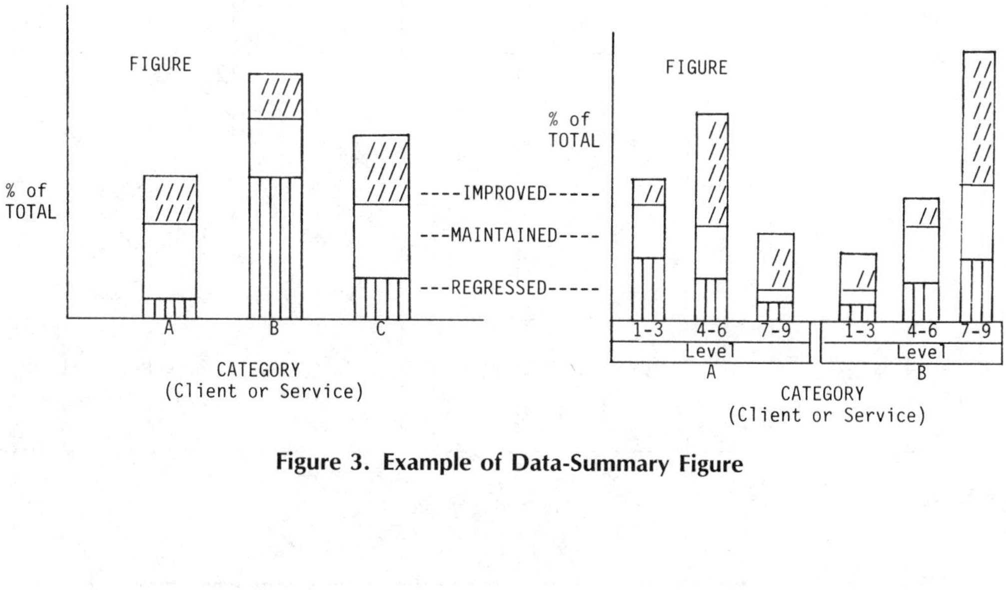

Figure 3. Example of Data-Summary Figure

Table 2. Episode Cost-outcome Results for Clients with Improvement Expected

No Prior Hospitalization/Ages 18–39

			Termination								
			Dysfunctional				Functional				
		END		5 $ 99	2 $325	10 $149	22 $133	22 $176	29 $219	12 $122	3 $199
INTAKE or READMISSION	START	Total 105 $170	1	2	3	4	5	6	7	8	9
DYSFUNCTIONAL	1	1 $323					1 $323				
DYSFUNCTIONAL	2	3 $120		3 $120							
DYSFUNCTIONAL	3	5 $331		2 $ 66	1 $163	1 $355		1 $606			
DYSFUNCTIONAL	4	14 $145				5 $105	1 $117	1 $249	5 $195	2 $ 81	
FUNCTIONAL	5	24 $155				2 $199	15 $ 84	2 $424	2 $366	2 $197	1 $ 88
FUNCTIONAL	6	36 $218			1 $488		4 $251	17 $121	7 $455	6 $110	1 $452
FUNCTIONAL	7	15 $ 78				1 $137	1 $217	1 $109	10 $ 45	2 $124	
FUNCTIONAL	8	6 $193				1 $169			5 $198		
FUNCTIONAL	9	1 $ 57									1 $ 57

52 Maintained @ $ 93.91
35 Improved @ 265.44
18 Regressed @ 202.51
105 @ $169.90

After you have completed the task for one of the questions, repeat the process for either one or both of the two remaining questions. The criteria for repeating the process is whether you can see yourself easily doing the task on the next replication. If you can easily perform the task, then move on. If the task still looks a little muddy, then repeat the process. But, if the task seems to be impossible, ask a friendly colleague to join you as a partner in the task. Be sure *not* to let your partner do all of the work. Otherwise, you will rob yourself of the confidence of ever having command of the concepts covered in this unit. That would be relinquishing too much management responsibility and control.

Remember, the best power of authority is the authority which comes with understanding, and being able to work with the concepts yourself.

6. CONSTRUCTING TABLES AND GRAPHS

Creating data summaries in the form of tables or figures is a combination of art and human engineering. Done properly, the summary can quickly convey the message relevant to the question without obscuring or exaggerating the critical features of the data. Most introductory statistics books provide a good review of the critical features of constructing good tables and figures. An excellent text is *Interpreting Graphs and Tables,* by Peter N. Selby, New York: John Wiley & Sons, Inc. 1976.

Do's & Don't's in Graphics

DO — Abstract the important information for the summary relevant to the question asked and the utility. You can provide the more detailed data listing or work table in an appendix.

DON'T — Use a numerical work table to summarize data. Too much data on a page obscures the message.

DO — Create a scale to make visually apparent any differences which are statistically or programmatically significant. By programmatic significance we mean that if such differences exist, then a decision of programmatic change might be needed.

DON'T — Expand a scale to blow up a slight difference or contract a scale to hide or diminish a significant difference.

DON'T — Confuse volume of a figure with number. Twice the size (volume) does not equal twice the number.

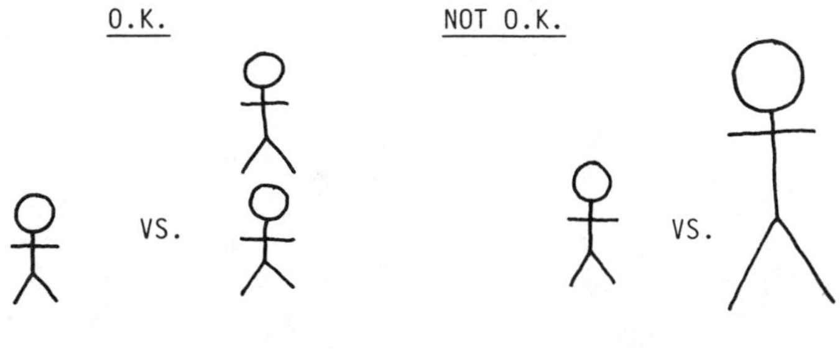

7. PROGRAM-IMPLEMENTATION STRATEGIES

At this point, you should feel comfortable with client-oriented questions and data summaries. Now the question is how to generate understanding throughout your program's management structure. If the double-edged sword is to work properly, all levels of your program (from line staff to board members) should ask questions about your program's products. Their questions and the data summaries ought to be appropriately tailored to their unique organizational levels and roles. A recommended strategy is similar to ones outlined in other chapters of the book (e.g., chapters 2 and 6):

(1) Assemble a small group of 4–8 friendly, middle-management colleagues to review and perform the exercises in this chapter. Ask them to do the exercises on their own and then come together for a group discussion. Raise such questions as:
   — Is asking an incomplete question by itself necessarily bad? (''No, but to raise only such questions without some integration can produce a negative management climate.'')
   — Are there positive and negative instances in your program?

(2) End the first friendly colleague session with a discussion of:
   — How will we train middle management and line staff? Who will be responsible for coordinating these tasks?
   — How will we train members of the board? Who will be responsible for coordinating these tasks?
   — What time commitments and resources will be needed?

After having oriented and trained the people involved in your program to the issues covered in this and earlier chapters, implementing a client-oriented cost-outcome system becomes a matter of technical development.

One area, however, may still raise some resistance among staff. Can costs be directly and usefully related to clinical activity, planning, and outcome? The following chapters deal with cost finding, cost outcome, and cost effectiveness for program analysis at all levels (from clinical supervisors to policy analysis and development).

SECTION VII

MANAGEMENT SUPPORT—PART II: DATA ANALYSIS FOR MANAGEMENT USE

We Are All Managers of Something and the Use of Data to Support our Decision Making Cuts the Line between Considered Decisions and Seat-of-the-pants Conjectures.

The first two of the four chapters in Section VII describe how client outcomes and cost data can be used together to help identify where strengths and weaknesses exist in clinical services (Chapter 21) and in program policies (Chapter 22).

The last two chapters focus on the design and analysis of planned studies of the relative cost effectiveness of two or more programs.

Chapter 21
Cost-Outcome Analysis of Clinical Services

How Much Does it Cost to Improve My Clients?
What Proportion of My Resources Were Consumed
by Lower Functioning Clients?
Who Are My High-cost Clients?
Who Are My High-risk Clients?
Are More Favorable Outcomes Associated with Special Combinations
of Services or Client Characteristics?

Putting client-service costs and outcomes together is the most popular feature of a client-oriented system. The system focuses on what happens to the client. It provides a means of analysis which integrates all clinical, management, and fiscal components in terms of the individual client's problems, goals, and outcomes. Almost all of the clinical and fiscal data needed is awaiting analysis by clinical staff and program managers.

Chapter 21 initiates a four-chapter series describing techniques for linking clinical outcome and cost data for the analysis of clinical services and program policies. This chapter focuses on clinical-service analysis and use of cost-outcome data for clinical supervision and utilization review. Chapter 22 focuses on program policies, and provides a means of analyzing the client cost-outcome data relative to the expectations raised by your program's policies. Together, these chapters provide you and your staff with the means of analyzing client characteristics, service efforts, and program policies in relation to varying levels of client outcomes and costs. Chapters 26 and 27 describe techniques to estimate which factors are most likely to lead to cost-effective services for each unique group of clients.

Stated in another way, the first two units provide a means of identifying which clinical factors may have influenced client cost and outcome results in the past. The last two chapters provide a means to isolate the most cost-effective factors, thereby providing guidance for revising clinical procedures and program policies.

The current chapter focuses on techniques for using cost-outcome data in clinical-service analysis. Specifically, the chapter will describe how to identify the relationships among client characteristics, service efforts, service costs, and cost-outcome results. The outline of the chapter is:

(1) COMBINING CLIENT OUTCOMES WITH SERVICE COSTS: Two issues are addressed: (a) Why combine cost and outcome data for clinical service and management analysis? and (b) What measures of client outcome and costs should be selected for this analysis? The first issue is one of identifying the potential products. The second issue will help focus on the relationship of client-cost and outcome data with clinical procedures and program policies.

(2) READING THE COST-OUTCOME MATRIX: This section provides instruction in the use of a single cost-outcome matrix for analysis of clinical services.

(3) IDENTIFYING CRITICAL CLINICAL ISSUES, USING THE COST-OUTCOME MATRIX: By contrasting the results of a number of cost-outcome matrices, relationships can be seen among a number of client and clinical service variables. When each matrix represents a different combination of client and/or service characteristics, research hypotheses can be formulated about what variables may be producing differences in client cost-outcome results.

(4) SUMMARIZING COST-OUTCOME RESULTS, USING A DECISION TREE: A *Decision Tree* provides an additional procedure for contrasting the client cost and outcome results across different subgroups of client and/or service characteristics.

(5) APPROPRIATE USE OF COST-OUTCOME ANALYSIS: Describes some of the technical limits on the descriptive analysis of cost-outcome results.

(6) APPLICATION AND IMPLEMENTATION STRATEGIES: This section provides a brief outline of the kinds of information needed, how to format and present cost outcome data for use by the clinical-service managers and staff.

The examples and exercises used throughout Chapter 21 will emphasize applications of client cost-outcome analysis to clinical-service management. Quality assurance and utilization review are highlighted. The analysis of cost-outcome data at this level will raise critical questions about both clinical procedures and program policies.

1. COMBINING CLIENT OUTCOMES WITH SERVICE COSTS

Why combine client behavioral data with service costs? Many professionals find the combination of client outcome with cost data to be both distasteful and distracting from the central concerns of client well-being and the provision of quality care. Yet, the combination of client outcome and cost data is, in fact, central to the theme of client well-being and quality care. According to all established professional standards, a treatment plan, and the actual clinical services provided to the client, are designed to help the client move toward his or her clinical goals and impact on their problems or deficits. A treatment plan is simply a means of budgeting clinical resources to assist in attaining treatment goals. Between 60% and 80% of a program's budget (resources) are clinical staff. Thus, each and every treatment plan commits part of the financial budget. Likewise, each budgetary decision by program management to allocate, or not to allocate, funds for clinical resources (e.g., staff) will directly influence treatment planning, services provided, and therefore affect client outcomes. Accordingly, if service efforts are considered to be influential on client outcomes, and program costs are directly related to service efforts, then client-service cost data and client-outcome data can help draw direct connections between service efforts and client problems and outcomes. By properly combining cost and outcome data, we can address clinical issues on quality of care, clinical service objectives, and the most effective use of limited clinical resources.

The second crucial question which must be addressed is the identification of "What are the appropriate measures of client outcome and service costs?" Here the best answer appears to beg the question. The most appropriate measures of client outcome and service costs are those reflecting the question being asked about client outcome and service costs. First, let us inspect the characteristics of an appropriate question and then we will inspect the characteristics of the measures of costs and outcomes.

If the question asked is a "client-oriented question" (see Chapter 20), then the measures must be sensitive to, and show relationships among:

— Client characteristics
— Service efforts
— Client outcome

Moreover, if the question asked is within the program context of a "client-oriented system" (see Chapters 2 and 3), then the measures must help relate service efforts to program goals for each specific target group. In summary, the appropriate measures will permit you to address questions which draw relationships among client characteristics, service efforts, and client outcome for specific target groups of clients and program-service goals.

The characteristics of the measures themselves can be briefly outlined as follows. The measures should:

— Be sensitive to changes in client behaviors as a function of service efforts (see Chapter 2).
— Be relatively consistent and dependable over time and among observers (see Chapter 14).
— Be verifiable (validated) by external criteria (see Chapter 14).
— Be adequately defined to identify what can and cannot be generalized from descriptive statistics involving the measures (see Chapter 14).
— Be cheaply obtained and easily used.
— Be sensitive to misuse, so that if misused or misinterpreted, such abuses are readily detected (see Chapters 12–15).

For many questions raised in client-oriented systems, a global level of functioning rating can provide an initial measure of outcome. For more detailed questions, more detailed measures on specific symptoms or behavior patterns are necessary. Routine measures obtained by clinical staff on global functioning and problem lists are the most relevant to clinicians, the easiest and the cheapest to obtain; but, they can only be considered as reliable, dependable, and valid if the precautions outlined in Section II (particularly the review procedures) and Section IV (particularly the staff-development and measurement procedures) are followed. Followup and observations by trained external interviewers are also needed, but these are more difficult and expensive to obtain. We recommend these outcome measures should be reserved for specific evaluation studies on issues of critical importance.

Similar issues exist with measures of cost. Cost data in a client-oriented system must reflect the kind and amount of effort and resources allocated on behalf of the client. The cost measures should be sensitive to differences in the type of clinical-service effort and the kind of backup support of the clinical effort provided on behalf of clients. More effort or more expensive (valued) efforts should be reflected in higher costs accumulated during a client's clinical episode. The unit-of-service cost finding procedures described in Section V have these features. Specifically, the linking of cost data to individual service efforts permits a summary description of service effort (cost) over the course of an individual client's clinical episode.

Cost and outcome data can be easily brought together to describe any part or all of the clinical episode if:

— A global level of functioning judgment is made at each clinical encounter (e.g., each visit for outpatient, each day on partial hospitalization or day care, and each shift for inpatient or residential care).
— Multidimensional measures of problems, strengths, and supports are obtained at intake, review, termination, and (for a sample of clients) at followup (in addition to the global level of functioning).

Up to this point, the issue of which measures of outcome to use still has not been addressed directly, and can be addressed now that we have reviewed the related issues. Initially, use the outcome measures most easily and cheaply obtained and interpreted (e.g., global level of functioning or depression or development); then, followup this initial analysis using an approach of successive approximations. Use more sensitive and expensively processed multidimensional outcome measures only when needed for more specific questions.

Initially, cost outcome data will be summarized in terms of episode (or 3–6 month time period) costs and global levels of functioning at two critical points in time.[1] We will see that a major objective of cost-outcome analysis techniques is to assist clinical service-management staff in formulating better questions and to identify where staff may look for better answers to these questions. By the time you complete Chapters 21 and 22, you may observe the moral of James Thurber's story about *The Scotty Who Knew Too Much*: ". . . It is better to know *some* of the questions than to know *all* of the answers."

Now we can turn to an exposition of the techniques of analysis; first, to the reading and use of a single cost-outcome matrix and then to the use of multiple matrices to identify the key issues needing review and study.

2. READING THE COST-OUTCOME MATRIX

We start the review of the techniques of cost-outcome analysis with the most general kind of summary of data for a single group of clients: mental-health adult clients, ages 18–40, whose treatment plans called for improvement over a 6-month period. Figure 1 on the next page summarizes what happened to 240 of this type of client admitted during a 6-month period, January 1 to June 30. The exercise questions following the figure will help you understand how to read and interpret the matrix of cost-outcome data.

---

[1] Other outcome measures besides level of functioning may be used. While the examples and exercises in Chapters 21–24 use a global level of functioning scale, any other measure may be used which is suitable to the client group, services, and program objectives under analysis.

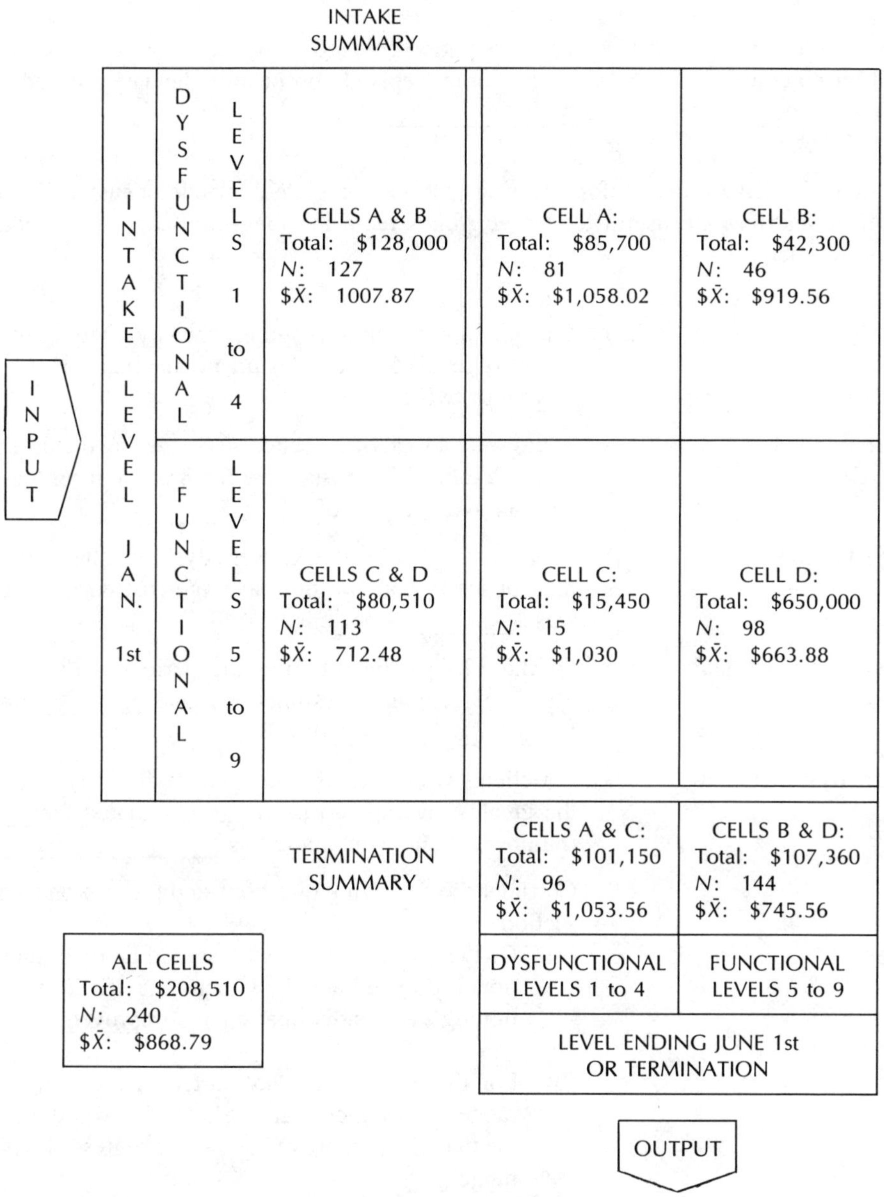

Figure 1. A Cost-Outcome Matrix for MH Adults, Ages 18–40

An Exercise on Reading a Summary Matrix

The following questions are based on Figure 1. The answers are provided in the left column. Please cover the solutions until you have entered your answer; then compare your answer before attempting the next question. Be sure to review any item where your answer and the suggested answer disagree.

Answer	*Question*
(1) June 30th or at termination	(1) The time period covered in the matrix starts at the beginning of the clinical episode on or after January 1st and ends on ________________.

You could have a matrix for covering just the completed episode or just a time period. Time period matrices are useful for target groups requiring long-term care, e.g., retarded or chronic-care clients.

(2) 1–4	(2) The nine-point scale was summarized by dividing functional clients of levels 5–9 and dysfunctional clients of levels ____ ____ into two groups.
(3) $868.79	(3) There were a total of 240 clients seen during the time period, whose total service costs were $208,510 during the period, with an average cost of $(\bar{X})$ = $_________ per client.
(4) $1,007.87	(4) There were 127 clients who were dysfunctional at the beginning of the period and their average cost during the period was $_________ per client.
(5) 81; 46; functional	(5) Of the 127 persons starting the period as dysfunctional, ________ remained dysfunctional and ________ improved to ________________ levels.
(6) 81; dysfunctional	(6) For clients who were *dysfunctional* at the end of the period, the greatest average costs were accumulated for ________ (number) clients who started as ________________.
	(7) Consider the following questions and then go on to the next section:
	(a) Of the 98 individuals who started and remained functional, do you know how many specific levels of functioning these individual clients improved?
(7a) No	Yes ________ No ________
	(b) For the 81 clients who started and remained in the range of dysfunctional levels (1–4), would it be possible that some improved and some regressed within this range?
(7b) Yes	Yes ________ No ________

From the answers to items 7a. and 7b., you might wish to conclude that this form of data summary is too crude to detect some important differences in costs and outcomes. This conclusion is essentially correct and, therefore, we recommend following up this level of analysis with a more detailed picture of a matrix involving all nine levels of functioning. But before leaving this data summary, let us review some of the rich interpretations this admittedly crude summary can provide.

Getting at Quality and Utilization

Armed with this simple matrix, several important quality assurance and utilization questions can be raised. Human-service managers are concerned about

— high clinical risks
— high clinical costs
— clinical puzzles (things that don't seem right)

These were the issues raised in the chapters on quality of care. Can the cost-outcome matrix help? Let's see.

Where Is the Greatest Clinical Risk? Probably those who started as functional and at the end of the period are dysfunctional (Cell C: 15 individuals who regressed, consumed $15,450 or $1,030 on the average). As a clinical manager, a review of these 15 cases is likely to be a first action.

Where Is the Highest Clinical Cost? Those in Cell A (dysfunctional both at time one and time two) are the most costly. They have consumed $85,700 of the $208,510 (or 41%) of the total resource. The average cost per client ($\bar{X}$ = $1,058.02) is also the highest. But as clinical managers, we know lower functioning levels are going to be expensive. If we are trying to identify where cost containment should start, Cell A (maybe Cell B also with an average of $919.56) might be a safer place to start.

Where Are the Clinical Puzzles? Probably Cell B is our target. How can clients move from dysfunctional to functional status at less cost than those remaining in Cell A (viz., $919.56 in Cell B vs. $1,058.02 in Cell A). While the answer isn't apparent from the matrix, clinical managers now have a better idea of where to look for potential answers.

Better Descriptions of Who Consumed How Much Resource. Besides helping us with quality assurance and cost utilization questions, we can better describe what happens to our resources *and* our clients. Contrast the two following service managers' explanations:

> Service Manager A (*without* a cost-outcome matrix):
> "We spent $208,510 of an average of $868.79 on our target-group clients during the first 6 months."
> Service Manager B (*with* a cost-outcome matrix):
> "We spent $208,510 or an average of $868.79 on our target-group clients during the first 6 months.
> "About 41% ($85,700/$208,510) of our resources were consumed by the 34% (81/240) of our clients who started and still remained dysfunctional. This resource intensive group consumed almost 22% more than our average client (viz. $1,058.02 vs. $868.79). Approximately 41% (98/240) of the clients were functional at the beginning and ending, however, they consumed only about 31% of the resources. This group consumed about three-quarters of the average client (viz., $663.88 vs. $868.79).
> "Fifteen clients regressed into a dysfunctional status and are the source of a current review."

Which is the better analysis? Remember, the only thing added was a simple dichotomy *between* functional and dysfunctional. Isn't the additional descriptive richness and improved managerial control startling? We think so. Imagine what can happen if all of the nine-point scale were used?

Before continuing, however, a note about the example and sample data is needed. While these data are fictitious, they have been designed to help highlight the major issues you might face when actually using cost-outcome data. The example uses the outcome measure of level of functioning, and the client data in the example entered within the range of levels 3–7. All clients in the example have treatment plans which recommend that improvement in either global level of functioning or symptom reduction (while maintaining their existing level of functioning) is possible within 6 months. We will see that these goals were apparent for 78% of the clients but not for the remaining 22%. We will also see that costs of services varied markedly among clients. The example illustrates how to use cost-outcome data to identify factors affecting costs and client outcomes.

Reading the Expanded Cost-Outcome Matrix: Self-study Exercise

Here are a series of statements and questions which will help you learn to read the matrix:

Totals. Over the six-month period, the

—total costs were $208,510
—number of clients were $N = 240$
—average[2] cost per client was $\bar{X} = \$869$ (rounded)

Find these data in Figure 2.

Marginal Totals. There were 71 people who started the period at Level 3, with a total cost of $72,500 and $\bar{X} = \$1,020$ per client.

Answer			
(8) $N = 56$	(8)	How many persons started at Level 4?	$N =$ ______
(9) $55,550	(9)	What were their total costs?	Total = $______
(10) $991	(10)	What was their average cost?	$\bar{X} =$ $______
(11) $N = 63$	(11)	How many persons ended at Level 5?	$N =$ ______
(12) $56,250	(12)	What were their total costs?	Total = $______
(13) $830	(13)	What were their average costs?	$\bar{X} =$ $______

The Cells of the Matrix. There were 56 persons who started at Level 4 and by June 30th, 15 had improved to Level 5 (4th row, 5th column). The total costs for these 15 people over the 6-month period was $130,000 with an average cost of $867 per person.

(14) $N = 18$	(14)	How many persons started and ended at Level 4 (maintained at Level 4)?	$N =$ ______
(15) $18,600	(15)	What were the total costs?	Total = $______
(16) $1,033	(16)	What were the average costs?	$\bar{X} =$ $______

[2]All average cost data have been rounded to the nearest dollar.

Answer		Question	
(17) $N = 36$	(17)	How many persons started at Level 3 and ended at Level 4 (improved to Level 4)?	$N =$ ______
(18) $34,150	(18)	What were the total costs?	Total = $______
(19) $949	(19)	What were the average costs?	$\bar{X} =$ $______
(20) $N = 7$	(20)	How many persons started at Level 5 and ended at Level 4 (regressed to Level 4)?	$N =$ ______
(21) $6,850	(21)	What were the total costs?	Total = $______
(22) $979	(22)	What were the average costs?	$\bar{X} =$ $______

Consider the expanded matrix of costs and outcomes in Figure 2. Clients grouped by initial level of functioning may be traced over time, with horizontal movement to the right of the shaded diagonal implying improvement, and movement to cells on the left of the diagonal implying regression. Total and average costs are accumulated by cell and by column and by row (viz., marginals).

LEVEL OF FUNCTIONING AT END OF PERIOD

LEVEL OF FUNCTIONING AT BEGINNING OF PERIOD		Level	INPUT	1 (Dysfunctional)	2 (Dysfunctional)	3 (Dysfunctional)	4 (Dysfunctional)	5 (Functional)	6 (Functional)	7 (Functional)	8 (Functional)	9 (Functional)
	DYSFUNCTIONAL	1										
	DYSFUNCTIONAL	2										
$128,000 127 $1007.81	DYSFUNCTIONAL	3	$72,500 71 $1,020.42		2,600 2 1,300	15,850 13 1219.23	34,150 36 948.61	15,300 15 1,020	4,600 5 920	IMPROVEMENT CELLS ARE ABOVE DIAGONAL		
	DYSFUNCTIONAL	4	$55,500 56 $991.07		3,900 3 1,300	10,600 9 1177.78	18,600 18 1033.33	13,000 15 866.67	7,750 9 861.11	1,650 2 825		
	FUNCTIONAL	5	$37,750 50 $725.96			3,700 3 1233.33	6,850 7 978.57	9,950 13 765.38	8,400 13 646.15	6,025 11 547.73	2825 5 565	
	FUNCTIONAL	6	$35,460 50 $707.20		REGRESSION CELLS ARE BELOW DIAGONAL		4,900 5 980	15,400 17 905.88	8,600 15 573.33	3,025 6 504.17	3,535 7 505	
$80,510 113 $712.48	FUNCTIONAL	7	$7,300 11 $572.73					2,600 3 866.67	2,600 4 650	1,200 2 600	900 2 450	
	FUNCTIONAL	8										
	FUNCTIONAL	9										
TOTAL: $208,510 240 $868.79					6,500 5 1,300	30,150 25 1206.00	64,500 66 977.27	56,250 63 829.86	31,950 56 570.54	11,900 21 566.67	7,260 14 518.57	

OUTPUT: DYSFUNCTIONAL $101,150 / 96 / $1,053.65; FUNCTIONAL $107,360 / 154 / $745.56

Figure 2. The Complete Cost-Outcome Matrix

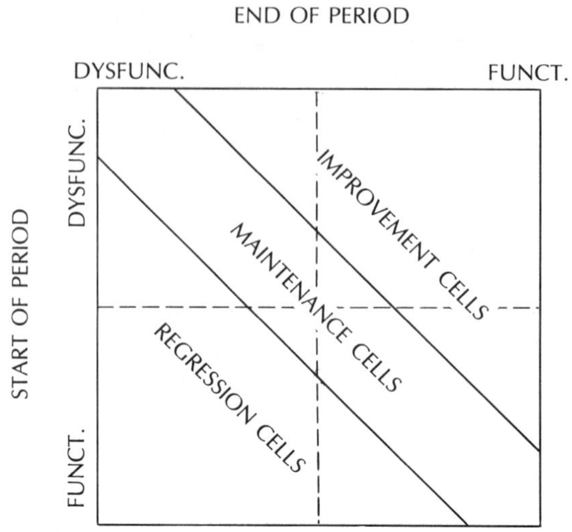

Figure 3. Global Picture of Client Movement

Looking at the Overall Picture

The matrix in Figure 2 can be viewed as a global picture of client movement over a specific time period. There are three general regions of cells in the matrix. As shown in Figure 3, these three general regions are cells representing improvement, maintenance, and regression. For a slightly more detailed overview, however, we could start with the understanding that both improvement and regression can occur within and across the dysfunctional (Levels 1–4) and functional ranges (Levels 5–9). Specifically, for those starting dysfunctional there are four possible outcomes, as shown in Figure 4. The clinical quality assurance issues raised within each of the four sectors of outcome differ. That is, followup courses of action by clinical or administrative staff would most likely differ.

Similarly, for those starting at a functional level, there are four sets of outcomes, as shown in Figure 5.

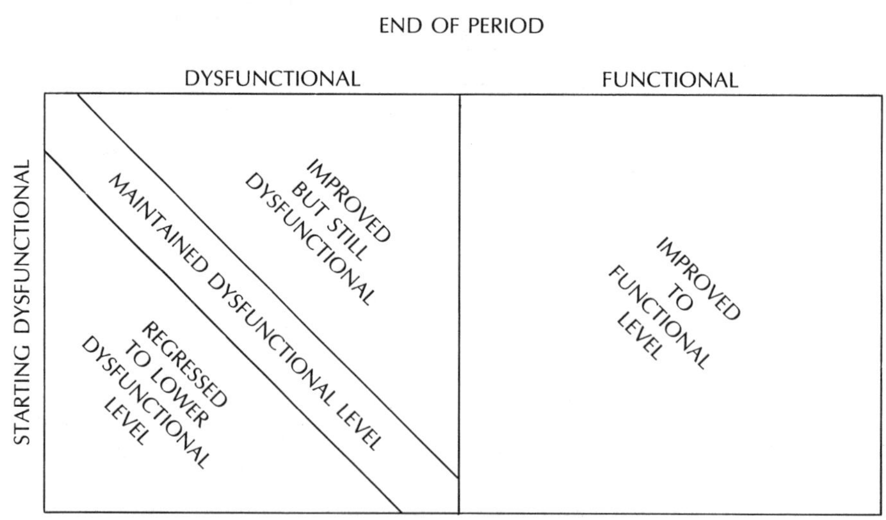

Figure 4. Global Picture for Clients Starting Dysfunctional

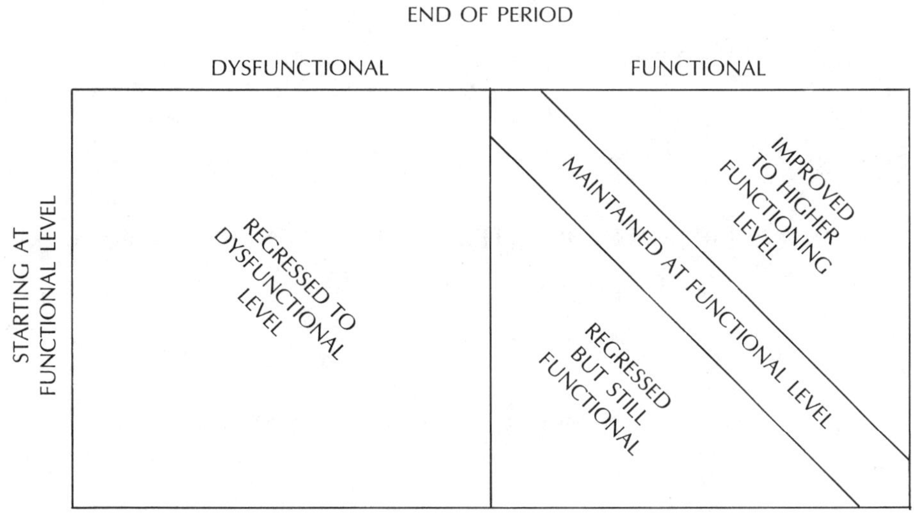

Figure 5. Global Picture for Clients Starting Functional

Thus, there are eight critical areas of the detailed cost-outcome matrix. Each of these eight areas of cost-outcome results raises unique clinical issues about the quality of care and allocation of clinical resources. Improved information results if each of these eight areas are summarized separately. In the following self-study exercise, you will see how the data are summarized and then be given some guidance on interpreting the data. The theme of the technique of data summarization is to assist in the formulation of better questions, i.e., questions which draw relationships among client characteristics, service efforts, and outcomes.

Self-study Exercise: Summarizing and Interpreting Cost-Outcome Results

The complete matrix does help you describe many of the critical issues which relate client characteristics and service efforts with outcomes. The exercise first shows how to summarize the data, and then suggests some of the interpretations made possible.

Summarizing the Cost-Outcome Data. The exercise uses the data on the clients who started at dysfunctional levels 1–4 as an example. The 127 clients who started the period dysfunctional can be described as ending the period in one of four categories: Regressed, maintained, improved but still dysfunctional, or improved to the functional levels 5–9. Compute the values of Total Costs, N, and average costs, $\$\bar{X}$, for each of these four categories.

Answers

REGRESSED (TO LOWER LEVELS)

(1) $17,100	(1) Total costs = $2,600 + $3,900 + $10,600 =	$______
(2) 14	(2) $N = 2 + 3 + 9 =$	______
(3) $1,221.43	(3) Average Costs, $\$\bar{X}$, = (Total $/$N$) = *Note:* Be sure that you use the cell total costs rather than the cell means for computing the average $\bar{X}$ over cells.	$______

MAINTAINED (AS DYSFUNCTIONAL)

(4)	\$34,450	(4)	Sum total \$ for cells 3-3 and 4-4 = Total \$ =	\$______
(5)	31	(5)	N =	______
(6)	\$1111.20 (\$1111)	(6)	$\$\bar{X}$ =	\$______

IMPROVED, BUT STILL DYSFUNCTIONAL (Less than Level 5)

(7)	\$34,150	(7)	Total \$ =	\$______
(8)	36	(8)	N =	______
(9)	\$948.61	(9)	$\$\bar{X}$ =	\$______

IMPROVED TO FUNCTIONAL LEVELS (5–9)

(10)	\$42,300	(10)	Total \$ =	\$______
(11)	46	(11)	N =	______
(12)	\$919.56 (\$920)	(12)	$\$\bar{X}$ =	\$______

The composite picture looks as follows:

	Client Initially Dysfunctional (N = 127)				
	To How Many?		At What Costs?		
What Happened?	N	% of Group	Total \$	% Total	$\$\bar{X}$*
Regressed	14	11.0%	\$17,100	13.4%	\$1,221
Maintained	31	24.4%	\$34,450	26.9%	\$1,111
Improved, Still Dysfunctional	36	28.3%	\$34,150	33.0%	\$ 949
Improved to Functional (5–9)	46	36.2%	\$42,300	33.5%	\$ 920
TOTAL	127	99.9%	\$128,000	99.9%	\$1,008

*Rounded to nearest dollar.

(13) Recall that all of these clients had treatment plans which called for improvement. With this in mind, what followup questions or actions might your pursue?

(13a) As a clinical supervisor or treatment-team leader?[3] ____________________

____

____

(13b) As a Utilization or Quality Assurance Review Committee chairperson? ______

____

____

[3] When cost-outcome matrices are produced for clinical staff use, it is necessary to provide a listing of clients (usually by I.D. numbers), grouped by cells within the matrix. Client confidentiality would require that only case numbers be used in these reports.

(14) The greatest percentage of clients improved to functional levels 5–9 and they had the lowest costs. What followup questions or actions might you pursue?
(14a) As a clinical supervisor or treatment-team leader? ____________________
____
____
(14b) As a Utilization or Quality Assurance Review Committee chairperson? ______
____
____

To Complete the Picture. We should next inspect what the summarized cost outcome results were for those who started service at the functional levels.

	Clients Initially Functional (N = 113) (Levels 5–9)				
	How Many?		At What Costs?		
What Happened?	N	% Funct.	Total$	% Total	$\$\bar{X}$*
Regressed to Dysfunctional	15	7.5%	$15,450	19.2%	$1,030
Regressed, But Still Functional	24	21.2%	$20,600	25.6%	$ 858
Maintained	30	26.5%	$19,750	24.5%	$ 658
Improved	44	38.9%	$24,710	30.7%	$ 562
TOTALS	113	94.1%	$80,510	100.00%	$ 712

*Rounded to nearest dollar.

(15) Again, the clients who regressed in their overall level of functioning consumed a larger proportion of the service costs. Which clients require immediate followup actions and what questions might you raise? ______________________________
____
____

(16) Only 38.9% of these intially functional clients actually improved, while just 26.5% were maintained. Again, what followup actions and questions might you raise?
(16a) As a clinical supervisor or treatment-team leader? ____________________
____
____
(16b) As a Utilization or Quality Assurance Review Committee chairperson? ______
____
____

(17) Overall, 156 of the 240 clients showed the expected improvement in functioning. This represents just 65% of the clients to achieve their goals. This is hardly satisfactory. One way of dealing with this poor showing is to try to determine what other variables (factors) may be influencing these outcomes. This can easily be done by inspecting the cost-outcome data matrices for subgroups of clients, where the subgroups may show differences in their patterns of cost-outcome results. Identify two or more client or service variables which you think may show differences in patterns of cost-outcome results.

Client Variables		Service Variables	
(1)	______________	(1)	______________
(2)	______________	(2)	______________
(3)	______________	(3)	______________

Answers to Items 13–17

(13) Regarding regressed and maintained clients:

(13a) Clinical Supervisor: Have records of the regressed clients pulled immediately and review with responsible clinicians, asking: "What is presently happening to and for these clients? Is immediate intervention needed? Were original goals realistic? Were services appropriate to clients' problems and situation? Were external influences evident? Was there any characteristic(s) peculiar to these clients relative to those who did not regress?" For the clients who maintained their level of functioning rather than improved, the same sorts of questions might be asked. An additional question would be: "Was improvement in any of the clients' problem areas evident, even though overall functioning was maintained?"

(13b) Utilization and Quality Assurance Review Committee Chairpersons: Meet with the clinical supervisors and research evaluation director to review: "Were there certain client characteristics or service factors which appear to differentiate the regressed and maintained clients relative to those who improved? If so, are changes in clinical standards and procedures recommended? Are follow-up client-care studies suggested?"

(14) Regarding improved clients:

(14a) Clinical Supervisor: Have a sample of records pulled to match what did occur with these clients relative to what was planned, and ask: "What was the match of client and therapist characteristics? Were services consistently applied to these clients? If not, what patterns were related to success? Were certain client characteristics peculiar to these clients?"

(14b) Utilization and Quality Assurance Review Committee Chairpersons: Meet with clinical supervisors and research evaluation director to review the same issues described in 13b, above. The emphasis here, however, is usually on affirming your existing clinical standards and procedures.

(15) Clients who started at the functional levels and regressed to the dysfunctional levels require immediate followup. Again we need to ask: "What is presently happening to and for these clients? Is immediate intervention needed? Were there client or service variables which were peculiar to this group of clients relative to those who maintained or improved their level of functioning?"

(16) When contrasting improved with maintained clients, some of the issues which could be addressed are as follows:

(16a) As a Clinical Supervisor: With responsible clinicians ask: "Was there improvement in particular problem or symptom areas for those who maintained their functional levels? What client or service-effort characteristics may have accounted for these differences in outcome?"

(16b) As Utilization and Quality Assurance Review Committee Chairpersons: Meeting with the clinical supervisors and evaluation research director, pursue the same line of questions raised in 13b, above. The issues raised here should be combined with those raised in the other items (i.e., 13b, 14b, and 15) to develop a coordinated followup action plan for client-care evaluation studies, as well as a review of existing clinical standards and procedures. Before pursuing such followup actions, a more detailed analysis of the cost-outcome results is needed.

(17) *Client Variables*: (a) Prior psychiatric hospitalization history; (b) Family or social supports; (c) Major presenting problems, e.g., psychosis, neurosis. *Service Variables*: (a) Individual, group therapy; (b) Chemotherapy, no chemotherapy.

3. IDENTIFYING CRITICAL CLINICAL ISSUES

The result of reviewing a complete cost-outcome matrix in the fashion just described usually leads to an attempt to understand the differences, or lack of differences, among clients by dividing up and grouping the clients' cost-outcome results according to different client and/or service characteristics. Again, the emphasis is on formulating better questions focusing on the relationships of client and service characteristics with outcome. An enriched view can be obtained by comparing two cost-outcome matrices. Finally, contrasting a number of client and service groupings of results is accomplished through the use of a decision tree. Together, these techniques of cost-outcome data analysis will assist in the formulation of a series of sharper questions to be tested in a formal evaluation study.

Self-study Exercise: Contrasting Cost-outcome Matrix Results

After reviewing the overall (9 × 9 cell) cost-outcome matrix and addressing the issues raised in the last exercise, a natural consequence is to wish to review the cost-outcome matrices of various client subgroups to determine what factors might be related to different patterns of cost-outcome results. For a first step, suppose we review the results of two subgroups, e.g., clients with:

— No Prior Psychiatric Hospitalization History
— Prior Psychiatric Hospitalization History

We divide the 240 clients into these two subgroups and find:

N (No) = 130 clients, with *no* prior hospitalization
N (Yes) = 110 clients *with* prior hospitalization.

Figure 6 provides the matrices for these two subgroups, with the *NO Prior Hosp.* group cost-outcome data represented in the upper matrix and the *YES Prior Hosp.* group cost-outcome data represented in the lower matrix. A quick viewing of these two matrices may, at first, feel overwhelming. The exercise questions which follow the matrices will describe a strategy for working your way into and using the cost-outcome data constructively.

The recommended approach is similar to that of eating many fruits and vegetables—you start working your way *from the outside to the inside,* contrasting the two matrix results as you do so. Specifically, we usually start our analysis by reviewing the overall cost data, then the marginal totals at intake and at the end of the period, and finally the cell entries within the respective sectors of the matrix representing entry level of functioning and outcome in terms of regression, maintenance or improvement.

NO PRIOR HOSP. HISTORY

STARTING LEVEL				END OF PERIOD: DYSFUNCTIONAL 2	3	4	FUNCTIONAL 5	6	7	8
DYSF.	3	$71,450 72 $ 992	$41,400 41 $ 1,110	2 1,300	8 1,225	21 914	8 1,004	2 875		
DYSF.	4		$30,050 31 $ 969	1 1,300	5 1,140	12 1,033	8 838	4 813	1 700	
FUNCT.	5		$17,600 24 $ 733		1 1,300	4 1,000	6 758	5 680	6 567	2 475
FUNCT.	6	$41,510 58 $ 716	$20,710 29 $ 714			3 1,000	10 930	8 563	4 481	4 496
FUNCT.	7		$ 3,200 5 $ 640				1 900	2 600	1 700	1 400
No Prior Hosp. Hist. OVERALL				3,900 3 1,300	16,800 14 1,200	38,600 40 965	29,500 33 894	14,100 21 671	6,725 12 560	3,335 7 476
Total $112,960 N = 130 $\bar{X}$ $869				$59,300 57 $1,040			$53,660 73 $735			

Figure 6. Cost-outcome Matrices for Clients with No Prior Hospitalization and with Prior Hospitalization

(1) What were the differences in the overall average costs between the two groups? ______

____

(2) Now consider those who entered dysfunctional and those who entered functional across the two groups. Were their average costs equivalent? If not, how do they differ? _____

____

(3) Consider the output side, i.e., the *end of period* data. Were there any group differences evident here? ______________________________

____

(4) For those clients who entered dysfunctional (72 and 55 for the two groups, respectively), what were the proportions to show some improvement for each of the two groups.

(4a) ________% for the No Prior clients?

(4b) ________% for the Yes Prior clients?

YES PRIOR HOSP. HISTORY				DYSFUNCTIONAL			FUNCTIONAL			
STARTING LEVEL				2	3	4	5	6	7	8
DYSF.	3	$56,550 55 $ 1,028	$31,100 30 $ 1,037		5 1,225	15 997	7 1,036	3 950		
	4		$25,450 25 $ 980	2 1,300	4 1,225	6 1,033	7 900	5 900	1 950	
FUNCT.	5	$39,000 55 $ 709	$20,150 28 $ 720		2 1,200	3 950	7 771	8 625	5 525	3 625
	6		$14,750 21 $ 702			2 950	7 871	7 586	2 550	3 517
	7		$ 4,100 6 $ 683				2 850	2 700	1 500	1 500
Yes Prior Hosp. Hist. OVERALL				2,600 2 1,300	13,350 11 1,214	25,900 26 996	26,750 30 892	17,850 25 714	5,175 9 575	3,925 7 561
Total $95,550 N = 110 $\bar{X}$ $869				$41,850 39 $1,073			$53,700 71 $756			

Figure 6. ***continued***

Now calculate whether these proportions were the same for those who improved from the dysfunctional (3 or 4) to the functional.

(4c) ________% for the No Prior clients?

(4d) ________% for the Yes Prior clients?

(4e) Give a narrative description of these results ____________________

____

____

(5) Next, with just a visual inspection of the mean cost data for initially dysfunctional clients who improved to the functional levels (5–7), describe the kinds of differences in mean costs between the two groups for these clients.

(5a) ____

____

____

While there was approximately the same proportion of initially dysfunctional clients to improve but remain dysfunctional (i.e., 21/72 = .292 and 15/55 = .273), the mean costs differed. How so?

(5b) ____

____

____

(6) Now inspect what occurred for those who started service at the functional levels, 5 and above. A quick inspection of these data suggests that there were little differences in the patterns of cost-outcome results, except for those clients who showed improvement. Describe these differences in results between the two groups. ____________________

____

____

(7) The overall picture for these two subgroups still leaves us in the same dilemma. That is, a large proportion of both subgroups did not improve as expected. The cost data, however, does suggest that there were some differences in costs and, therefore, in amount or type of service. What service patterns would you suggest might account for these differences? _

____

____

Answers

(1) None.

(2) A slightly greater difference between dysfunctional and functional clients at intake for those who had a prior hospitalization history; but even these differences were not very large, $1,028 vs. $992 and $709 vs. $716, respectively.

(3) Here we inspect the output marginal totals. The differences between the two groups was small. However, those who had no prior hospitalization history tended to have less service costs if they ended the period at the higher levels of functioning.

(4) (4a) 61% for the *No Prior* clients.
(4b) 69% for the *Yes Prior* clients.
(4c) 32% for the *No Prior* clients.
(4d) 42% for the *Yes Prior* clients.
(4e) There was a greater proportion of the clients to improve overall in the *Prior Hosp.* group; however, this difference, while still great, was lessened when considering the percentages of those who improved to the functional levels 5 and above.

(5) (5a) The mean costs were lower in each cell.
(5b) Again, the mean costs were lower for those with no prior hospitalization history.

(6) The outcomes representing improvement to level 8 were all showing lower average costs for the *No Prior Hospitalization clients.* While these results are not conclusive by themselves, they do suggest that clients with no prior hospitalization histories do consume less resources in their improvement to level 8 of functioning. This raises the issue, once again, of what were the differences in services provided between the two groups.

(7) Service patterns which may be related to the observed differences in costs between the two groups are:

— Individual vs. Group Therapy
— Day (Partial Hospitalization) Treatment vs. Outpatient only

A brief review of the clinical records "Flow Sheets" for a sample of clients from each group would indicate which service variable to follow up.

4. SUMMARIZING COST-OUTCOME RESULTS USING A DECISION TREE

We now have better questions, but not answers. The cost-outcome analysis using the detailed matrices has been useful in identifying some specific issues which need to be followed up. In summary, the detailed matrices, when contrasting the two client groups, suggested that there were lower average service costs for the clients with no prior hospitalization history. Typically, the next step is to make a quick inspection of the clinical records Flow Sheets (see Chapter 10) for a sample of clients from both groups which should suggest possible differences in type and amount of services provided. The type of service listed on the Flow Sheet would suggest differences in unit-of-service costs accumulated for a client. Moreover, the costs increase with the amount of each type of service listed on the Flow Sheet.

Suppose a review of the Flow Sheets suggested day treatment was fairly constant across both groups when clients were at levels 3 and 4 of functioning; however, the amount of service costs appeared to be related to the use of group therapy. Suppose, further, that clinical policy was to graduate clients from the day-treatment program if they could constructively participate in group therapy. This policy could be related to the decrease in service costs for clients receiving group therapy, *but,* were these reduced costs also influenced by whether the clients had a history of prior psychiatric hospitalization? To follow this issue up, we could then partition the two prior hospitalization groups in terms of whether they had participated in group therapy or just had individual therapy.

The path of inquiry has now proceeded along three steps, which can be described as branches in what is called a *decision tree* (see Figure 7).

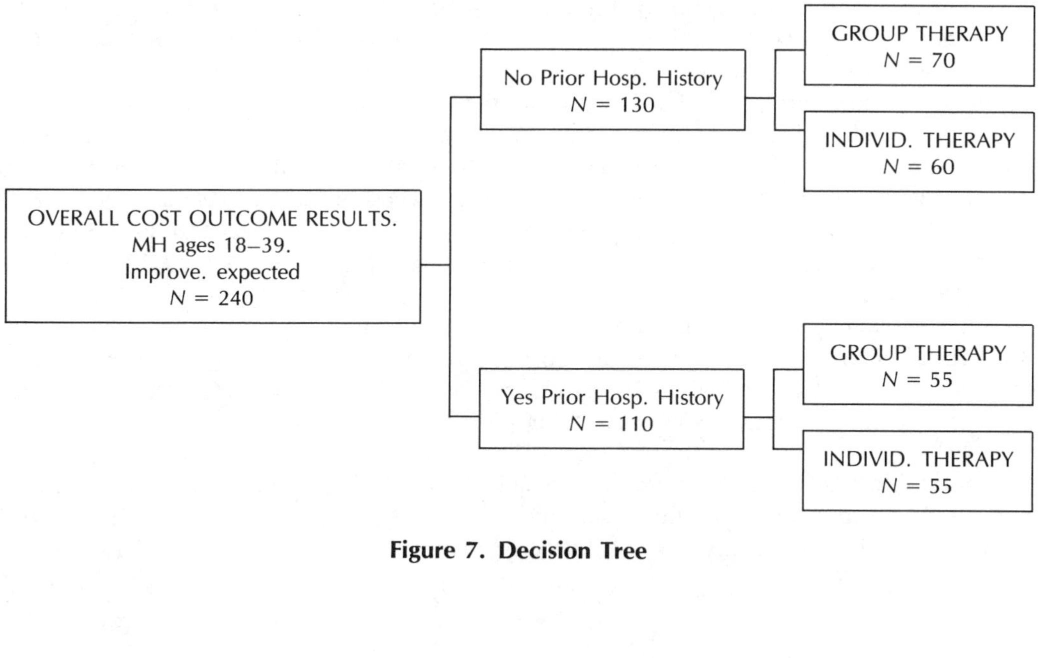

Figure 7. Decision Tree

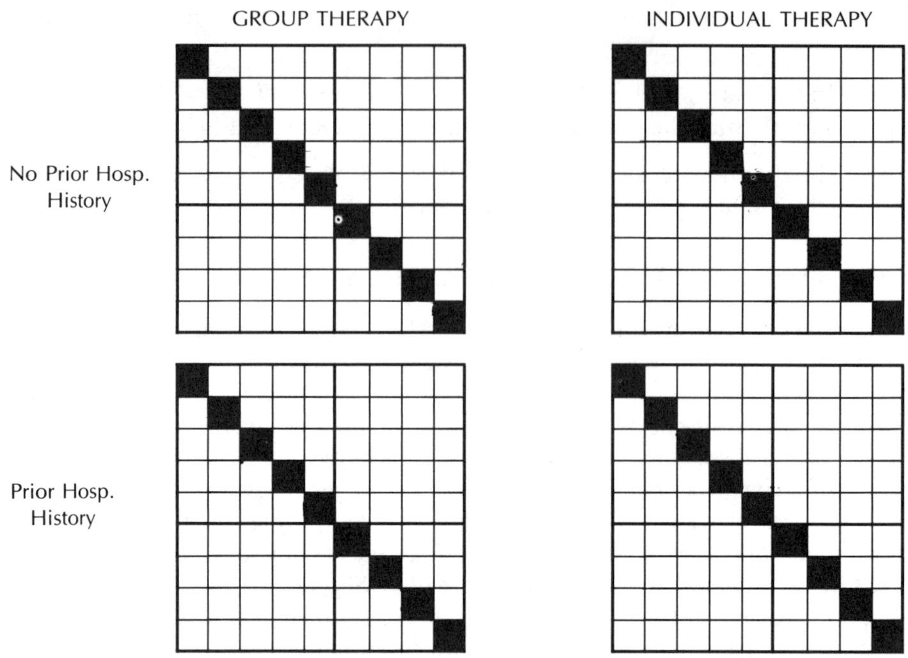

Figure 8. Cost-outcome Matrices for Hospital and Service History

To analyze the cost-outcome data you have two major choices in the form of analysis. One way would be to prepare four detailed, 9 × 9 cell, cost outcome matrices and inspect these four matrices accordingly, as shown in Figure 8.

This detailed approach is useful, but often cumbersome since so much data is reviewed at once. Another approach is to use a summary table of the data which reflects the logic of the decision tree.

The data in the upper portion of Table 1 summarize the final step of the decision tree. The rows represent the four combinations of prior psychiatric hospitalization history and therapeutic services (individual vs. group therapy). The columns are organized according to both entry and exit levels of outcome (level of functioning in the present example). The cells of the table provide the number of clients and the average costs rounded to the nearest dollar. The rationale for organizing the columns of the table is based upon the types of clinical and managerial decisions needed to be made in followup. The types of questions and issues raised because of differences within a column (over client subgroups) will be uniquely different from those issues raised by data within other columns. The self-study exercise which follows Table 1 will provide examples of this feature.

The remaining tables on the page represent the earlier steps in the decision-tree analysis. The two center tables provide the cost-outcome data for the single variables of service and prior history, and the bottom table gives the grand total. The following self-study exercise will help you see how this decision-tree descriptive analysis will formulate better questions.

Self-study Exercise. This exercise is designed to provide some experience with reviewing cost-outcome data in a decision-tree descriptive analysis. The emphasis is on how this form of analysis can help you identify and clarify the issues which need to be addressed for clinical service management.

Table 1. Cost-outcome Results for the Interaction of Two Variables: Prior Hospitalization History and Services Including Group Therapy

(EXAMPLE OF DECISION TREE)

Branches of Decision Tree		Started Dysfunctional (Levels 1–4)				Started Functional (Levels 5–7)				Totals
Prior Hosp. Hist.	Services Includes Group Therapy	Regressed	Maintain.	Improved Dysfunc.	Improved to Funct.	Regressed Dysfunc.	Regressed Func.	Maintain.	Improved	Service by Prior Hosp.
NO PRIOR	INDIVID.	4 $1,250	12 $1,142	9 $1,000	7 $ 979	5 $1,060	7 $893	7 $750	9 $667	60 $948
	GROUP	4 $1,150	8 $1,063	12 $ 850	16 $ 850	3 $1,000	6 $858	8 $563	13 $446	70 $794
YES PRIOR	INDIVID.	4 $1,300	7 $1,150	8 $1,075	9 $1,072	4 $1,025	7 $829	7 $771	9 $683	55 $963
	GROUP	2 $1,150	4 $1,050	7 $ 907	14 $ 871	3 $1,017	4 $850	8 $575	13 $500	55 $775
SINGLE VARIABLE RESULTS	SERVICE RESULTS									
	INDIVID. THERAPY	8 $1,275	19 $1,145	17 $1,035	16 $1,031	9 $1,044	14 $861	14 $761	18 $675	115 $946
	GROUP THERAPY	6 $1,150	12 $1,058	19 $ 871	30 $ 860	6 $1,008	10 $855	16 $569	26 $483	125 $786
	PRIOR HISTORY									
	NO	8 $1,200	20 $1,110	21 $ 914	23 $ 889	8 $1,038	13 $877	15 $650	22 $548	130 $869
	YES	6 $1,250	11 $1,113	15 $ 997	23 $ 950	7 $1,021	11 $836	15 $667	22 $575	110 $869
	GRAND TOTALS	14 $1,221	31 $1,111	36 $ 949	46 $ 920	15 $1,030	24 $858	30 $658	44 $562	240 $829

(1) What differences in cost-outcome results are apparent for clients who started service at dysfunctional levels 1–4 and improved? Attend to the relative proportions to improve to higher levels of dysfunction or to the functional levels of 5–9. Also note the relative costs for these two levels of improvement.

(2) What issues should be addressed in followup to the analysis described in question 1, above?

(3) The middle two tables describe cost-outcome results in terms of the two major variables singly. Review the data for the initially dysfunctional clients who improved within these

single variable tables and ask: "Were the single variable tables adequate to show the effects seen in the topmost table?" ______________________________

____

____

____

(4) Return to the topmost table and review the cost-outcome data for the clients who started at the functional levels. Identify at least two trends and issues which are apparent here.
(a) ______________________________
____
(b) ______________________________
____

(5) Did these two variables fully explain the high proportions of clients to either maintain or regress in their levels of overall functioning? ______________________________

____

____

____

____

Answers

(1) Re: Clients starting dysfunctional and improving:
- (a) The proportions to improve but still be dysfunctional were about the same (.13 to .17), but the average costs were lower for those receiving group therapy, particularly those with no prior hospitalization history.
- (b) The most noticeable differences in proportions were among those to improve to the functional levels, 5 and above. The average costs for both prior history groups were the lowest.

		Improved Still Dysf.	Improved to Funct.
No	Individ.	9/60 = .15 @ $1,000	7/60 = .12 @ $979
	Group	12/70 = .17 @ $850	16/70 = .23 @ $850
Yes	Individ.	8/35 = .15 @ $1,075	9/35 = .16 @ $1,072
	Group	7/55 = .13 @ $907	14/55 = .25 @ $871

(2) Some followup issues which might be addressed are:
—Were the family or social support systems of the clients equivalent? For example, one might expect family/social support to accentuate the differences between group and

individual therapy, particularly if the groups emphasized social support within their sessions.

—Were the clients with prior hospitalization histories also differentiated by family/social supports? Moreover, were those with no such supports influencing the cost differential the most?

—What were the major presenting problems which might further differentiate those who improved the most?

(3) No.

(4) For clients who started at functional levels 5 and above:

(a) There is an interaction of outcomes, service mode, and service costs. For clients who maintained or improved, clients receiving group therapy cost much less than individual therapy clients. These cost differences were greatly diminished, almost equal for those who regressed. These trends did not appear to be influenced by prior hospitalization history.

(b) There is also a greater proportion of regressed clients who had received individual therapy relative to those who had received group therapy.

(5) Maybe, but we may also try additional decision-tree analyses for clients with different levels of

—Family or social support

—Principal presenting problem

5. THE APPROPRIATE USE OF COST-OUTCOME ANALYSIS

We need to identify how the foregoing cost-outcome procedures can be used to their fullest advantage, without misusing the techniques or being misled. In brief, what can and cannot be accomplished with these procedures? The descriptive cost-outcome techniques of this chapter also fit with those described in Chapter 22 on policy analysis, and in Chapters 23 and 24 on cost effectiveness and evaluation-research design.

The approach is to identify critical *issues* emerging from our technical assistance efforts and to offer a *reply* summarizing our technical response to the issue. There are three major issues with specific questions within each category.

(a) Outcome scale sensitivity to change

— Will any outcome measure be equally sensitive to change for all clients?

— What is the appropriate measure for cost-outcome analyses?

— Shouldn't multivariate measures be used to describe outcome, rather than simple univariate measures of outcome?

— Will a unit of change on any behavioral outcome measure have the same meaning at all levels of the scale? Can statistical procedures requiring interval scales be applied?

(b) Costs as a process and an outcome measure

— Do costs reflect process or outcome or both?

— What are some of the relationships of costs with client and service variables?

— What kinds of costs are not covered in typical cost-outcome analyses?

(c) Cause and effect or chance outcomes

— What conclusions can be drawn on existing data?

— What changes in behavior can be expected by chance, natural causes and/or by regression toward the mean?

Each issue is addressed in turn.

(A) Outcome Scale Sensitivity to Change

ISSUE: Will any outcome measure be equally sensitive to change for all clients?

REPLY: No, and they should not be. From the very beginning, emphasis has been placed on tailoring measures and procedures to the clients served and to the programs providing the service. The measure (or measures) must be relevant to the relationships among clients' problems, goals, and service efforts. While the unit illustrates the use of cost-outcome analyses with a global level of functioning scale, the global scale is only appropriate for an overview of how overall program goals are met for clients with similar demographic and diagnostic characteristics. Global measures provoke followup inquiry.

ISSUE: What is the appropriate measure for cost-outcome analyses?

REPLY: The selection process proceeds sequentially by first identifying the major client and service characteristics. Psychometricians refer to this process as the domain or universe of measurement. The decision-tree shown in Figure 9 helps to identify the appropriate domain of measurement. These steps are actually the framework provided in Chapters 2–8 covering program goals and clinical-service design.

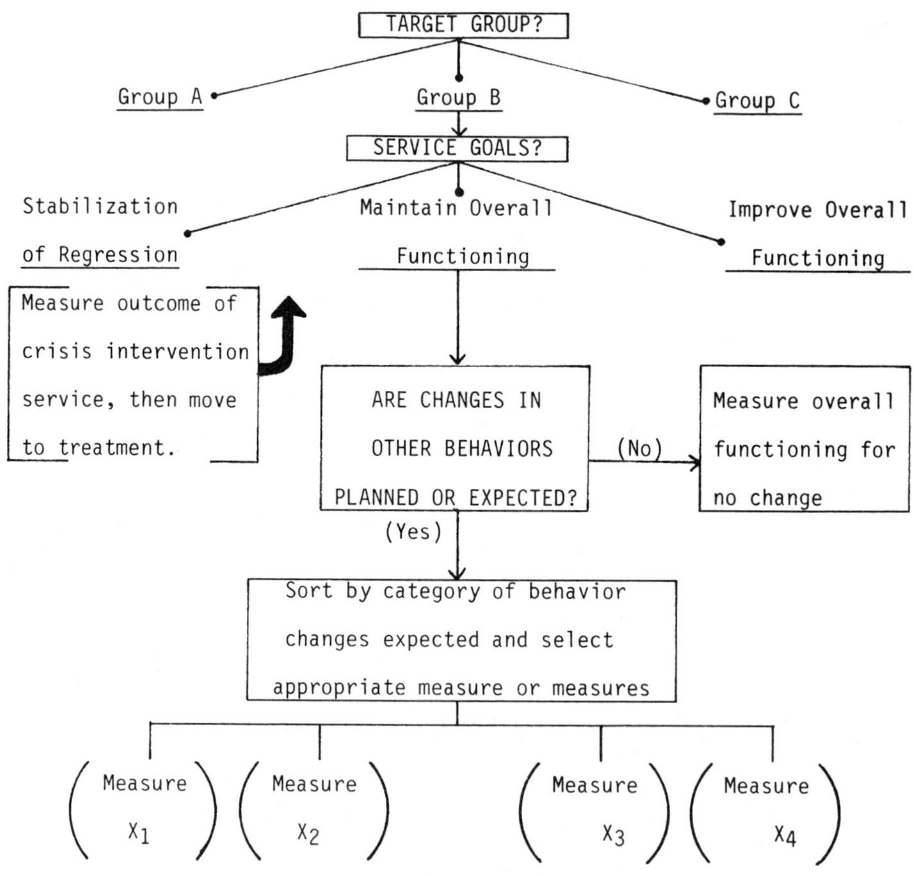

Figure 9. Selecting of Outcome Measures

ISSUE: Shouldn't multivariate measures be used to measure outcome rather than simple, single-dimension measures of outcome?

REPLY: Usually both are needed, but the measure depends upon the potential decisions and actions. Decisions and actions require the decision maker consider multidimensional (many faceted) data and integrate the multidimensional information to make unidimensional judgments and decisions. Like the preceding question, a branching process is required, but in reverse. While the general process is described below, the detailed procedure requires complex analytic and computing techniques. Some evidence suggests experienced and trained observers do reliable information processing and integration. Steps in the process include:

(1) Sort relevant from irrelevant information.

X_1 X_2 X_3 X_4 X_5 X_6	Y_1 Y_2 Y_3 Y_4
Relevant	Irrelevant

(2) Identify major categories and sort small bits of information by major categories (clusters), e.g.,

X_1 X_2	X_3 X_4 X_5	X_6
C_1 Vocational	C_2 Emotional Stress	C_3 Family Support

(3) Identify the formal rules for integrating the categories of information for the decisions to be made. Usually, relative weights or importance, of the categories of information are related to the decision. Let w_i ($i = 1, 2, 3$) be the weightings for categories C_1, C_2, and C_3; then the integrated decision, D, would be:

$$D = w_1C_1 + w_2C_2 + w_3C_3 + \text{(Error of measurement)}$$

While the research findings of psychometricians are needed to identify the relevant categories of information for a particular target group's behavior, experienced clinical staff can be trained to report their observations of multivariate problems and integrated univariate functioning with a fair degree of reliability and validity, assuming clinical supervision and review are employed (see Chapters 2 and 14). Please recall earlier chapters:

Chapter 2 identifies unitary and multivariate dimensions relevant to each target group by asking "What does the research literature suggest?"

The chapters in *Section II* identify the client categories of concern and prioritize the concerns for each category of client by asking "What does the research literature suggest?"

Sections III and IV identify the data elements to be collected by category of clients and services, reliable procedures for data collection (Chapters 10 and 11) and estimates of the data's reliability, validity, and generalizability (Chapters 12–14).

ISSUE: Will a unit of change on any behavioral outcome measure have the same meaning at all levels of the scale? Can statistics requiring interval scales of measurement be applied?

REPLY: No. Moving from level of functioning 2 to 3 or 6 to 7 on a 9-point scale does not have the same meaning either clinically or programmatically. While this differential response will limit statistical procedures, it does not restrict statistical techniques using an interval scale.

Return to the foregoing example. Moving from level 2 to 3 is more dramatic than moving from level 6 to 7. In other words, the response rate of the client is *not* a linear function as suggested by the cost-outcome matrix. Someone who moves from level 2 to 3 has accomplished more than someone who moves from level 6 to 7. First, the higher functioning person often has more personal and social resources at his or her disposal to accomplish the change. As many

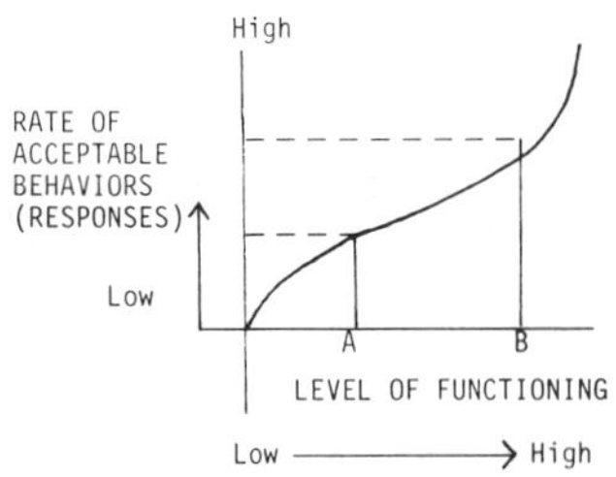

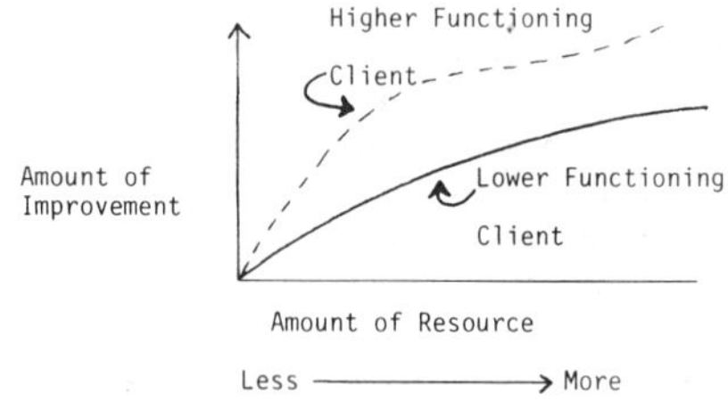

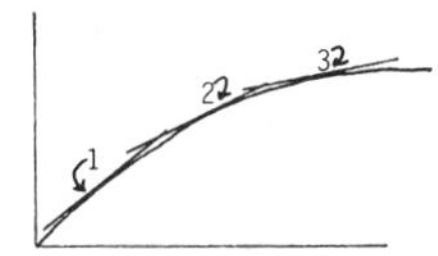

Figure 10. Relationship of Behaviors and Level of Functioning

Figure 11. Relationship of Resources, Functioning, and Improvement

Figure 12. Estimating Curvilinear Relationships

researchers have observed, the client's capability to behave (respond) appropriately is generally inverse to the client's level of functioning. Graphically speaking, the behavioral response function looks like Figure 10.

Clients A & B operating at two levels of functioning show varying appropriate response rates. At the lower end of functioning, the response rate is lower but at the high end of functioning the response rate is much higher.

A parallel issue exists for the amount of resources required to obtain improvement. Generally, more resources are required to move a lower functioning client than a higher functioning one.[4] Figure 11 plots the relationship.

The cost-outcome matrix and the decision tree can accomodate these observations by *segmenting* the functioning continuum. If, for example, all 1s, 2s and 3s are grouped, the variability of the improvement response is likely to be reduced. Behavioral scientists often fit linear functions (straight lines) to curvilinear ones. Figure 12 examines how a complex curve can be approximated with straight lines.

If three straight lines can be estimated, then a more complex curve can be estimated with minimal error. In brief, the population is segmented; by looking at groups of clients with common initial levels of functioning, distortions are minimized. Many statistical procedures requiring an interval scale of measurement can now be applied if clients are grouped by their initial levels of functioning. (Statistical procedures will be reviewed in Chapters 23 and 24.)

(B) Cost as a Process and an Outcome Measure

ISSUE: Do costs reflect process or outcome or both?

REPLY: Both. A treatment plan represents a budgeted estimate of clinical-service resources and resources to be allocated to a client in achieving treatment goals. At the time of review, clinical-process costs may be reviewed in terms of resources consumed by the treatment plan and resources available for the next phases of treatment. Costs provide a quantitative estimate of the treatment process. At termination of an episode (or even at critical decision points in the treatment process), costs reflect the resources expended as a *result* of prior decisions. Now costs reflect an outcome measure of the prior resource-allocation decisions.

[4] The exception, of course, is with some long-term clients requiring medication to maintain a stabilized middle-to-upper level of functioning. These clients sometimes require a simple adjustment in their medication, but have regressed to a very low level of functioning before the problem is detected. Often, a relatively small amount of resources is required to move them up to an appropriate level again.

ISSUE: What are some of the relationships of costs with client and service variables?

REPLY: Costs of service, of course, will vary according to client problems, circumstances, and goals. These latter variables describe the domain of services needed for the client. Therefore, costs as a measure of process and outcome require the same considerations as outcome measures; the four issues discussed in part (A) of this portion of the chapter also apply to costs as a measure of outcome.

ISSUE: What kinds of costs are not covered in the typical cost-outcome analysis?

REPLY: The typical costs used in cost-outcome analysis are those supplied by the agency providing the service. There are other monetary and nonmonetary costs which are not accumulated. Monetary costs to the client, the family or friends, and other health and social institutions are not often included. Nonmonetary costs of personal anguish and leisure time of friends and family consumed are not often accounted for in these analyses. But, they could be, and, for some issues, these cost measures should be used. For example, in the provision of community-support services for the chronic client, an analysis of other health and social-agency costs would be appropriate for a cost outcome analysis. Examples of these types of measures are described in several references (see Yates & Newman, 1980a,b).[5]

[5]The references on these topics are listed at the end of the book.

(C) Cause and Effect or Chance Outcome

ISSUE: What conclusions can be drawn on pre-existing data?

REPLY: Only tentative conclusions may be drawn from an analysis of pre-existing data. Relationships found in old data may or may not be either stable or true relationships. The relationships would not be stable if they do not occur again on several repeated samplings. The relationship may not be a true one if it does not hold up when certain supposedly irrelevant factors are controlled. To estimate whether a relationship among variables is stable and/or true is to perform repeated samplings under a variety of circumstances.

Consider the following economical ways of sampling to assess the relative stability of a relationship.[6]

(1) Take small samples of past time periods for different combinations of clients and services. Sample sizes between 10–50 clients should be sufficient. The sample size would depend upon the type of question. Often, three samples of 20 clients are better than one sample of 60 clients. The timeframes could be 3–6 month periods going back in time sequentially. If the relationships hold up under two or more samples, and irrelevant factors have been controlled, the relationship may have been stable in the past. But what of the future?

(2) A prudent action is a prospective sample, where the relationship is predicted to hold in a future time period. Replication through two future time samplings is better than one, but is also more expensive. The level of costs of sampling and the costs of *not acting* (to client or to service) need to be considered here as well. The design for prospective sampling studies is described in Chapter 24.

(3) Sequential sampling, either forward or backward in time, should be statistically analyzed with the techniques described in the last portion of Chapter 14. Generally speaking, as data are added, the evidence of support for the relationship should grow stronger if the confidence interval and the error terms become smaller.

ISSUE: What changes in behavior can be expected by chance, natural causes, and/or by regression toward the mean?

REPLY: Much of the positive impact of mental-health (or any health or social-service) intervention is because of factors other than the therapeutic technique applied. The human being, like most organisms, has internal biological and psychological mechanisms promoting survival. When imbalance or disability occurs, homostatic biological and psychological factors appear to play a role in returning the person to a more normal status, even if little else is done. Sometimes the only therapy needed is a little attention and rest. The hypothetical process of movement in functioning of someone where our biological and psychological mechanisms were most instrumental in a "return to normalcy" is shown graphically in Figure 13.

[6]Words like "stable" and "true" are relative rather than absolute terms. Absolute "stability" or "truth" are unrealistic goals for the current stage of technological development.

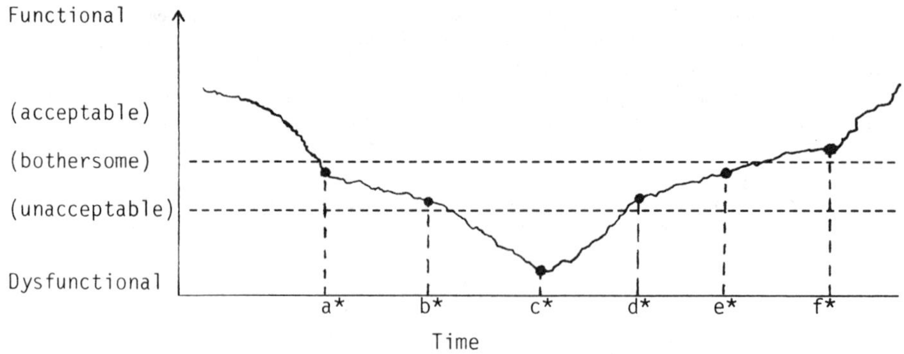

Figure 13. Interventions and Levels of Functioning

* See Table 2.

The letters a, b, . . . , f along the baseline of the figure represent events occurring with either a technical or nontechnical intervention. Both nontechnical and technical explanations might account for the movement of a person from a functional to dysfunctional level and back to a functional level (See Table 2).

Some evidence suggests general positive effects cut across both technically sound therapeutic and supportive nontechnical (e.g., friends and relatives) interventions (Strupp & Hadley, 1979; Yates & Newman, 1980a,b). The issue is whether the therapeutic interventions or other factors caused change in the client. There is no way one can adequately review existing data to determine what therapeutic service or client variables actually produced or retarded the

Table 2. Nontechnical and Technical Interventions

Event	Intervention and Explanation: Nontechnical	Intervention and Explanation: Technical (Therapy)
(a) Feeling distressed and depressed.	(a) Talk with friend.	(a) Talk with family physician (clergy).
(b) More depressed.	(b) Withdraws and sleeps a lot, but does talk with friend and uncovers some of the person's "real" fears.	(b) Physician or clergy refer to Mental-Health Center and person meets with a therapist. Client and therapist uncover "actual" problems and fears.
(c) Very distressed, clearly dysfunctional.	(c) Friend, at first moves in with person and then the two go off on a camping retreat.	(c) Therapy is intensively applied.
(d) Some improvement to acceptable level, but still distressed.	(d) Returns from camping retreat and starts work again, part-time.	(d) Therapy is "working" but needs to continue.
(e) No noticeable improvement, but still feeling some distress, and growing impatient with lack of progress.	(e) Takes up a new hobby which will divert attention from own problems.	(e) Tries a shift in therapeutic approach.
(f) Everything is OK, feels fine.	(f) It worked, thanks to the friend and the new hobby.	(f) It worked, thanks to the therapist.

outcomes. By tracing the branches of the decision tree, factors may appear to be related or not related to better or worse outcomes. But such analysis cannot determine actual cause and effect. A retrospective analysis of existing data may suggest what causal factors may be eliminated. If the cost-outcome data may be partitioned by a particular variable, and no appreciable differences appear, then either the outcome measurement technique is insensitive, or the variable has no significant effect.

Except for the elimination of "other explanations," definitive cause-effect conclusions are not warranted, even if relationships discovered in the past are studied in the future via a controlled experiment. But, more confidence in plausible explanations of possible cause and effect can follow if prospective experimental studies are performed. The design of these studies is described in Chapter 23.

Before leaving the issues of cause and effect, a brief note of explanation about a phenomenon of *regression toward the mean effects* is required. Sometimes significant behavioral changes are associated with clinical services where such is not the case. If a sample of scores (observations, measures) differ appreciably from the overall average, repeated sampling will typically result in some mean scores coming closer to the overall average. The sample means will regress toward the overall population mean with repeated sampling. In mental health, low deviation scores are more likely and improvement toward "normalcy" may be, in part, an effect of regression of the repeated samples mean toward the overall "normal" population's mean. Prospective studies contrasting the progress of comparable groups of clients with different treatment procedures (or placebo procedures) are more likely to eliminate some alternative causal explanations.

6. APPLICATION AND IMPLEMENTATION STRATEGIES

Figure 14 summarizes how cost-outcome analysis fits into the overall client-oriented cost-outcome system. The figure is organized in three columns: "Stage," "Process," and "Actions." Relevant chapters of the text are listed in the first column. So Figure 14 serves as a referral index for administrative actions or evaluation-research questions.

Certain guidelines are offered to facilitate the development of a cost-outcome system:

— If a global level of functioning is used, be sure that:
   (a) The judgments are made regularly by all clinical observers at all meaningful clinical encounters, not just at intake and termination, to avoid other confounding effects (see Chapters 2, 12, and 13).
   (b) Use the ratings of clinical encounter shortly *after* intake and shortly *before* termination.
   (c) Have other behavioral measures taken at critical points in time (e.g., at intake, review, termination, and, for a random sample, in followup).
   (d) There are review and staff-development procedures.

— Format data for the decisions staff are required to make (see Chapter 20). Examples include:
   (a) For clinical staff, include client I.D. number. A printout of the data might appear as in Figure 15.
   (b) For administrative staff and boards, use either decision-tree data or figures. Examples of some useful figure formats are shown in Figure 16. None of the individual client data and identification numbers should go to administrative and policy levels.

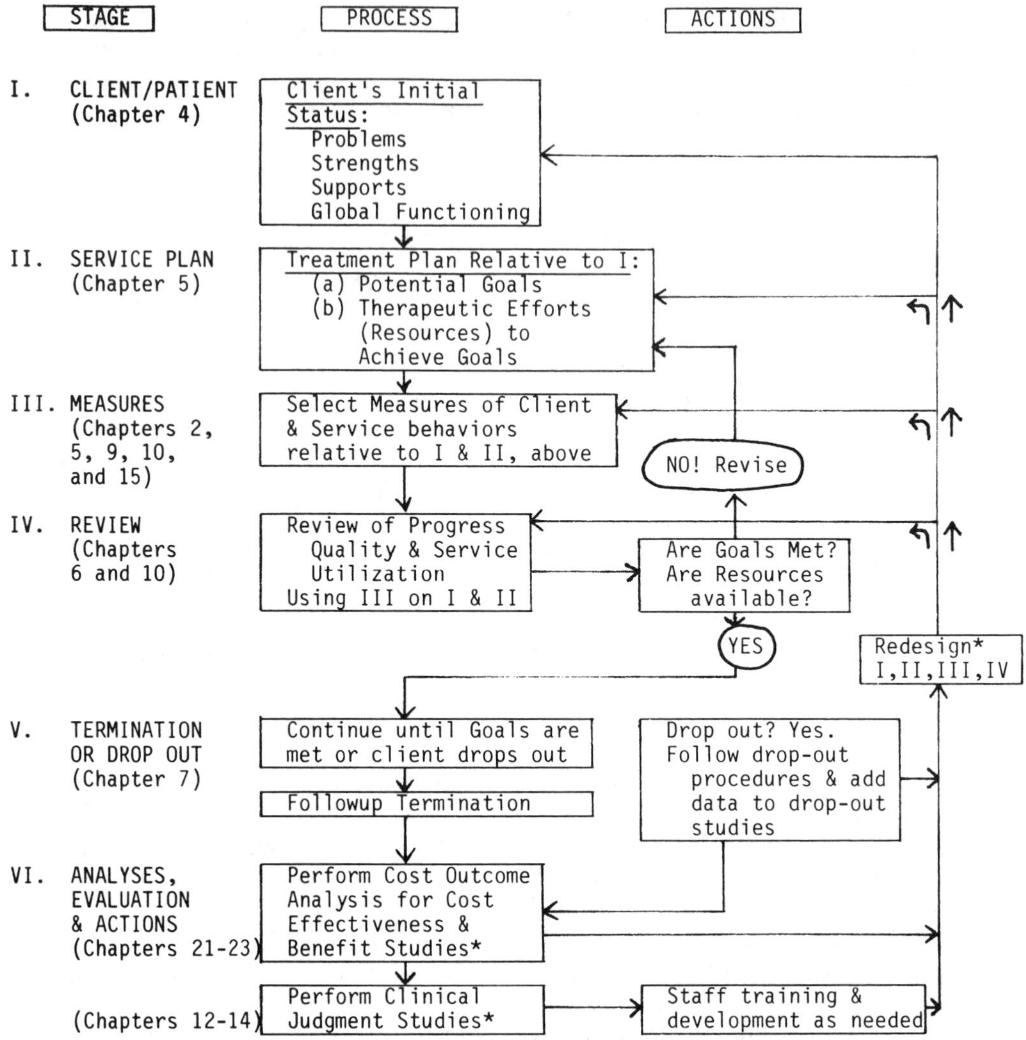

Figure 14. Client-Oriented Cost-outcome System (COCOS) Model for Service Management and Evaluation Research

* Studies called for in these instances should, wherever possible, use experimental or quasi-experimental designs contrasting different groups (see Chapter 23).

Finally, the Client-Event File consolidates cost-outcome data. The Client-Event File (e.g., a 5″ × 8″ card in a manual system; full-page sheets in a McBee system; or an event file in a computer system) has the relevant demographic, diagnostic, and financial liability information, followed by a chronological listing of all relevant service information, both chargeable and nonchargeable. Minimal service information recorded on a manual system-ledger card is illustrated in Figure 17.

The first five column entries come directly from the Staff-Activity Analysis. Entries in the ‘‘Cost’’ column are taken from one of two kinds of cost tables: One which lists costs by type of

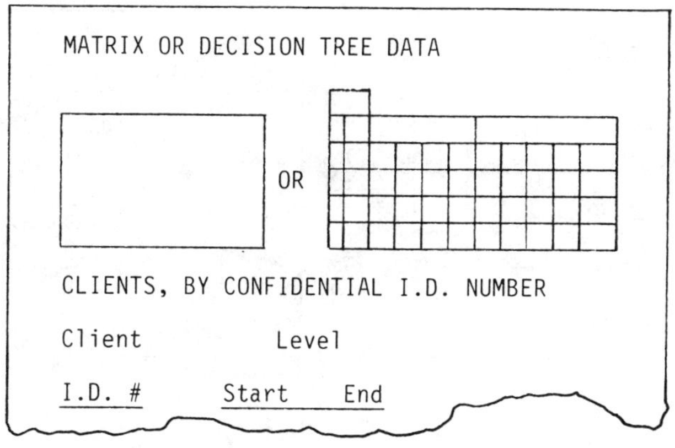

Figure 15. Layout of Data for Clinical Staff

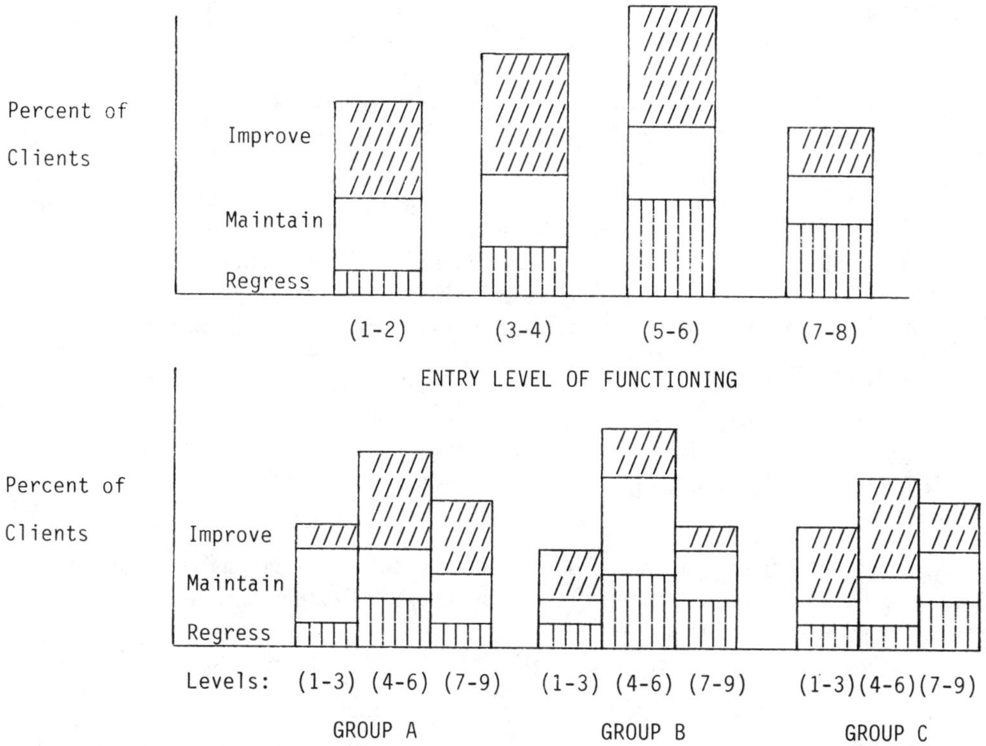

Figure 16. Type of Client (or Service) by Entry Level of Functioning

service and time; another which lists costs by staff category (Psychiatrist, Psychologist, Social Worker, etc.) and time. Whichever method used, the costs are entered for each chargeable service event. These cost tables are periodically updated. The "Charge" information also comes from a table listing the charges permitted for each service activity for each category of client financial liability. Using the information from Figure 17, (which is a manual system), the following issues can be addressed:

CLIENT ID
DEMOGRAPHIC DATA
FINANCIAL LIABILITY

DIAGNOSTIC & SERVICE GOALS, e.g.
Sustenance or Growth Plans

Date	Level of Functioning	Service Rendered	By Whom	Time	Cost	Charge	Pay ments	Balances Charges-Payments	Costs-Charges
2/9/79	4	313	440	1:30	$ 90	$ 60	$ 60	$0.00	-30.00
⋮	⋮	⋮	⋮	⋮	⋮	⋮	⋮	⋮	⋮
6/3/79	7	317	221	1:00	40	40	40	0.00	0.00
			TOTALS	=	$550	$400	$400	$0.00	$150.00

(Adapted from William Underhill)

Figure 17. Example of a Client-event File

FISCAL SOLVENCY

Potential balances provide a basis for discussion with program funding agencies and third-party payors. (The numbers are from the example.)
—(Charge − Paid) = Amount to be collected ($0.00)
—(Costs − Charges) = Net costs beyond or over charges ($150)
—(Costs − Paid) = Net costs relative to amount paid ($150)

UTILIZATION REVIEW

Cost outcome analysis for the individual client
—By episode, sum costs over episode, and list entry and termination level of functioning (Entry Level 4, Termination at 7, costs $550)
—Over course of episode or for any time period during the course of service

PROGRAM ANALYSIS

Cost outcome analysis for groups of clients or services
—Utilization and review
—Client-care evaluation studies

At this point, all the pieces for performing the cost outcome-analyses have been described. Applications of these techniques to policy analysis (Chapter 22) and cost-effectiveness analysis (Chapters 23 and 24) follow.

Chapter 22
Cost-outcome Analysis of Program Policies

Are Client Outcome and Service Costs Related to Program Policies and Goals?

This chapter illustrates how client cost-outcome data can be used to evaluate program policies and goals. The chapter has three major sections:

(1) RATIONALE AND PROCEDURAL DESCRIPTION—The general procedures for using cost-outcome data for program policy and goal analysis are described.
(2) EXAMPLE—A demonstration of the procedures is provided.
(3) PROGRAM IMPLEMENTATION STRATEGIES.

1. RATIONALE AND DESCRIPTION OF PROCEDURES

Program policies and goals represent the reasons for a program's existence. Collectively, program policy and goal statements provide the program's mission, the direction of effort, and the identification of acceptable products and results. Thus, client-oriented cost-outcome data would be useless unless results could be related to a program's policies and goals.

Chapter 22 provides program managers, Citizen Board members, and regulatory agencies with a simple means for evaluating program policies and goals with client-oriented cost-outcome data. Before describing the procedures, however, the characteristics of policies and goals should be clearly specified.

Definitions and Examples of Policies and Goals[1]

Policy. A statement of philosophy and direction guiding the conduct of the organization; a ''mission statement.''

Examples (from Chapter 2):

(a) Provide services to help adult citizens attain their highest level of psychosocial functioning in their ordinary community.

[1] The fine distinction between a policy and a goal statement was not made in Chapter 2 for simplicity of instruction. In this chapter, however, we require more concise goal statements to be drawn, thus finer distinction is drawn.

(b) Provide services to help children achieve optimal functioning and growth rate in their ordinary family, community, and educational setting.

Goals. A specific problem-oriented statement of the results an organization seeks to achieve. A goal statement serves to bring an observable direction or outcome for service efforts provided to a specific target group.

Examples (from Chapter 4):

(a) Improvement in psychosocial functioning should be obtained for 70% of the clients if a "growth" treatment plan is recommended.
(b) Improvement or maintenance in psychosocial functioning for 80% of the clients should occur if a "sustenance" treatment plan is recommended.

While this chapter is restricted to policy and goal analysis, the same techniques could be extended to the analysis of specific program objectives within each goal, e.g., objectives which specify what kind of change in specific types of treatment.

Self-Study Exercise

(1) Give an example of a *policy* statement other than the two given above.

____
____
____

(2) Give an example of a *goal* statement other than the two given above.

____
____
____

Overview of Policy Analysis Procedure

The procedure consists of five major steps.

Step 1. For each client-related policy and goal statement, prepare a set of outcome objectives related to the policy and goal statement.

Example: Using the combination of the first policy and goal example above (adults with growth treatment plans):

(1.1) Services with the greatest proportion of dysfunctional clients to improve are desirable.
(1.2) Low costs for improvement of the initially dysfunctional clients to the functional levels are desirable.
(1.3) Services with the greatest proportion of functional clients to improve are desirable.
(1.4) Service costs to improve dysfunctional clients are expected to be more than service costs to improve functional clients.

Step 2. Develop a rank order of the outcome statements in Step 1. Let the rank of "1" represent the best outcome. Assign the values to each branch of the decision tree.

Example: Regarding outcome statement (1.1), above, let the rank of "1" be the branch in the decision tree (Table 1) which has the greatest proportion of improved clients among those who started dysfunctional. For each of the other three rules,

Table 1. Hypothetical Decision Tree Data*

Branches of Decision Tree	Started Dysfunctional				Started Functional				n
			Improved		Regressed				
	Regressed	Maintained	Still Dysf.	To Funct.	To Dysf.	Still Funct.	Maintained	Improved	
A	5 $2,000	16 $1,200	4 $1,050	1 $1,050	2 $1,500	5 $800	15 $600	3 $625	50
B	2 $2,000	8 $ 800	6 $ 775	9 $ 750	0	5 $700	10 $525	10 $450	50
C	4 $1,500	10 $1,000	5 $ 950	2 $1,000	1 $2,000	8 $800	10 $575	6 $600	50
D	3 $1,500	9 $ 900	7 $ 875	6 $ 900	0	5 $775	12 $525	8 $525	50
E	3 $2,000	11 $ 950	6 $ 900	5 $ 925	1 $1,750	10 $800	12 $550	2 $550	50
F	4 $1,750	12 $ 900	6 $ 850	3 $ 875	0	6 $750	12 $525	7 $500	50

*Cell entries give number of clients, and average costs per client-service episode.

(1.2) Let 1 = group(s) of initially dysfunctional clients with the lowest average costs for improvement.

(1.3) Let 1 = group(s) of initially functional clients to show the greatest proportion of improvement.

(1.4) Let 1 = group(s) where the proportion of improved dysfunctional clients relative to the number of improved functional clients is the greatest.

Step 3. Tabulate the sum of the ranks assigned each branch of the decision tree by each rank ordering rule given in Step 2, and evaluate the policy and goal by the sum of the ranks,[2] where,

— The branch with the lowest rank sum has had the *best* outcomes
— The branch with the higest rank sum has had the worst outcomes.

Table 2. Summing the Ranks and Ranking the Sums

Branches of Decision Tree	Rank Order Rules (1.1)	(1.2)	(1.3)	(1.4)	Sum of Ranks	Rank of Sums	
A	6	5	5	6	22	6 *worst*	A
B	1	2	1	1	5	1 *best*	B
C	5	6	4	5	20	5	C
D	2	1	2	3	8	2	D
E	3	4	6	4	17	4	E
F	4	3	3	2	12	3	F

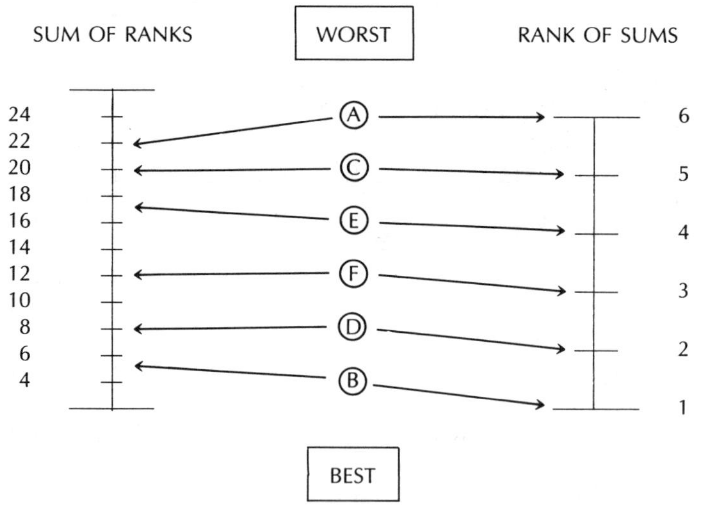

Figure 1. Evaluating the Rank of Sums

[2] *Technical Note*: After reviewing Table 2 and Figure 1, note that we are assuming that ranked data can be added. Usually this is a safe assumption, if you only interpret the rank of the sums (the right side of the figure) and not the sum of the ranks (the left side of the figure).

Step 4. Interpret the results of Step 3 and propose followup actions.

Example: Branches B, D, and F achieved better outcomes than branches A, C, and E. Therefore, the following lines of inquiry should be addressed;

- What characteristics were common to branches B, D, and F, and not to A, C, and E?
- Were the characteristics common to the better outcome branches factors we can control by
  - Reallocating resources?
  - Staff training and development?
- Were the results so clear that appropriate administrative action can and should take place without further study?
- If further study does seem warranted
  - What should be studied?
  - What criteria of outcome performance would lead to administrative decisions?
- What variables should be controlled?
- What time frames and expense ought to be devoted to the study?
- What decisions would you make with the results?

Step 5. List followup actions along with monitoring and review procedures to insure followup actions were performed as prescribed and achieved the desired results.

Example: A report reviewed and endorsed by participants in the followup actions be submitted to the Citizen Board. The report should provide a brief (two-page) summary of problem, actions taken, results, and recommendations. Appendices to the report can provide the appropriate details.

2. EXAMPLE DEMONSTRATION OF PROCEDURE

Try applying the procedures yourself. Use the data in Table 3 and proceed through the five steps.

Step 1: List three outcome objectives for the policy statement: "To provide services for the purpose of helping adult citizens attain their highest level of psychosocial functioning in their ordinary community setting."

(1.1) ____________________

____

(1.2) ____________________

____

(1.3) ____________________

____

Step 2: Give a rank ordering rule for each of your outcome objective statements. Let the rank of 1 = Best results.

(2.1) ____________________

____

(2.2) ____________________

____

(2.3) ____________________

____

Step 3: Tabulate the sum of the ranks across the three outcome objectives and then rank the sums.

Branches of Decision Tree			Outcome Objectives			Sum of Ranks	Rank of Sums (1–8)
Prior Hosp. Hist.	Family Social Support	Therapy: Indiv. or Group	2.1	2.2	2.3		
NO	GOOD	Indiv.					
		Group					
	POOR OR NONE	Indiv.					
		Group					
YES	GOOD	Indiv.					
		Group					
	POOR OR NONE	Indiv.					
		Group					

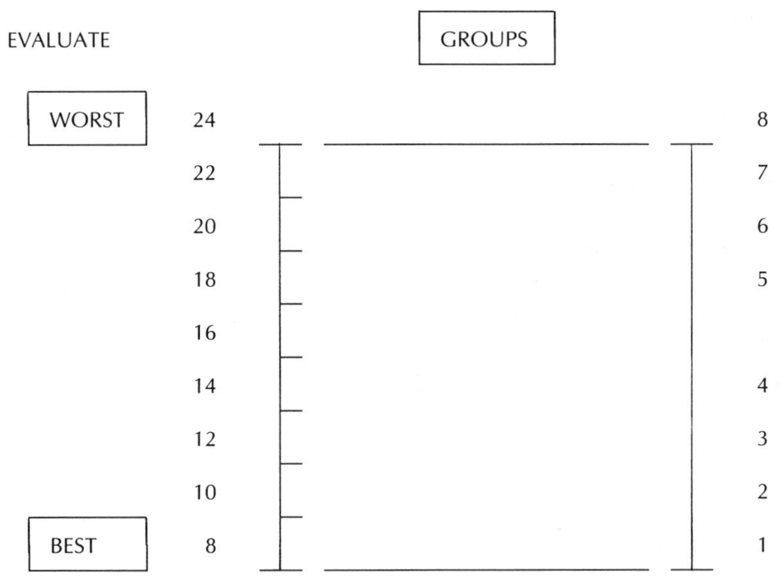

Step 4: Interpret results.

Step 5: List followup actions.

A More Sophisticated Approach: Value Weighting of Policies

Not all policies and not all outcomes have the same values to policy makers. Suppose, in the example above, that rules (1.1) and (1.3) were considered to be twice as important as rules (1.2) and (1.4). Value ratings may be incorporated in Step 3.

Step 3A Assign value ratings to each rule, multiply the rankings by each rule's respective value rating. Then proceed to sum the weighted ranks.

Branches of Tree	Rules, Values, and Ranks						Sum of Wtg. Ranks	Rank of Wtg. Sums	
	(1.1) × 2		(1.2) × 1	(1.3) × 2		(1.4) × 1			
A	6	12	5	5	10	6	31	6	A
B	1	2	2	1	2	1	7	1	B
C	5	10	6	4	8	5	29	4.5	C
D	2	4	1	2	4	3	12	2	D
E	3	6	4	6	12	4	26	3	E
F	4	8	3	3	6	2	29	4.5	F

Results: Note that by adding the value weighting to the rules, the final rank of the weighted sums changed the final ordering of the branches of the decision tree. Specifically in the ranks 3–5.

	RANKS	1st	2nd	3rd	4th	5th	6th
RANKS OF	Weighted Sums	B	D	E	Tied-C&F		A
	Simple Sums	B	D	F	E	C	A

Table 3. Decision Tree of Episode Results* for 18–40 Clients with Growth Treatment Plans

Branches of Decision Tree				Clients Started Dysfunctional				Clients Started Functional				
						Improved		Regressed				
Prior Hosp. Hist.	Family Social Support	Therapy: Indiv. or Group†		Regress	Maint.	Still Dysf.	To Funct.	To Dysf.	Still Funct.	Maint.	Improv.	#
NO	GOOD	Indiv.	A	2 $1200	2 $1100	3 $980	3 $960	2 $1000	2 $850	3 $730	3 $625	20
		Group	B	2 $1100	2 $950	6 $750	8 $775	1 $1000	2 $775	3 $500	6 $450	30
	POOR OR NONE	Indiv.	C	2 $1200	10 $1150	6 $1000	4 $1000	3 $1100	5 $900	4 $750	6 $675	40
		Group	D	2 $1200	6 $1100	6 $950	8 $925	2 $1000	4 $700	5 $600	7 $480	40
NO	GOOD	Indiv.	E	2 $1300	3 $1150	4 $1050	5 $1050	2 $1000	4 $850	4 $750	6 $675	30
		Group	F	1 $1100	2 $1000	3 $850	8 $850	1 $1050	2 $800	5 $560	8 $500	30
	POOR OR NONE	Indiv.	G	2 $1300	4 $1150	4 $1100	4 $1100	2 $1050	3 $800	4 $800	3 $700	25
		Group	H	1 $1200	2 $1100	4 $950	6 $900	2 $1000	2 $900	3 $600	5 $500	25

*Entries within each cell are number of clients, n, and average episode costs, $\$X$. Total costs equal n times $\$\bar{X}$.

†Where a family or social network exists and is willing to participate in therapy, then the group interaction was actually family or social-network therapy. Thus, for all clients with "good" family or social supports, family or network therapy was employed. Furthermore, one to three sessions of individual therapy often preceded the family or group therapy sessions.

3. PROGRAM IMPLEMENTATION STRATEGIES

The material in this chapter provides an excellent basis for joint workshops for Citizen Board members and program staff. The workshop goals would be to help both staff and Citizen Board members understand how cost outcome can be used in policy analysis. Moreover, the staff may come to better understand the functions of the Citizen Board. The workshop could also surface and clear up any misunderstanding Board members may have about their roles.

In preparation for such a workshop, consider the following outline:

(1) Announce the intention to provide the workshop at both a staff meeting and a Board meeting. Initiate group discussion on some of the potential products and pitfalls of the workshop to help identify potential hidden agenda items.

(2) Distribute Chapter 22 (or an adaptation of it) to all potential attendees, requesting they complete the exercise portions of the chapter.

(3) At the scheduled meeting, focus group discussion on individual responses to the exercises and on followup strategies to the policy and goal analyses.

(4) Next, schedule a meeting where the joint group will perform the same tasks with actual data from your own program. End the session with clear identification of which followup actions are administrative responsibilities and which are Board policy responsibilities.

Chapter 23

Cost Effectiveness and Evaluation Research Design

> Which Services Are the Most Cost Effective for Each Client Group? How Can You Design Cost-Effectiveness Studies to be Most Useful to Management Decision Making?

With the billions of dollars spent on mental-health services each year, ineffective services cheat the mental-health consumer and funder. Burdening limited resources to pay for ineffective services or to spend more than is needed to provide effective service should be avoided. The goal of a cost-effectiveness procedure is to choose the most effective therapeutic service with the least cost for a given client group. The bottom line of cost effectiveness is a set of recommendations to clinical managers and/or policy makers regarding the relative costs and effectiveness of services. In summary, the design of cost-effectiveness studies must be molded for decision making. The results of the study should be useful for analysis of and decisions about client cost and outcome data relative to program goals (Chapter 2), service processes (Section II), and management's organizational structure (Section IV).

Chapter 23 is constructed to assist service managers and evaluation research staff to work together in designing, conducting and analyzing cost-effectiveness studies for ongoing program decisions. That is, management's concerns are translated into technical procedures used by the evaluator to conduct the cost-effectiveness study.

The chapter has two major sections:

(1) THE RELATIONSHIP OF COST OUTCOME TO COST-EFFECTIVENESS STUDIES describes how the cost-outcome studies discussed in Chapters 21 and 22 set the stage for the more formal, critical and expensive studies of cost effectiveness.

(2) THE DESIGN AND PLAN FOR CONDUCTING THE STUDY describes the procedures needed by decision makers (clinical service managers or policy makers) to work with evaluation research staff in planning and conducting a cost-effectiveness study. The emphasis is on guiding the decision maker through a series of choices in planning the study so the results will be useful to the decision makers.

Then, in Chapter 24, we will provide a review of the major statistical procedural options which can be used in the analysis of cost-effectiveness data. The emphasis of Chapter 24 is on the usefulness of the different procedures for management and policy-level decisions.

1. THE RELATIONSHIP OF COST OUTCOME TO COST-EFFECTIVENESS STUDIES

Cost-outcome analysis is a set of techniques for *asking questions* while cost-effectiveness analysis is a set of techniques for making formal decisions with cost-outcome data. Cost-outcome analysis precedes and sets the stage for cost-effectiveness studies. The two forms of analysis may be contrasted by the questions addressed by each form of analysis. Two basic types of questions characterize cost-outcome analysis. Note the historic emphasis of cost outcome for each question.

(1) *Problem Identification and Analysis*—In the past, which client or service variables (facets) have been related to consistent differences in cost-outcome results? (See Chapter 21.)
(2) *Policy and Standards Analysis*—Are the cost-outcome results in the recent past for specific groups of clients aligning with the expected clinical standards or program policies? (See Chapter 22.)

For cost-effectiveness analysis the same two sets of questions become more formal and emphasize concerns of how to maximize service effectiveness while minimizing costs. Moreover, the emphasis is on what probably will occur in the future. The preceding questions are rephrased:

(1) *Problem Identification and Analysis*—Which combinations of client characteristics and service efforts will result in the better client/patient outcome with the least cost?
(2) *Policy and Standards Analysis*—For a given set of program policies or clinical standards, what combination of service efforts, when applied to a particular group of clients, will be most cost efficient in meeting or exceeding those policies or standards?

Cost-effectiveness analysis leans toward decisions selecting or investing in particular service efforts because they maximize client/patient outcome while they minimize costs. The decision is based upon predictable and replicable data.

Cost-effectiveness analysis must be relevant to ongoing management. Studies are done *in vivo,* and not in the laboratory or in an academically controlled clinical setting. Thus, the context of the service setting and the clinical process must be acknowledged in the design of the study. Analysis of the clinical system facilitates identification of the factors to be manipulated or controlled in the formal study of cost effectiveness. Figure 1 provides an overview of the client-oriented system and how its component parts can be identified for evaluation research in general, and cost-effectiveness research in particular.

The design of a study of cost effectiveness requires isolation of primary and secondary variables of interest to the study. The outline provided in Figure 1 can serve as a guide for reviewing the system to be considered in the study. Each component addresses specific questions:

(I) What are the initial client characteristics? Seldom will any therapeutic technique or program policy be all things to all clients. Thus, the types of clients to be studied must be specified.
(II) What services or service policies are influencing the potential outcomes? The services provided, along with client characteristics, are the two focal issues of most studies. Section II on clinical process echoes this viewpoint by encouraging treatment planning by types of clients and clinical concerns.

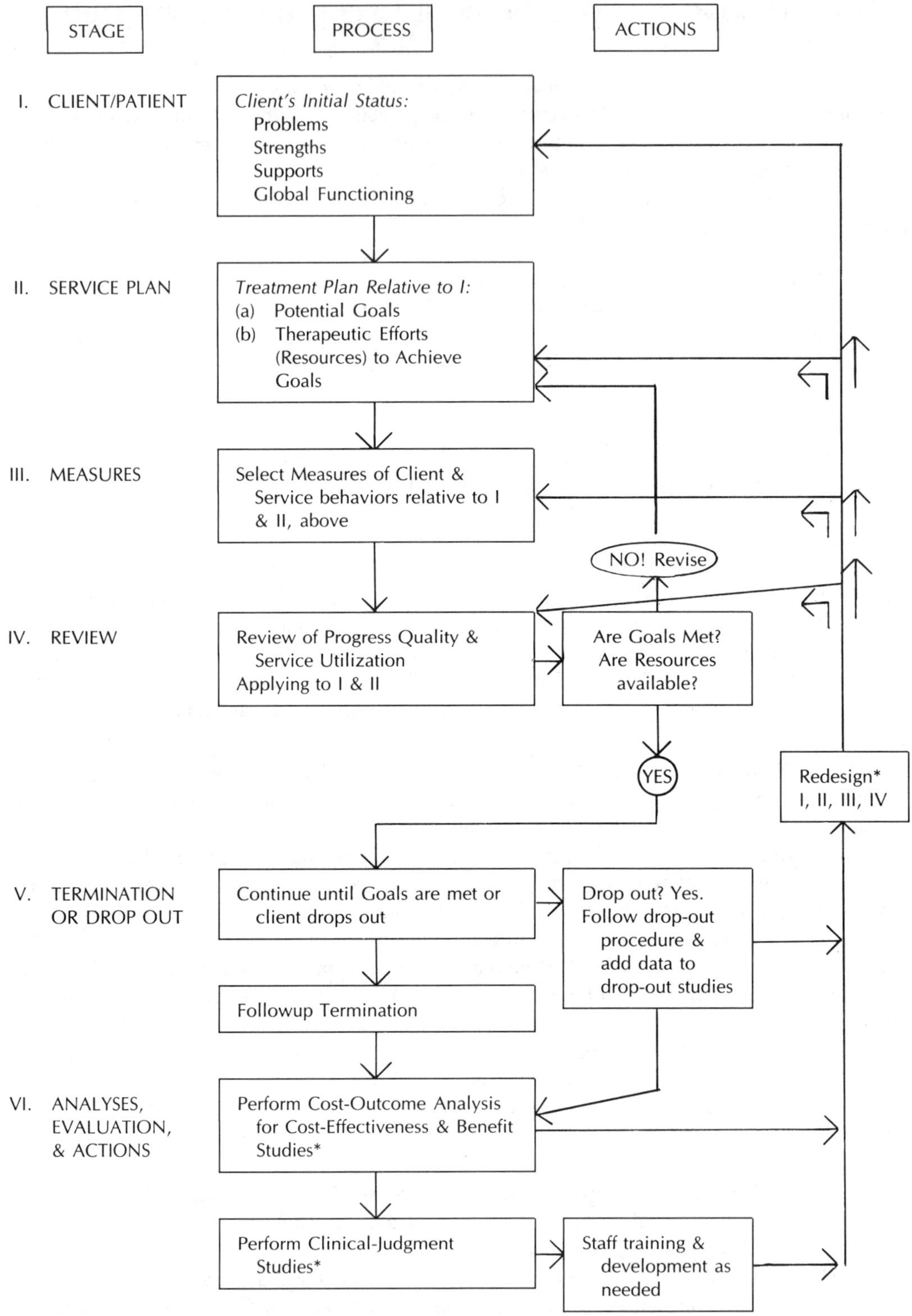

*Studies called for in these instances should, wherever possible, use experimental or quasi-experimental designs contrasting different groups.

Figure 1. Client-Oriented Cost-Outcome System (COCOS) Model for Service Management and Evaluation Research

(III) What measures of client behavior are clinically useful as feedback in review and followup evaluation?

(IV) What are the procedures for observing progress during the therapeutic process and will these review procedures influence the outcome of therapeutic effort?

(V) & (VI) What termination and followup procedures will be routinely employed to estimate the short and long term impact of the therapeutic effort?

Together these five questions will help set the stage for the study design.

While establishing explicit cause and effect relationships between service effort and client/patient outcome and costs may not always be possible, the cost-effectiveness analysis should eliminate the plausible alternative explanations with some degree of confidence. Next we need to address the issues of how to design a study of cost effectiveness to eliminate plausible alternative explanations, and how to choose the most effective and least costly services.

2. THE DESIGN AND PLAN FOR CONDUCTING A COST-EFFECTIVENESS STUDY

Designing and planning a cost effectiveness study can be described in twelve (12) steps (Table 1). The technical level of the discussion is geared toward facilitating a dialogue between an experienced program manager and a program evaluator with two semesters of graduate-level statistics and research design. The emphasis is on encouraging the manager to take an active role in the design, implementation, and interpretation of the study.

Steps (1)–(3) formulate the basic rationale for the study. Typically, a cost-outcome analysis of existing data has suggested that certain client or service variables appear to be consistently related to differences in outcome or costs or both. But management level concerns needs to emerge before initiating the expense of a cost-effectiveness study. Steps (1) through (3) provide the formal definitions of these issues: (a) What variables do clinical and program managers feel should be studied? (b) What kinds of observations (measures) are to be made as indicators of costs and outcomes? and (c) What are the criteria for identifying differences in cost or effectiveness results leading to changes in policy or resource allocation or both?

For *Step (1),* the principal consideration is to identify the characteristics of the client groups representing the variables to be studied. Suppose, for example, interest focused on the four combinations of the effects of two variables:

(A) Type of Service—Individual Therapy versus Group Therapy
(B) Level of Family/Social Support—Poor versus Good

Clearly stated definitions are needed so no ambiguity is experienced in the assignment of a client to one of the four combinations of type of service and level of family/social support. Definitions of levels must be meaningful in terms of the purpose of the study and the groups must be defined as mutually exclusive sets so a client will be identified as belonging to one and only one group. Meeting these two criteria is not always easy. Even with a variable as apparently clearcut as individual versus group therapy, ambiguity will arise. For example, most group therapy is preceded, and sometimes accompanied, by some individual therapy. Moreover, clients who have had prior episodes would have experienced either individual or group therapy or both. Definitions of the treatment groups must not run counter to the purpose of the study and thereby void the managerial utility of the results. An example would be to define group therapy as a condition where clients have had no prior experience with individual therapy and then to identify which intake and treatment planning sessions beyond the first session were individual

Table 1. The Design and Implementation of a Cost-Effectiveness Study

Step	Activity
(1)	IDENTIFYING ISSUES AND VARIABLES (TREATMENTS) OF INTEREST by using information from cost outcome, clinical-judgment studies, or consumer surveys.
(2)	SELECTING MEASURES TO BE USED which reflect the issues and variables of interest.
(3)	IDENTIFYING OUTCOME CRITERIA by differentiating critical points among levels of results.
(4)	IDENTIFYING EXTRANEOUS VARIABLES AND APPLYING EXPERIMENTAL AND STATISTICAL CONTROL TECHNIQUES to assure extraneous variables do not (a) unevenly influence one group relative to another, or (b) obscure important outcome effects.*
(5)	ASSURING THE TIME PERIOD AND NUMBERS OF CLIENTS TO BE INVOLVED are both sensitive to the treatment service effects of interest in Step (1) and timely to political managerial decision pressures.
(6)	OUTLINING TABLES OF DECISIONS TO BE MADE BY POSSIBLE OUTCOME by applying the general strategy comparing the cost-outcome results of two treatment groups, A and B:

		Costs		
	Result	A < B	A = B	A > B
OUTCOME EFFECTIVENESS	A > B	Choose A	Choose A	No Decision Possible
	A = B	Choose A	Choose Either A or B	Choose B
	A < B	No Decision Possible	Choose B	Choose B

Step	Activity
	The outcome effectiveness criteria in Step (6) are those specified in Step (3).
(7)	ESTABLISHING PROTOCOLS FOR COLLECTING AND ANALYZING THE DATA and assuring the data collection and analysis procedures reflect Steps (1)–(6).
(8)	OUTLINING LIMITATIONS (CONSTRAINTS) OF STUDY by defining what can and cannot be said with the measures [Step (2)], criteria [Step (3)], techniques [Step (4)], amount of data sampled [Step (5)], and procedures for collecting and analyzing the data [Step (7)].
(9)	COLLECTING AND ANALYZING THE DATA as specified in Step (7), recording any deviations from the protocols, and reconsidering the limitations given in Step (8).
(10)	PREPARING A REPORT tailored to the target audience of decision makers, and summarizing the results relative to Steps (6)–(9).
(11)	APPLYING THE RESULTS FOR DECISION MAKING by recording what decisions were and were not made relative to those recommended by the data.
(12)	REVIEWING THE VALUE OF THE STUDY by examining the decisions made and preparing recommendations for followup studies.

*Experimental and statistical control techniques will be detailed later in this chapter. Experimental control is a systematic effort to evenly distribute extraneous variables across groups in an unbiased fashion, and statistical control is a technique for systematically partitioning (subtracting out) the influence of extraneous variables to maximize the likelihood of observing any treatment effect which may exist.

therapy sessions. Such a definition would preclude all but the most clearcut cases, as it would select only those with no prior individual therapy experience in prior episodes in the study.

Identifying treatment groups requires more than unambiguous definitions. The management question must be clear as well. There must be a contrast between a treatment group or groups of interest and an established standard, a comparable control group, or one or more other therapeutic procedure groups which will draw sharp enough distinctions for decision making. The final product of a cost-effectiveness study is a decision on whether differences in treatment outcomes among groups are sufficient for labeling one approach as more cost effective than another. Table 2 provides examples of 16 types of between-group contrasts which fall into three categories. The first is ''Naturalistic Comparisons'' of people treated versus those not selected,

Table 2. Three Types of Contrasts of Therapeutic Effectiveness

Contrast Operations	Question/Issue
1. *Naturalistic Comparisons** 1.1 Candidates/Noncandidates	How are those people who are candidates for therapy different from other patient groups or nonpatient groups?
1.2 Selected/Rejected	How are the people selected for therapy different from those not selected?
1.3 Remainers/Dropouts	How are people who drop out of therapy against professional advice different from those who remain in therapy?
1.4 Successful/Unsuccessful at Termination	How are people who are successful at termination different from people who are not?
1.5 Successful/Unsuccessful at Followup	How are people successful at followup different from people unsuccessful at followup?
2. *Treatment Effect vs Controls* 2.1 *No Treatment* Controls 2.1.1 Normals (Randomly selected from population)	How do untreated, randomly selected people from the general population, differ from those involved in treatment?
2.1.2 Waiting List	How do those in need of and motivated to receive treatment, but held from treatment for the period of treatment, differ from those in treatment? Is there spontaneous or self-induced improvement for these waiting patients?
2.2 *Attention* 2.2.1 Listening for and/or accepting advice from nonprofessional	Will simple attention from an actively untutored listener and advisor produce the same results as professional treatment?
2.2.2 No advice, but a pseudo-psychotherapeutic task, e.g., relaxation, jogging	Will noncognitive tasks with apparent benefits be as beneficial as a treatment intended to affect the cognitive, emotional and/or intrapsychic processes?
2.3 *Counter Therapy* 2.3.1 "This won't work for a long time" (specify time)	Will treatment effects be observable even when client/patient has been told not to expect results for a certain time period?
2.3.2 "This will have negative effects at first"	Will treatment effects be observable even when the client/patient is told to expect negative effects?
2.4 *Alternative Forms of Treatment* 2.4.1 Standard vs. New	Will the new treatment show effects different from the standard therapeutic practices?
2.4.2 Same treatment but with minor variations	Will one facet of a therapeutic activity make a difference?

(*continued*)

Table 2. (*Continued*)

Contrast Operations	Question/Issue
3. *Program Intervention Activities* [These contrasts run parallel to the *Treatment Effect vs. Controls* but emphasize contingencies placed upon the circumstances and environment of the therapists rather than the therapies themselves.]	
3.1 Reimbursed *vs.* No Reimbursed Activities by third-party payor (e.g., telephone and second party interactions)	To what degree do monetary values affect therapeutic processes and outcomes?
3.2 Peer-Review Effects	Do the existence and type of peer review influence process and outcomes?
3.3 Treatment planning by principal therapist alone or by a treatment team	Does "ownership" of the treatment plan have an influence?

*Adapted from Kiesler. (1978). "Experimental Design in Psychotherapy Research." In Garfield & Bergin, *Handbook of Psychotherapy and Behavior Change: An empirical analysis* (2nd ed.). NY: Wiley.

or those treated unsuccessfully. These comparisons are usually prone to post hoc (after-the-fact) analyses and strong "cause and effect" conclusions cannot be drawn. Stronger conclusions are usually possible with the second kind of contrast, "Treatment Effect versus Control." Here the emphasis is directly on the distinguishing characteristics of the treatment itself and how the treatment can have a uniquely beneficial effect on clients when contrasted with the outcomes of clients who did not have the opportunity to experience that treatment. The third kind of contrast concerns the environment of the therapeutic intervention rather than the intervention itself, i.e., it focuses on "Program Intervention Activities" which could influence therapeutic outcome. The list of three categories and 16 contrasts provided in Table 2 is not exhaustive, but it presents the prevailing questions and contrasts currently popular in psychotherapy and mental-health research.[1]

For *Step (2)*, the critical issues are the selection and definition of one or more behavioral measures of outcome and service costs to differentiate the groups. Chapter 21 discussed four issues concerning outcome scale sensitivity to change:

— Will any outcome measure be equally sensitive to change for all clients?
— How does one select the appropriate measure for cost-effectiveness study?
— Shouldn't we be using multivariate measures to describe outcome, rather than simplistic univariate measures of functioning?
— Will a unit of change on any behavioral outcome measure have the same meaning at all levels of the scale? And if not, does this mean that statistical procedures requiring interval scales cannot be applied?

All of the observations made about cost outcome in Chapter 21 are equally applicable to cost effectiveness, so they are not repeated here.

---

[1] More detailed expositions are provided in Campbell and Stanley, 1963; Cook and Campbell, 1979; Craighead, Kazdin and Mahoney, 1976; Garfield and Bergin, 1978; Riecken and Boruch, 1974.

An additional classification scheme may help in the selection of outcome measures for any single target group. Three questions may be asked:

(a) What is to be observed?
(b) From whose perspective will the observation be made?
(c) When is the observation to be made?

Figure 2 illustrates the categorization scheme which can be applied to select the behavioral measures for a client target group.

What to measure and how to perform the measurements on the therapeutic process has been thoroughly reviewed in Waskow and Parloff (1975). While continued research is still required, Waskow and Parloff will be useful for our exposition (and will probably serve as a basis for future work in the field). Measurement is viewed from three basic domains: (1) *What is to be observed about the client*? (2) *From whose vantage point are observations to be made*? and (3) *When should the observations be made*?

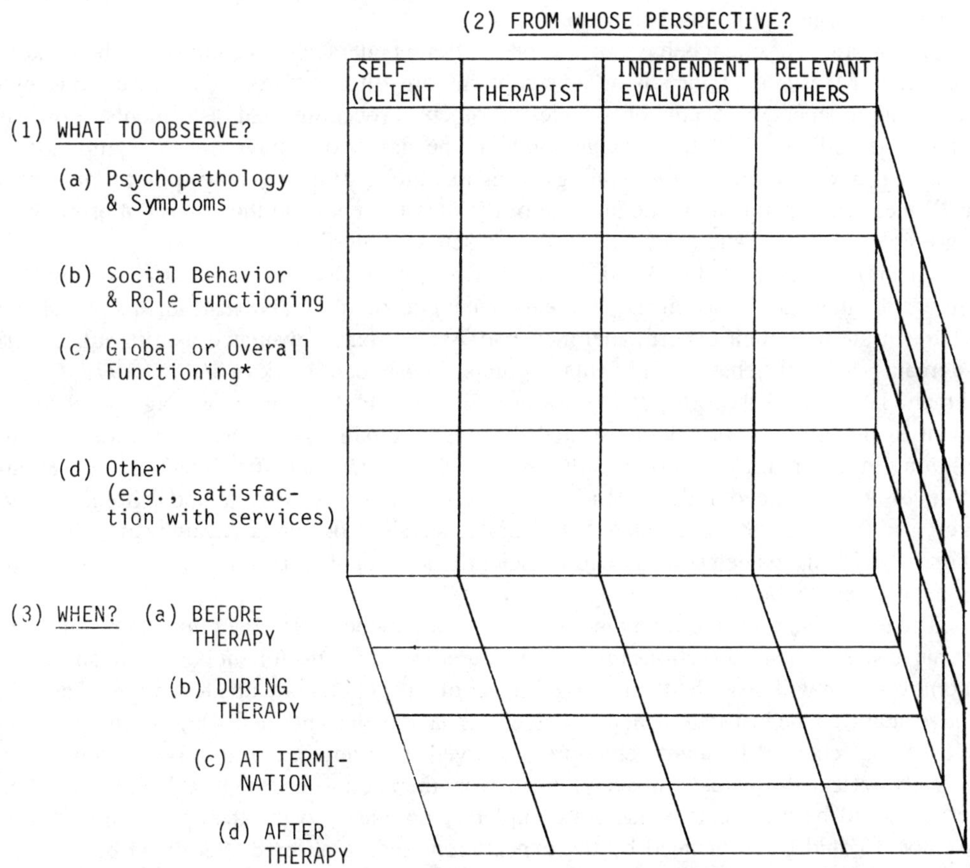

Figure 2. Schematic Describing the Three Basic Measurement Domains

* Global functioning was not considered to be an adequate form of instrumentation by an expert panel in 1975, but recent progress in overcoming the empirical difficulties of global scales suggests they can be useful (Newman, 1980).

The three major classes of client variables are identified across the horizontal rows of Figure 2. The vertical columns identify the four vantage points of observation. The third dimension represents the time the observations are taken during the clinical episode.

"What is to be observed about the client?" addresses the issue of the components and degrees of mental health or mental illness. The three classes of behaviors described are not independent classes, but they can be, nevertheless, measured separately. For example, somatic symptoms such as tics or stuttering have effects on social behavior and role functioning. Likewise, social behaviors can influence symptoms. A third category of observation, the global measurement of functioning describing the clients' ability to function in their ordinary community setting, given their multidimensional problems, strengths and circumstances (Luborsky, 1962; Newman, 1980; Spitzer, Endicott et al., 1970), serves as an integration of the other two categories of observation and has been shown to be positively related to both role functioning measures and symptom measures during the course of the clinical episode (Mintz et al., 1979; Newman, 1980; Steer & Henry, 1978). The global scale can provide a measure of the clients' overall functioning, which is the overriding goal of most psychotherapies. The global measure could also serve as one critical index of a psychotherapy's effectiveness when used in conjunction with the target complaint behaviors.

Observations of client behaviors take on a different character depending on who makes the observation. Measures of the client's perceptions are different from the perceptions of the therapist, an independent evaluator, or relevant others. Procedures and instruments of measurement vary according to both the vantage point and the classes of behaviors (i.e., symptoms, role functioning, or overall global functioning) being examined. Which vantage point represents the "best" measure depends upon the purpose of the measurement and the criteria of effectiveness being employed. The issue of criteria will be discussed later.

The monograph edited by Waskow and Parloff (1975) does an excellent job of summarizing the strengths and weaknesses of measurement techniques and instruments which were available at the time their expert panel met in 1970. The panel evaluated instruments covering the domains of client behavior and vantage points. Subsequent work (Bigelow, 1979; Ciarlo & Reihman, 1977; and Ellsworth, 1979) has provided information on the vantage point of independent evaluators and has demonstrated sufficient reliability and validity under specified conditions in community mental-health settings. Moreover, specific behavioral observation techniques using trained independent observers (e.g., Yates, Haven and Thoresen, 1979; Seigert and Yates, 1980) and other behavioral analysis procedures (Craighead, Kazdin and Mahoney, 1976) have been shown to be sufficiently dependable for estimating overall effectiveness of the therapeutic intervention.

The third domain is the time the observations are made during the clinical episode. In the most naive sense, the observations made in the other two domains (client behaviors and vantage points) over time will describe the relative impact of a psychotherapeutic technique. The reason we have qualified the last statement as "naive" is that one does not really know whether change (or absence of change) in client behaviors, observed from any one of the four vantage points, will really reflect the actual impact of the psychotherapeutic effort. The behavioral change observed could be the result of factors completely unrelated to the therapeutic efforts themselves, or it could be influenced by the expectations of the observer (Gottman & Markman, 1978). These are issues related to the third set of critical questions—how to detect the effect due uniquely to one type of mental-health intervention (Gottman & Markman, 1978)?

The strengths and weaknesses of any of the observational (measurement) techniques taken from different vantage points need to be understood before they can be used in estimating the effectiveness of mental-health treatment. The measurement instruments proposed by the panel of experts in the Waskow and Parloff monograph, the behavioral assessment procedures described by Yates et al. (1979), and the followup measures of Bigelow (1979), Ciarlo & Reihman (1977), and Ellsworth (1979), have been shown to have sufficient elements of reliability and validity under the conditions in which they were tested. But will these techniques be generalizable for application in cost-effectiveness and policy studies? The results obtained with any one of these instruments or procedures will very likely be reliable and valid when generalized to the specific types of client populations, with the sets of specific symptoms, physical conditions, and socioenvironmental circumstances under which the instruments were tested. The question is, can we estimate the extent to which these behavioral measures are invariant across different environmental circumstances?

In *Step (3),* the identification of outcome criteria brings systematic administrative and political considerations into the design of the study. If the study is to be focused for management decision making, then preliminary decisions about the criteria leading to final management decisions need to be outlined. The critical issues are risk and expense. Strict criteria are warranted if the choice among two or more services or treatments presents high risk to clients, to staff, or to the organization. Strict criteria are recommended if high costs or intensive efforts are involved. If little risk and/or expense is involved, looser criteria may be acceptable. Examples of loose and strict criteria are characterized in Figure 3. The low risk–loose criteria example is shown in the upper part of Figure 3 and the high risk–strict criteria example is shown in the lower part. A program manager and evaluator may proceed through Step (3) by identifying the potential assets and liabilities of making a decision in favor of one group or treatment over another. Once these considerations are listed, then a level of confidence in decision making should be set. An example of strict criteria would be: "I choose treatment A over B if $P(A > B) = 0.99$."

Step (4) outlines the design and plan for conducting the study. Here the goal is to assure the study clearly addresses the issues intended without contaminating or obscuring influences from extraneous variables. Specifically, factors or variables not of direct interest to the purposes of the study (i.e., extraneous variables) should not be permitted to (a) influence one group relative to others involved in the study, or (b) obscure the important outcome effects.

The technical terms applied in Step (4) are *experimental* and *statistical* control. Experimental control exists when contaminating extraneous variables are evenly distributed in an unbiased fashion across all treatment groups. For example, even distributions of the frequency or proportions of client and/or staff characteristics across treatment groups would assure that client or clinician influences on treatment or cost outcomes are equally distributed across the groups. Experimental control efforts are typically applied before the study. Statistical control, however, is exerted in the analysis of the data after the data are collected.[2] Here the extraneous variables are identified and partitioned out of the results so that differences between treatment groups can be viewed without the influence of the contaminating extraneous variables. Statistical control usually takes the form of reducing the variability of scores about each treatment group's mean, thereby accentuating the mean differences among groups. In Figure 4, the effects of statistical control are shown as a subtraction process which reduces the variance of scores within a group.

Usually, variability of scores within the groups are reduced by statistical regression techniques. These techniques reduce the variability by subtracting out any consistent (systemat-

---

[2] Of course, prior to collecting data there may have been plans to exert statistical control, but the actual operation of exerting statistical control is applied after the data are collected.

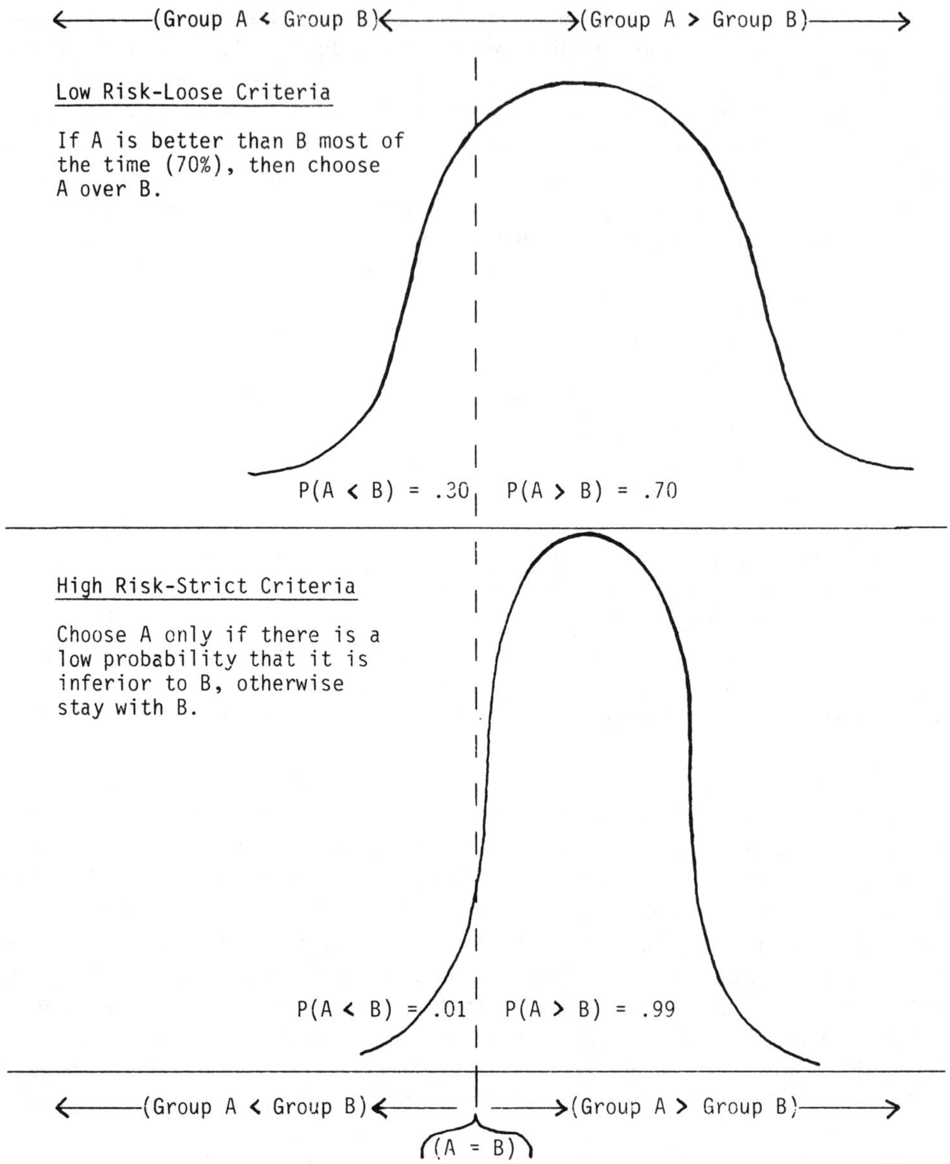

Figure 3. Comparing "Loose" and "Strict" Outcome Criteria

ic) differences related to the treatment variables of interest, thereby accentuating remaining differences.

The following example describes the techniques of experimental and statistical control. If we were comparing the average effects of three therapeutic procedures for adult clients, our basic interest would be in whether the variability among treatment group means is significantly greater than error variability. This comparison is often done by means of a statistical technique called an *F*-ratio. We will use the logic of the *F*-ratio to explain and contrast experimental and statistical control procedures.

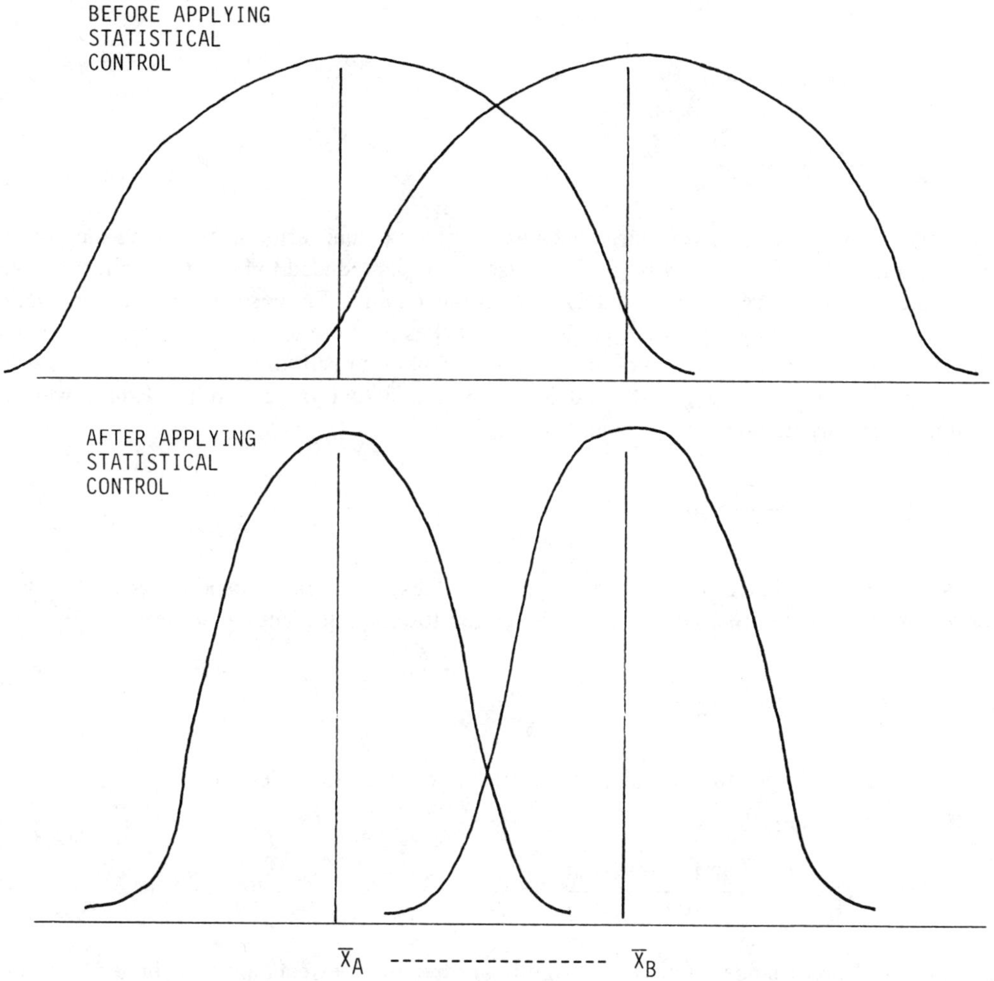

Figure 4. Statistical Control Characterized as a Subtraction Process

$$F = \frac{(\hat{\sigma}^2_{\text{Treatment Group Means}} + \hat{\sigma}^2_{\text{error}-1})}{\hat{\sigma}_{\text{error}-2}} = \frac{\hat{\sigma}^2_{\bar{X}} + \hat{\sigma}^2_{e_1}}{\hat{\sigma}^2_{e_2}}$$

where

$(\hat{\sigma}^2_{\bar{X}} + \hat{\sigma}^2_{e_1})$ = The variance among the treatment group means is inflated by the error variance inherent in sampling group means.

$\hat{\sigma}^2_{e_2}$ = The error variance in estimating each group's mean averaged across treatment groups.

The average within group variance ($\hat{\sigma}^2_{e_2}$) is assumed to be an unbiased estimate of error variance of sample means ($\hat{\sigma}^2_{e_1}$). Thus, $\hat{\sigma}^2_{e_2} = \hat{\sigma}^2_{e_1} = \hat{\sigma}^2_{e}$. Given this assumption, the *F*-ratio provides a valid test of differences among treatment group means. If there are actual differences among treatment group means, then $\hat{\sigma}^2_{\bar{X}} > 0$ and the ratio becomes greater than 1:

$F > 1.00$, if $\hat{\sigma}^2_{\bar{X}} > 0$, and conversely

$F = 1.00$, if $\hat{\sigma}^2_{\bar{X}} = 0.00$, i.e.,

$$F = \frac{\hat{\sigma}^2_{\bar{X}} + \hat{\sigma}^2_e}{\hat{\sigma}^2_e} = \frac{\hat{\sigma}^2_e}{\hat{\sigma}^2_e} = 1.00$$

Thus, as $\hat{\sigma}^2_{\bar{X}}$ becomes very large because there are actual differences among the groups, then the value of F becomes very large. Likewise, as $\hat{\sigma}^2_e$ is reduced to be very small, then even a very small value of $\hat{\sigma}^2_{\bar{X}}$ can be detected with the F-ratio. Suppose there were, in fact, a difference among three therapeutic treatment approaches in average outcome, so that on a 100-point behavioral scale the actual amount of improvement as a result of the respective therapeutic approaches were: $\mu_1 = 7$, $\mu_2 = 10$, and $\mu_3 = 13$. The actual value of $\hat{\sigma}^2\mu$, if there were no sampling error variance ($\sigma^2_e = 0$), would be

$$\sigma^2_\mu = \frac{3^2 + 0^2 + 3^2}{3} = 6$$

As the error variance, σ^2_e, assumes varying values, the F-ratio responds accordingly. If error variance is small, treatment effects are judged to be significant. Assume:

$$\sigma^2_e = 1 \qquad F = \frac{\sigma^2_{\bar{X}} + \sigma^2_e}{\sigma^2_e} = \frac{6 + 1}{1} = 7.00$$

If error variance is large, then no significant treatment effects are detected.
Assume:

$$\sigma^2_e = 100 \qquad F = \frac{6 + 100}{100} = \frac{106}{100} = 1.06$$

By reducing error variance, statistically significant treatment effects are highlighted. The purpose of exerting experimental and/or statistical control is to attempt to reduce error variance (σ^2_e) *in a meaningful way.*

Experimental control can reduce error variance in two ways. The first is to insure the major extraneous variables are evenly or proportionately distributed over the treatment groups of interest so their contribution to outcome variance can be studied systematically. These major factors may be clients' age, sex, marital status, etc. The second way is to insure that all extraneous variables are random factors which ought to be distributed among treatment groups in an unbiased fashion. Usually, random selection of clients and/or random assignment of clients to treatment groups will assure that extraneous variables are not unduly influencing one treatment group more than another.

Exerting systematic control over the major extraneous variables will concretely identify their contributions (if any exist) to the differences among groups. Consider an example where we would wish to evenly, or proportionately, distribute clients by gender and marital status across three different treatment groups, and to review the changes in behavior for those clients starting treatment at a middle level of functioning (46–55 on a 100-point scale). To assure that only the treatment variables were systematically influencing outcome, clients with these characteristics would be randomly and sequentially assigned until the three major treatment groups had

Table 3. Sources of Variance

Source of Variance	Expected Mean Squared Variance for Each Component of Variance*
MAIN EFFECTS	
Treatment (T)	$cgm\ \sigma^2_T + \sigma^2_e$
Gender (G)	$ctm\ \sigma^2_G + \sigma^2_e$
Marital Status (M)	$ctg\ \sigma^2_M + \sigma^2_e$
INTERACTION EFFECTS	
T × G	$cm\ \sigma^2_{TG} + \sigma^2_e$
T × M	$cg\ \sigma^2_{TM} + \sigma^2_e$
G × M	$ct\ \sigma^2_{GM} + \sigma^2_e$
T × G × M	$c\ \sigma^2_{TGM} + \sigma^2_e$
ERROR TERM	
Clients within the T × G × M combinations (C/TGM)	σ^2_e

**Technical Note:* One or more coefficients precede all variance terms except the error term, σ^2_e, where g = # of groups, m = # of levels of marital status, t = # of treatments and c = # of clients within each level of gmt. All of these terms are considered to be fixed effects in a factorial design and the coefficients represent the number of levels the fixed effect was summed across as a constant, i.e., the sum of a constant is the constant times the number of terms being summed.

proportionate numbers of males and females and proportionate numbers from each category of marital status. The sources of variance may be broken out as illustrated in Table 3.

By employing the statistical estimation procedures found in standard texts (e.g., Myers, 1979; Winer, 1971), the expected mean squares for each component of variance could be estimated and tested for significant effects by the *F*-ratio. For example, the test for a significant treatment effect would be:

$$F_{\text{observed}} = \frac{cgm\ \hat{\sigma}^2_T + \hat{\sigma}^2_e}{\hat{\sigma}^2_e}$$

and if the value of F_{observed} is greater than expected by chance[3], then the treatment ($\sigma^2{}_T$) effect is considered to be a significant effect. Other variables may be evaluated as "Main Effects," or in combinations as "Interactions." The interaction terms describe whether and how the whole array of effects may be greater than the sum of its parts.

The analysis can be extended by evaluating the generalizability of the treatment effects. The process is similar to analyzing the factors influencing clinical judgments. For example, consider the effects of the different treatments relative to the influence of gender as a main effect and gender in combination with treatment variance, i.e.,

$$\frac{cgm\ \hat{\sigma}^2_T}{cgm\hat{\sigma}^2_T + ctm\ \hat{\sigma}^2_G + cm\ \hat{\sigma}^2_{GT} + \hat{\sigma}^2_e}$$

[3] As discussed in Chapter 14, expected values of *F* by chance or random error are compiled in tables in standard texts and are consulted to determine levels of significance, given the null hypothesis of no differences among group means.

This describes the proportion of variance accounted for by the treatment effects relative to the combined contributions of treatment and gender effects (singly and as an interaction) along with random error, $\hat{\sigma}^2_e$, but omitting marital-status effects. As that ratio becomes large, the treatment effect should be considered as a more important influence relative to the other factors identified in the ratio.

Employing experimental control in a study of treatment effectiveness permits systematic estimation and review of the relative influences of the major extraneous factors that might influence outcomes for each of the treatment groups. While simple tests of significance (the *F*-test in the example) describe only the significant effect of a variance component (e.g., $\sigma^2{}_T$), the use of generalizability ratios provides additional insight by describing the significant effect's influence relative to the influence of specific extraneous variables. In general terms, the ratio of generalizability would be[4]:

$$\frac{C_K\hat{\sigma}^2_{\text{Treatment}}}{C_K\hat{\sigma}^2_{\text{treatment}} + \hat{\sigma}^2_{\text{error}} + [\Sigma C_{K'}\sigma^2_{(\text{important extraneous variable})}]}$$

As more variables are systematically controlled, greater flexibility can be achieved in computing different generalizability ratios describing the differences in treatment-outcome effectiveness relative to the combined domains of treatment, extraneous, and random-error variance.

Statistical control can provide similar forms of analysis. For example, regression techniques (available on most standard statistical computer packages) can estimate accounted for variance as systematic controls or partitions are applied. The logic of the typical applications of statistical control relative to experimental control, however, does change. For example, a typical statistical-control procedure focuses on an effect after the relationship between the extraneous variable and the outcome measure has been subtracted (partitioned) from the overall outcome variance. The emphasis is on the *relationship.* What is often subtracted from the final analysis is the variance due to the relationships of the extraneous variables to the treatment variable of primary concern to the study. Thus, the conclusions drawn would have to be about the treatment variable as it is *unrelated to* (i.e., unaffected by) the extraneous variable(s). Often an important loss of information hinders use of the study results. Consider an example of statistical control at its worst, i.e., using the analysis of covariance to examine outcome level of depression by adjusting for entry level of depression as the extraneous covariate. Here, outcome depression level scores are adjusted by entry level of depression so that the outcome levels are not contaminated by differences among entry levels of depression. Two major problems exist. First, control exerted by covariance procedures have an important statistical assumption, i.e., the treatment and the controlled covariate *do not interact systematically.* In treating depression, for example, there is good reason to believe that entry levels of depression and treatment approaches do have a systematic interaction. In fact, such an assumption is the principal rationale for many therapeutic treatments.

Second, there is a logical problem with statistical-control procedures such as covariance analysis. The problem is one of interpretation. Rhetorically, we can ask, "Would you dare apply any treatment of depression without knowing the entry level of depression?" Probably not, since the interaction of treatment and entry level is of concern along with the main effect of

---

[4] The coefficients C_K and $C_{K'}$ will vary according to the experimental design employed. In general, they represent the number of levels of other factors involved in the particular study performed.

treatment. What statistical-control procedures such as covariance analysis do is to both subtract out and logically disallow the covariate's relationships with the outcome measure. Generally speaking, any statistical-control procedure seeking to partition or subtract out extraneous sources of variance should be viewed with caution. The most general caveat is to *not* use any statistical-control procedure which takes out any information typically used in making a clinical or management decision. This caveat would avoid controls which subtract initial levels of problem behavior or variables considered important in the development of a treatment plan or quality assurance review. Ask yourself, "Would I make a clinical *or* management decision without knowing anything about the level of the extraneous variable?" Finally, the caveat also applies to experimental- control procedures fixing and partitioning consideration of any variables crucial to the clinical or management decisions. The most prudent strategy is either to make use of random selection and assignment to ensure extraneous but important variables are included in an unbiased fashion, or to systematically partition the effects of variance due to the extraneous variables and include these effects in a generalizability ratio, i.e.,

$$\frac{C_K\hat{\sigma}^2_{\text{Treatment}}}{C_K\hat{\sigma}^2_{\text{Treatment}} + \hat{\sigma}^2_{\text{error}} + [\Sigma C_{K'}\hat{\sigma}^2_{(\text{extraneous variable of interest})}]}$$

Step (5) addresses the pragmatic considerations of specifying the time period and the numbers of clients to be involved in the study. The boundaries of time and numbers are set by the guidelines of timeliness for decision making on the one hand, and by insuring there are sufficient time and numbers for treatment outcome to be demonstrated as effective or ineffective, on the other hand. Major management decisions usually need to be made annually as part of the budget planning process. Time periods are not likely to be more than 9 to 12 months. While many cost effectiveness studies could be completed within this time frame, some client groups and treatment regimes will not be expected to produce significant behavior changes in less than 12 months. Cost effectiveness often focuses on estimating both cost and outcomes during a 6, 12, or 18 month followup period (after an initial discharge from service). Formal cost-effectiveness studies have an expense in both time and dollars. In summary, the major considerations in specifying the time period are:

— What is the expected time course of a treatment's impact on client behaviors or situation?
— Are followup time samples needed to answer the questions being addressed?
— When would program managers need the data to use in their decision making?

Specifying the numbers of clients within each treatment group is part of a practical compromise. For most studies, having between 20 and 40 clients within each major treatment group is sufficient. The more clients within each group, the greater the sensitivity of the study to show among-treatment group differences, because the error term, $\sigma^2{}_e$, usually decreases in direct proportion to sample size. Thus, increasing sample size increases the possibility of detecting small differences between treatment-group means.[5] Two important problems emerge when increasing sample size. First, is the required number of clients available in the time period addressed by the cost-effectiveness study? The second problem is one of logic as well as practicality. If a favorable treatment effect is so variable (inconsistent) that it can only be

[5] *Technical Note*: Increased sample size also, according to the central limit theorem, assures that the statistical assumptions of normality and homogeneity of variance (germane to many statistical procedures) are more nearly met.

demonstrated by reviewing a large number of clients, then the treatment effects may be too small or too inconsistent to be of any practical importance. A sufficient number of clients in a treatment group, however, assures the results are not accidental.

Step (6) specifies the decisions to be made given the outcome criteria described in Step (2). Step (6), along with Step (3), is the most critical in distinguishing between cost-outcome and cost-effectiveness studies. A formal cost-effectiveness study requires advance specification of the criteria for distinguishing differences among the groups that will determine the decisions made, given a particular outcome. The decision matrix of cost results relative to outcome results, shown under Step (6) in Table 1, states the circumstances under which four decisions could be made:

— Choose A
— Choose B
— Choose either
— No data-based choice is possible

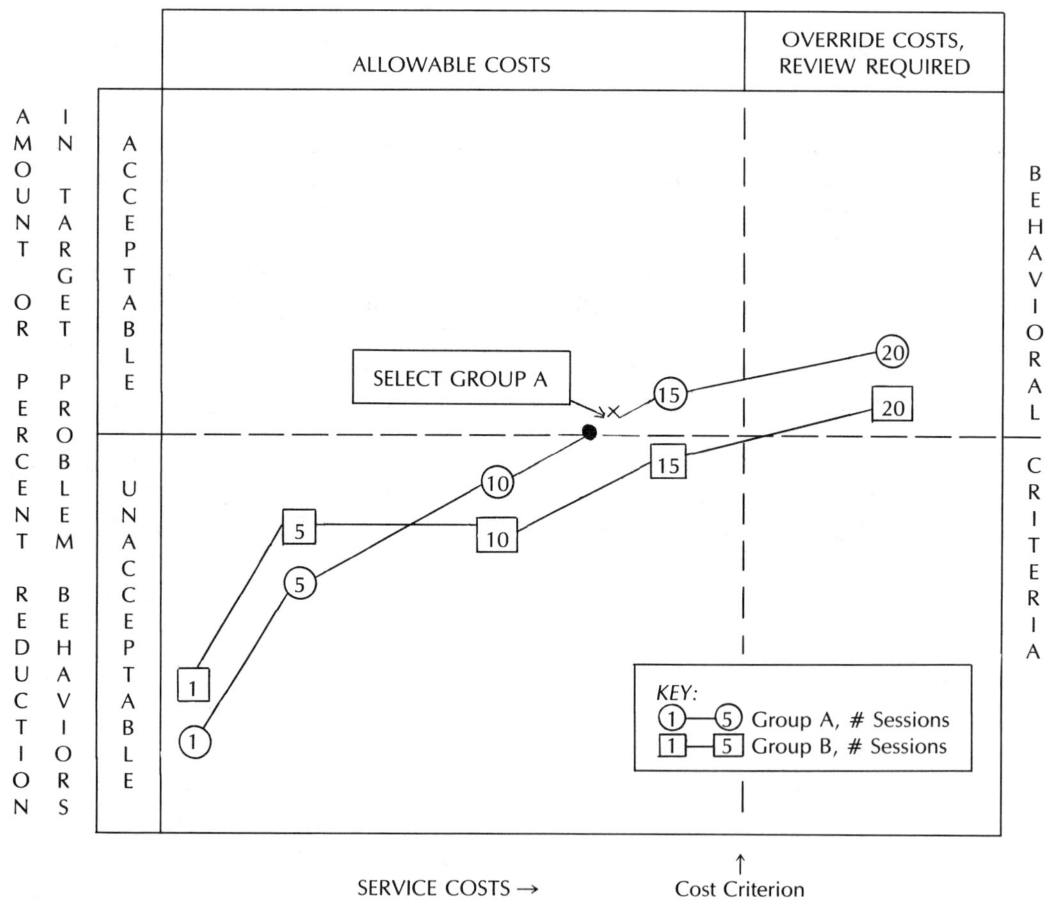

Figure 5. Plotting and Selecting among Treatment Groups According to Amount or Percent Reduction in Problem Behaviors and Service Costs

Other types of decision strategies are possible. Another example is Figure 5. Treatment groups are plotted according to the amount, or percent, of reduction in target problem behaviors (vertical axis), the cumulative service costs, and the number of treatment sessions. Note that two criterion lines are drawn: one where target behaviors are at an acceptable level to consider termination from treatment (the horizontal criterion line); the other decision line, the vertical line, represents allowable and "override" costs. Often, when treatment costs cross the override cost-criterion line, a utilization review procedure is needed to assess if further services of the same or of a different kind are needed. Either individual client or treatment group behaviors can be plotted for ongoing decision making or for group analysis. The decision criterion here would be to select the group to cross the "acceptable behavior" line at the lowest cost. The example shown in Figure 5 is the simplest form of multiple criteria or "Resource-Constraint-Process-Outcome Analysis." This technique will be described further in Chapter 24.

Steps (7) and (8) are straightforward but essential. Too often the protocol for collecting and analyzing the data (7) and the limitations or situational constraints (8) are not documented clearly. Failure may occur because the procedures used did not match the purposes of the study or because the study limitations are so great as to preclude any managerial utility.

Steps (9)–(12), while perfunctory, need to be executed with the care and involvement of both managers and evaluators. The interactive involvement of manager-decision maker with evaluator is particularly important at these last steps, since final decisions and the use of the study is what makes the expense of doing the study worthwhile.

Chapter 24

The Analysis of Cost-Effectiveness Studies

What Alternatives Exist for Analyzing the Results of Cost-Effectiveness Studies?

The final chapter of Section VII provides a technical review of the statistical procedures which could be applied in the analysis of cost-effectiveness studies. The emphasis is on the questions being addressed in the study, i.e., on selecting and applying statistical techniques which best suit the cost-effectiveness analyses required by the management questions which gave rise to the formal study. For the most part, we will assume that the reader has access to statistical texts which contain the computational procedures for the analyses discussed. The exceptions will occur only when such computational procedures do not exist in a readily accessible form elsewhere.

Three kinds of procedures will be discussed. The first is the *variance/generalizability* analysis procedures. The second is the *best* or *optimal case* approaches which contrast actual outcome to an idealized model of cost outcome. The third is the *multiple criteria* or *component-resource-constraint-analysis* techniques. It is particularly important that the three kinds of procedures be seen as potentially overlapping. Each cost-effectiveness study will be an application of technology to your unique circumstances and, therefore, will most likely require some special mixture of the three kinds of procedures.

VARIANCE/GENERALIZABILITY ANALYSIS

These procedures attempt to contrast the effectiveness and cost results of two or more treatment groups in terms of the amount or proportion of variability accounted for by the variables of interest to clinical or management decision making. In fact, it is the domain of clinical or management questions and decision making which serves as the focus of a variance/generalizability analysis. When there is a clear understanding of the major facets (variables) which comprise the domain of the different questions and decisions, there is little difficulty in designing the analysis.

To identify the major facets, we again call upon the client-oriented focus to provide guidelines. In the clinical design section (Section II), we emphasized that treatment planning and review procedures need to be partitioned by categories of clients presenting unique clinical concerns, questions and decisions which justify unique approaches to treatment planning and review. The same problem and its solution apply here: the variables which need to be identified and partitioned are those which would influence unique client-related concerns, questions, and decisions.

The typical factors of concern are similar, if not identical to, those which were identified in the clinical design sections on treatment planning, review, and termination. Some examples are:

(1) Client's initial functioning status as related to presenting problems, problem severity, and social and economic supports.
(2) Demographic characteristics, e.g., age or sex.
(3) Service history, e.g., types of services rendered in previous episodes.
(4) Legal status and level of client cooperativeness with treatment regime.

Thus, one would attempt to restrict the cost-effectiveness question and the domain of decision making to the cost effectiveness of a particular treatment with clients of similar

— Initial functioning and/or problems and/or supports
— Demographic characteristics
— Prior service history
— Level of cooperativeness with treatment

These considerations could also be described in a probability or likelihood statement, e.g., for a particular treatment, X_1,

Likelihood (Outcome | Initial functioning, Demographics, History, Cooperativeness, and Treatment X_1)

These four variables would all be "Between-Subject" variables in an analysis of variance; but they would be more generally known as independent variables for analysis by either regression, variance, discriminant, or path analysis.

A single probability or likelihood statement about a particular therapeutic treatment is not, however, sufficient for a study of cost effectiveness. As we emphasized earlier, two or more groups should be contrasted so that the likelihood or probability statement can offer a contrast useful for a decision, e.g.:

> Select A over B, since the likelihood of better or more cost-effective outcome is higher with A than with B.

Thus, most studies of cost effectiveness will need to consider controlling at least five "Between-Subject" variables.

(1) Therapeutic treatment
(2) Initial level of functioning or problem areas and severity
(3) Demographic and social-support characteristics
(4) Prior service history
(5) Level of cooperativeness

As discussed in Chapter 23, control over these variables can be either experimental or statistical. Moreover, the control can be exerted to partition these five variables as major sources of variance, or to attempt to assure their random and unbiased distribution over groups. The approach we favor is to experimentally control and thereby fix the major sources of variance wherever possible. This will permit you to use a coefficient of generalizability to estimate the impact of a particular treatment relative to the major facets which could be influencing outcome.

The alternative approach is to partition the sources of variance which are practical (and easy) to partition and to plan a regression or path analysis statistically controlling the important variables which cannot be practically partitioned. Step-down and partial correlation techniques can offer an analysis similar to a coefficient of generalizability. The logic of the regression analysis follows directly from the likelihood statement described earlier. Consider the logic of each along side the other.

(i) Likelihood (Outcome | Initial functioning, Demographics, History, Cooperativeness).

(ii) (Relationship of Outcome to Treatment) | (Relationships of outcome to Initial functioning, to Demographics, to History, and to Cooperativeness).

The only caveat to be aware of in using regression techniques is that one must remember to note the relationships controlled in the interpretation of the results of analysis.

The bottom line of using variance/ generalizability analysis procedures is still a decision, i.e., to make a selection among alternatives. The approach for making such a decision still follows what was outlined in Chapter 23. Specifically, after applying the variance/generalizability analysis to both cost and outcome data, the matrix of possible decisions is as follows:

		COSTS OF A RELATIVE TO B		
		A < B	A = B	A > B
OUTCOME EFFECTIVENESS	A > B	Choose A	Choose A	No Decision Possible (Effective but inefficient)
	A = B	Choose A	Choose Either A or B	Choose B
	A < B	No Decision Possible (Efficient but ineffective)	Choose B	Choose B

BEST OR OPTIMAL CASE APPROACH

One of the most popular features of the client-oriented cost-outcome system has been the use of a cost-outcome matrix to describe the relative impact of specific treatments on a particular group of clients over the course of their clinical episodes (or over any two points in time). But a cost-outcome matrix, by itself, is only descriptive. Specifically, the matrix simply describes the numbers of clients who exhibit certain degrees of improvement, maintenance, or regression in their level of functioning or symptom severity over time. What is needed for cost-effectiveness analysis is a procedure for comparing two or more matrices to estimate whether one set of factors leads to more effective results than another. The procedure described here can be used to contrast two or more outcome matrices or to contrast the average cell costs within pairs of matrices.

The technique, an extension of χ^2 procedures, contrasts observed outcomes with expected outcomes. The particular extension used here requires that the evaluator and the decision maker generate a "hypothesis matrix" which describes the relative outcomes which would lead to a decision such as "Treatment A is more effective thant Treatment B." Consider an example in which more improved clients would be expected from Treatment A as compared with Treatment B. This is illustrated by entering a value of "1" or "0" in the cells of a blank outcome matrix to describe where the proportions of Treatment A clients are greater than ("1"), equal to ("0"), or less than ("0") Treatment B clients. In this case, the "1" identifies the cells where greater improvement is predicted.[1] Thus, the hypothesis matrix would take the following form:

	Termination Levels			
Intake Levels	(1–2)	(3–4)	(5–6)	(7–9)
(1–2)	0	1	1	1
(3–4)	0	0	1	1
(5–6)	0	0	0	1
(7–9)	0	0	0	0

The cells with a value of "1" represent those cells where the expected outcomes should be contrasted between Treatment A and Treatment B clients. Specifically, we will contrast for both groups the proportions of clients to terminate at a particular cell level relative to the numbers of clients who started at that cell's level. Table 1 gives sample results of two groups in terms of:

(a) The observed frequency of clients in each cell
(b) The proportion of clients to terminate at a particular level (column level) relative to the total number to start at that particular level (row sum).
(c) The difference of cell proportions of Treatment A minus Treatment B cell proportions.

Note that matrix (c) in Table 1 provides a good description of the outcome of the study of effectiveness. Positive values of differences in proportions ($P_{Aij}-P_{Bij}$) predominate the upper right half of the matrix above the "maintenance" diagonal. This is the area where the hypothesis of more improvement by A over B occurs in the hypothesis matrix, i.e., the cells with "1" entries. Thus, a visual inspection of the signs of the differences suggest that the hypothesis is confirmed, i.e., five of the six cells are positive.

To test the hypothesis that Treatment A produces greater proportions of improvement than Treatment B, we only need to contrast proportions of those cells with "1" values in the hypothesis matrix. Two statistical tests are possible: the sign test and the Θ-technique. The easiest to perform (but the less powerful) is the sign test, which simply computes the proportion of positive cell entries relative to all nonzero cells (five of six cells in the present example). Most statistics texts have tabled values for the sign test and exact proportions for various combinations of (+) and (−) can be found there. For a quick reference for the significance test of number of (+) signs, the values given below list the numbers of cells required to obtain significance at $p < .05$.

[1] Examples of other hypothesis matrices are given later in the chapter.

Table 1

(a) Observed cell frequencies

	Termination Levels									
	Treatment A					Treatment B				
Intake Levels	(1–2)	(3–4)	(5–6)	(7–9)		(1–2)	(3–4)	(5–6)	(7–9)	
(1–2)	1	3	4	2	10	3	4	3	1	11
(3–4)	1	4	8	4	17	2	8	5	1	16
(5–6)	0	1	5	10	16	0	5	8	3	16
(7–9)	0	0	4	2	6	0	2	4	1	7
	2	8	21	18	49	5	19	20	6	50

(b) Observed cell proportion relative to total number at that level at intake (row total).

	Treatment A (P_{Aij})				Treatment B (P_{Bij})			
	(1–2)	(3–4)	(5–6)	(7–9)	(1–2)	(3–4)	(5–6)	(7–9)
(1–2)	.100	.300	.400	.200	.273	.363	.273	.091
(3–4)	.059	.235	.470	.235	.125	.500	.313	.062
(5–6)	0	.062	.313	.625	0	.313	.500	.187
(7–9)	0	0	.667	.333	0	.286	.571	.143

(c) Difference in cell proportions ($P_{Aij} - P_{Bij}$)

	(1–2)	(3–4)	(5–6)	(7–9)
(1–2)	−.172	−.063	+.127	+.109
(3–4)	−.066	−.265	+.157	+.173
(5–6)	0	−.251	−.187	+.438
(7–9)	0	−.286	+.096	+.190

# of Nonzero Cells with "1" Values	# Positive Cells p < .05	# Nonzero Cells with "1"	# Positive Cells p < .05
5	5	21	15
6	6	22	16
7	7	23	16
8	7	24	17
9	8	25	18
10	9	26	18
11	9	27	19
12	10	28	19
13	10	29	20
14	11	30	20
15	12	31	21
16	12	32	22
17	13	33	22
18	13	34	23
19	14	35	23
20	15	36	24

Since outcome matrices and corresponding hypothesis matrices will seldom have more than 36 cells with values of "1," the Table of Values given above will be sufficient for the sign tests. There is, however, a problem with using the sign test. It is only sensitive to differences in the relative number of (+) and (−) cells and is *not* sensitive to the magnitude of differences in the proportions. Moreover, for small matrices (e.g., 10 or fewer cells with "1" values), the occurrence of zero entries or at least one negative sign value [e.g., −.063 in cell row (1–2), column (3–4)] will lead to a nonrejection of the null hypothesis (H_0). While it may be a correct conclusion (i.e., do not reject H_0), the power of the sign test to correctly reject H_0 is relatively low and gets lower as cell numbers decrease. Moreover, we would want a test which is also sensitive to the magnitude of differences.

The Θ-technique (proposed by Ross, in press; Ross, 1977; Ross & Klein, 1979) appears to suit our purposes. Before detailing the methods for computing Θ, let us describe its logical features in terms of a study designed to contrast the effectiveness of two treatments (A vs. B). The index $\hat{\Theta}$ represents a measure of the differences in patterns of client outcomes for those initiating the two treatments, at measured levels of intake functioning or problem severity, relative to a hypothesized pattern of outcomes. Recall that the hypothesis matrix discussed earlier assigns values to each cell as "1" or "0" to describe whether we are predicting the difference in proportions of clients starting each treatment at a particular behavioral level and terminating at each outcome level to be +, 0, or −. The cells with "1" entries, under the Θ-technique, would contain the greatest proportion of clients entering treatment at a particular level, if that treatment is to be considered the more effective of the two treatments under consideration. While many different hypotheses can be tested using the Θ-technique, in our example the hypothesis is that Treatment A will result in greater proportions of improvement at all levels of intake. The value of $\hat{\Theta}$ can vary between 1.00 and 0.00, where 1.00 implies that Treatment A resulted in greater proportions of improvement over all improvement cells. A value of 0.00 would mean that the results were completely reversed from the predicted pattern. The value of $\Theta = \frac{1}{2}$ is expected if there are no differences in outcome patterns.[2]

The test statistic for significance is a χ^2 with one degree of freedom,

$$\chi^2_{(1)} = (\hat{\theta} - \tfrac{1}{2})^2/\hat{\sigma}^2_{\hat{\theta}}$$

The value of $\hat{\theta}$ is computed as

$$\hat{\theta} = \tfrac{1}{2}\left[\sum_{j=1}^{Int.} (P_{..j}) \sum_{i=1}^{Ter.} W_{ij}(P_{Aij} - P_{Bij})\right] + \tfrac{1}{2}$$

—P_{Aij} and P_{Bij} are the proportions of clients within each group to end the period or terminate the episode at level i having initiated at level j.
—$P_{..j}$ is the proportion of clients to start either treatment at level j.
—w_{ij} is the value "1" or "0" from the hypothesis matrix for the ij^{th} cell.

---

[2] *Technical Note*: The expectation of $\theta = \frac{1}{2}$ assumes that when contrasting the same cell in any pair of matrices [e.g., cell (4,4) of Group A vs. cell (4,4) of Group B], the probability of the difference in the proportion of clients between groups being ≥ is ½. This also assumes random assignment to each group or no initial fixed bias between groups in their intake level of functioning. If there is an initial bias, it should be estimated and the expected value of θ should be reassigned to assume the estimated value.

The value of $\hat{\sigma}^2_\theta$ is computed as:

$$\hat{\sigma}^2_{\hat{\theta}} = 1/4\left(\frac{1}{N_A} + \frac{1}{N_B}\right)\sum_j^{Int.}\sum_i^{Ter.}\frac{n_{Aij} + n_{Bij}}{N_A + N_B}(w_{ij} - \bar{w}_{.j})^2$$

where the newly introduced terms are defined as:

—n_{Aij} and n_{Bij} are the number of clients in each cell of the matrix A and B, respectively.
—N_A and N_B are the numbers of clients in treatments A and B, respectively.
—$\bar{w}_{.j} = \left(\frac{1}{P_{..j}}\right)\sum_{i=1}^{Ter.} w_{ij}(P_{Aij} + P_{Bij})$

An inspection of the equations given above along side of the hypothesis matrix

0	1	1	1
0	0	1	1
0	0	0	1
0	0	0	0

would show that the computations will only involve the 12 cells covered by the first three rows of intake levels. That is, the computations will only involve the cells of rows with at least one nonzero entry.

An example application of the θ-technique is given in Table 2. Note that where the sign test did not result in a significant difference ($p > .05$), the $\hat{\theta}$-technique did ($p < .001$). Thus, we have shown that the $\hat{\theta}$-technique can be (and typically is) more sensitive to differences in the two patterns of outcome. In the example, the value of $\hat{\theta}$(.6441) gives the estimated proportion of clients whose outcomes would be better with Treatment A than with Treatment B, with an estimated $\sigma_{\hat{\theta}}$ of $\sqrt{.001} = .0316$.

There are other hypothesis matrices which can be generated when using the θ-technique. Here are some examples.

(a) Treatment A will result in greater maintenance and improvement than Treatment B.

	Termination Levels			
Intake Levels	(1–2)	(3–4)	(5–6)	(7–9)
(1–2)	1	1	1	1
(3–4)	0	1	1	1
(5–6)	0	0	1	1
(7–9)	0	0	0	1

(b) Treatment A will result in greater maintenance and improvement for functioning at level 6 or below.

Intake Levels	(1–2)	(3–4)	(5–6)	(7–9)
(1–2)	1	1	1	1
(3–4)	0	1	1	1
(5–6)	0	0	1	1
(7–9)	0	0	0	0

Table 2. Example Computation of a Test for ($\theta = \hat{\theta}$) (Using Data in Table 1)

$$\hat{\theta} = \tfrac{1}{2}\left[\sum_{j=1}^{Int.} (P_{..j}) \sum_{i=1}^{Ter.} w_{ij}(P_{A_{ij}} - P_{B_{ij}})\right] + \tfrac{1}{2}$$

where for $P_{..j}$, using part (a) of Table 4.7.1

$$P_{..1} = (10 + 11)/(49 + 50) = \frac{21}{99} = \frac{7}{33},\ P_{..2} = \frac{33}{99} = \frac{1}{3},\ P_{..3} = \frac{32}{99},\ P_{..4} = \frac{13}{99}$$

For the values of $(P_{A_{ij}} - P_{B_{ij}})$ use part (c) of Table 1. Since there are only six values of 1.00, we can compute

$$\hat{\theta} = \tfrac{1}{2}\left[\frac{7}{33}(-.063 + .127 + .109) + 1/3(.157 + .173) + \frac{32}{99}(.438)\right] + \tfrac{1}{2}$$

$$= \tfrac{1}{2}[.212(.173) + .333(.330) + .323(.438)] + \tfrac{1}{2}$$

$$= [(0.5)(0.0367 + 0.1100 + .1415)] + 0.5 = [(0.5)(0.2882)] + 0.5$$

$$\boxed{\hat{\theta} = 0.6441},$$

$$\hat{\sigma}^2_{\hat{\theta}} = \tfrac{1}{4}\left(\frac{1}{N_A} + \frac{1}{N_B}\right) \sum_{j=1}^{Int.} \sum_{i=1}^{Ter.} \left(\frac{n_{A_{ij}} + n_{B_{ij}}}{N_A + N_B}\right)(w_{ij} - \bar{w}_{.j})^2$$

for $\bar{w}_{.j} = \sum_{i=1}^{Ter.} w_{ij}\left(\frac{n_{A_{ij}} + n_{B_{ij}}}{n_{A_{.j}} + n_{B_{.j}}}\right)$, as $j = (1, 2, 3, 4)$ and where $w_{ij} = 1$

$$\bar{w}_{.1} = \frac{(3 + 4 + 2) + (4 + 3 + 1)}{10 + 11} = \frac{17}{21},\ \bar{w}_{.2} = \frac{(8 + 4) + (5 + 1)}{17 + 16} = \frac{18}{33} = \frac{6}{11},$$

$$\bar{w}_{.3} = \frac{10 + 3}{16 + 16} = \frac{13}{32},\ \bar{w}_{.4} = 0$$

$$\hat{\sigma}^2_{\hat{\theta}} = \tfrac{1}{4}\frac{1}{49} + \frac{1}{50}\left\{\left[\frac{4}{99}\left(0 - \frac{17}{21}\right)^2 + \frac{7}{99}\left(1 - \frac{17}{21}\right)^2 + \frac{7}{99}\left(1 - \frac{17}{21}\right)^2 + \frac{3}{99}\left(1 - \frac{17}{21}\right)^2\right]\right.$$

$$+ \left[\frac{3}{99}\left(0 - \frac{6}{11}\right)^2 + \frac{12}{99}\left(0 - \frac{6}{11}\right)^2 + \frac{13}{99}\left(1 - \frac{6}{11}\right)^2 + \frac{5}{99}\left(1 - \frac{6}{11}\right)^2\right]$$

$$\left. + \left[\frac{0}{99}\left(0 - \frac{13}{32}\right)^2 + \frac{6}{99}\left(0 - \frac{13}{32}\right)^2 + \frac{13}{99}\left(0 - \frac{13}{32}\right)^2 + \frac{13}{99}\left(1 - \frac{13}{32}\right)^2\right] + [0.0]\right\}$$

$$\hat{\sigma}^2_{\hat{\theta}} = (0.25)(0.0404)[(0.0265 + 0.0026 + 0.0026 + 0.0011)$$

$$+ (0.0090 + 0.0360 + 0.0271 + 0.0104) + (0.0 + 0.0100 + 0.0217 + 0.0463) + (0.0)]$$

$$\hat{\sigma}^2_{\hat{\theta}} = (0.00505)[(0.0328) + (0.0825) + (0.0780)] = (0.0101)(0.1933)$$

$$\boxed{\hat{\sigma}^2_{\hat{\theta}} = 0.0019523}$$

Thus to test ($\theta = \hat{\theta}$)

$$\chi^2 = (\hat{\theta} - \tfrac{1}{2})^2/\hat{\sigma}^2_{\hat{\theta}} = (0.6441 - 0.5)^2/(0.0020)$$

$$\chi^2 = \frac{(0.1441)^2}{(0.002)} = 10.3824,\ \text{significant } p < .001 \ (\text{df} = 1).$$

Thus, Treatment A results in a significantly greater proportion of clients to improve across the various levels of initial functioning.

The acceptable pattern of "1" and "0" values in the hypothesis matrix is limited by one logical restriction: One can only predict an outcome pattern for the more effective treatment as maintenance or improvement or both. This means that you cannot hypothesize a curvilinear relationship such as the one below when using the θ-technique since a linear pattern is one of the statistical assumptions underlying θ.

Intake Levels	(1–2)	(3–4)	(5–6)	(7–9)	
(1–2)	0	1	1	0	NOT PERMISSIBLE!
(3–4)	0	0	1	0	
(5–6)	0	0	0	1	
(7–9)	0	1	1	0	

Using θ-Technique for Multiple Comparisons—One can run as many pair-wise comparisons, using θ, as there are degrees of freedom in the design. Each θ-statistic consumes one degree of freedom.

MULTIPLE CRITERIA TECHNIQUES

Multiple criteria techniques provide a means of simultaneously considering a number of facets in the analysis. For example, when analyzing the relative cost and effectiveness of two or more therapeutic approaches, we might wish to consider the following:

— behavior change relative to entry level
— behavior change relative to agreed upon goals
— costs of professional time and support
— personal and psychological costs (stigma) to client
— ethical limits of intervention and control

Professor Brian Yates' definition text, *Improving effectiveness and reducing costs in mental health,* details a model for manipulating techniques which permit multiple facets to be considered successfully or simultaneously when selecting among alternatives.[3] An adaptation of Yates' model is diagrammed in Figure 1. Let us examine the major features of the Resource-Constraints-Process-Outcome (RCPO) model:

— *Resources* are the elements which can be initially identified. These elements can be categorized in any fashion which is convenient to the cost-effectiveness question being addressed. In Figure 1, the resources are categorized by the logic of mental-health systems followed throughout this book. Note that the model considers what the client brings to the situation as a resource. To quote Professor Yates, client "dysfunctions, or at least their potential of developing in the community, are a necessary resource because without dysfunction the existence of mental health services cannot be justified" (p. 94).
— *Constraints* on resource elements and on the technology of therapeutic intervention are the elements of reality which influence the entire process, and often result in less than suc-

[3] The Yates (1980) text, chapter 5, is the basic reference. Our discussion only provides a general review of the techniques.

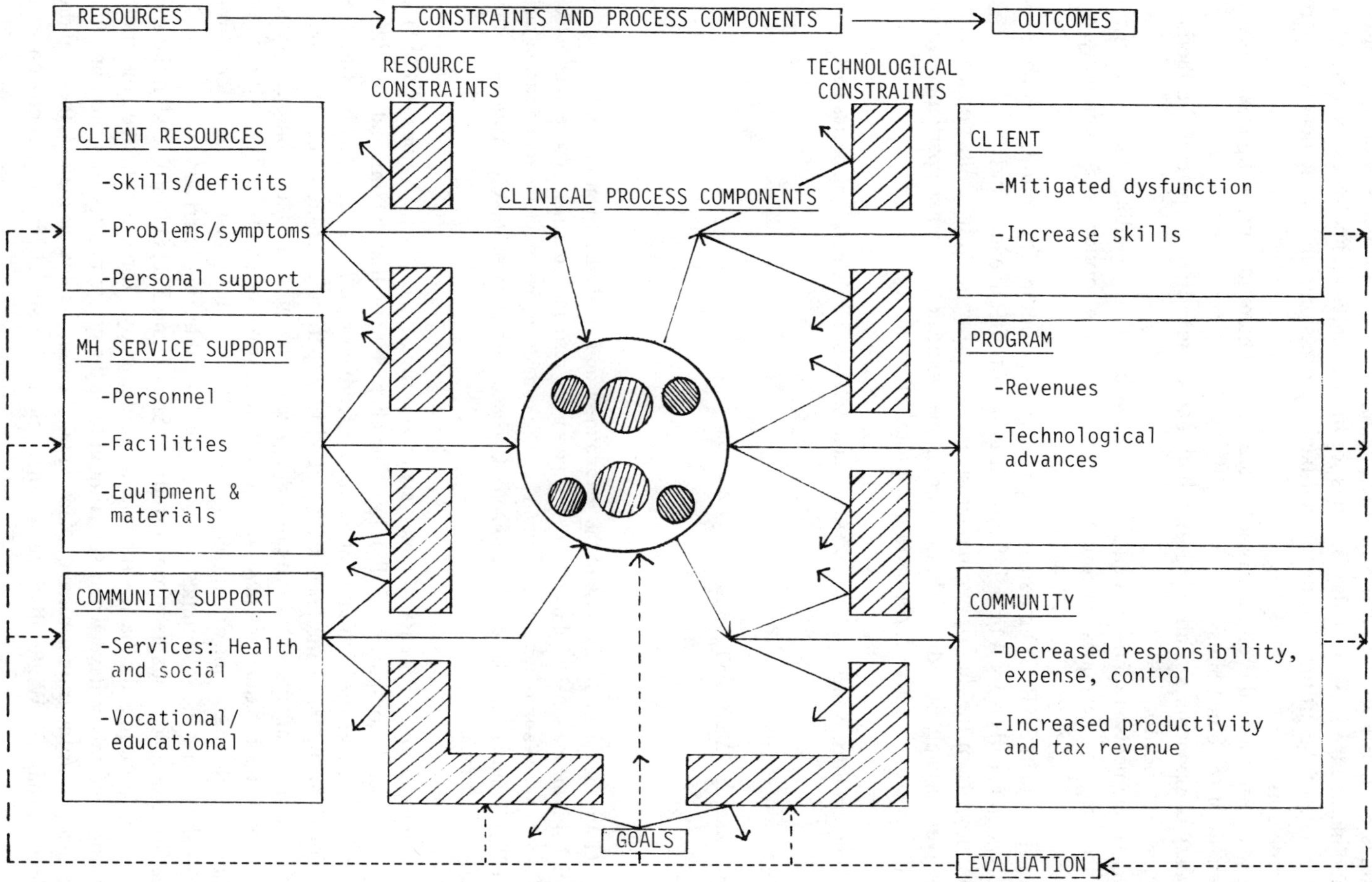

Figure 1. The RCPO Analysis Model (Adapted from Yates, 1980)

cessful outcomes. Examples of client resource constraints are the limits in the clients' abilities to understand or deal with their problems or deficiencies. Service constraints would include the lack of funds, facilities, or trained staff. Technological constraints refer to the state-of-the-art limits of the mental-health professions' abilities to deal with particular problems.

— *Goals* filtering into the clinical process are those which are agreed upon and possible, given all of the constraints.
— *Process* components are all of those which can be identified as part of the therapeutic process (see Section II).
— *Outcome* elements are those which are selected as useful for deciding whether to terminate services, to draw revenues, or to evaluate the impact on services and community

The major strength of the RCPO model is that it provides an outline for detailing which elements are to be systematically varied or held constant in a cost-effectiveness study.

The move from the descriptive model (as shown in Figure 1) to a functional model for cost-effectiveness analysis is direct. For example, one would consider that a particular treatment program (T_j) is cost effective for a particular group of clients if:

$$(\text{Program Effectiveness of } T_j) \geq \Sigma(\text{Acceptable levels of all RCPO})/\text{components of } T_j)$$

or

$$E(T_j) \geq \sum_{i=1}^{n} [\Delta E(T_{ij}) P(T_{ij})]$$

where

$E(T_j)$ is the total effectiveness of the jth treatment on a particular client group.
$E(T_{ij})$ is the marginal level that the ith component (of resource, constraint, process, or outcome) can have in order for an alternative to be considered as acceptable to a decision maker.
$P(T_{ij})$ is the amount of the ith component needed to maximize the effectiveness of the jth treatment.

Thus, the purpose of the RCPO analysis is to estimate the ''best'' values of $P(T_{ij})$. The ''best'' levels of each component, $P(T_{ij})$, have the characteristic that in combination with other components will render the jth treatment as most effective or, at least, acceptably effective for selecting the jth treatment as therapeutically sound for a particular group of clients. The techniques of quantitative analysis for estimating $P(T_{ij})$ values are all related to techniques (systems) of solving simultaneous equations involving two or more unknown values.[4] We will not review the mechanics of these methods here (see Yates, 1980 for details). Instead, we offer a graphic example to show how the techniques can be applied for selecting alternatives.

The first example is adapted from a study by Siegert and Yates (1980). The initial step in the analysis is to outline the basic components in the study. Table 3 describes the multiple considerations one might have when selecting among three alternatives in a program (plus a contact control group) to train parents of ''acting out'' children to better manage their children's inappropriate behavior. While all three alternatives used a social learning approach to help

[4] Two examples are simplex solutions and linear programming. Many of the popular estimation techniques are available in computer programs.

Table 3. Matrix Identifying RCPO Components

Resources	Individual-in-Home	Individual-in-Office	Group-in-Office	Contact Controls	Resource Constraint
—Therapist salaries —Travel expenses —Allocated personnel overhead (e.g., staff development, supervision)	Time costs per client in home	Time costs per client in office	Time costs per group in office	Time costs per client in home	Budget limit on total time costs for all clients
Facility use, e.g., office, secretary, equipment	Overhead allocated per client without office costs	Overhead allocated per client with office costs	Overhead allocated per client with office costs	Overhead allocated per client without office costs	Budget limits on total office space and hours available
Psychological costs to client (stigma)	Scaled amount on a survey & drop-out rate	Scaled amount on a survey & drop-out rate	Scaled amount on a survey & drop-out rate	Scaled amount on a survey & drop-out rate	Ethical limit on total amount tolerable (e.g., a relative frequency of drop-out ≤ .20, and reduction in problem behaviors of ≤ 15%)
	Success probability or reduction in target (problem) behavior frequency	Success probability or reduction in target (problem) behavior frequency	Success probability or reduction in target (problem) behavior frequency	Success probability or reduction in target (problem) behavior frequency	
	OUTCOME EFFECTIVENESS				

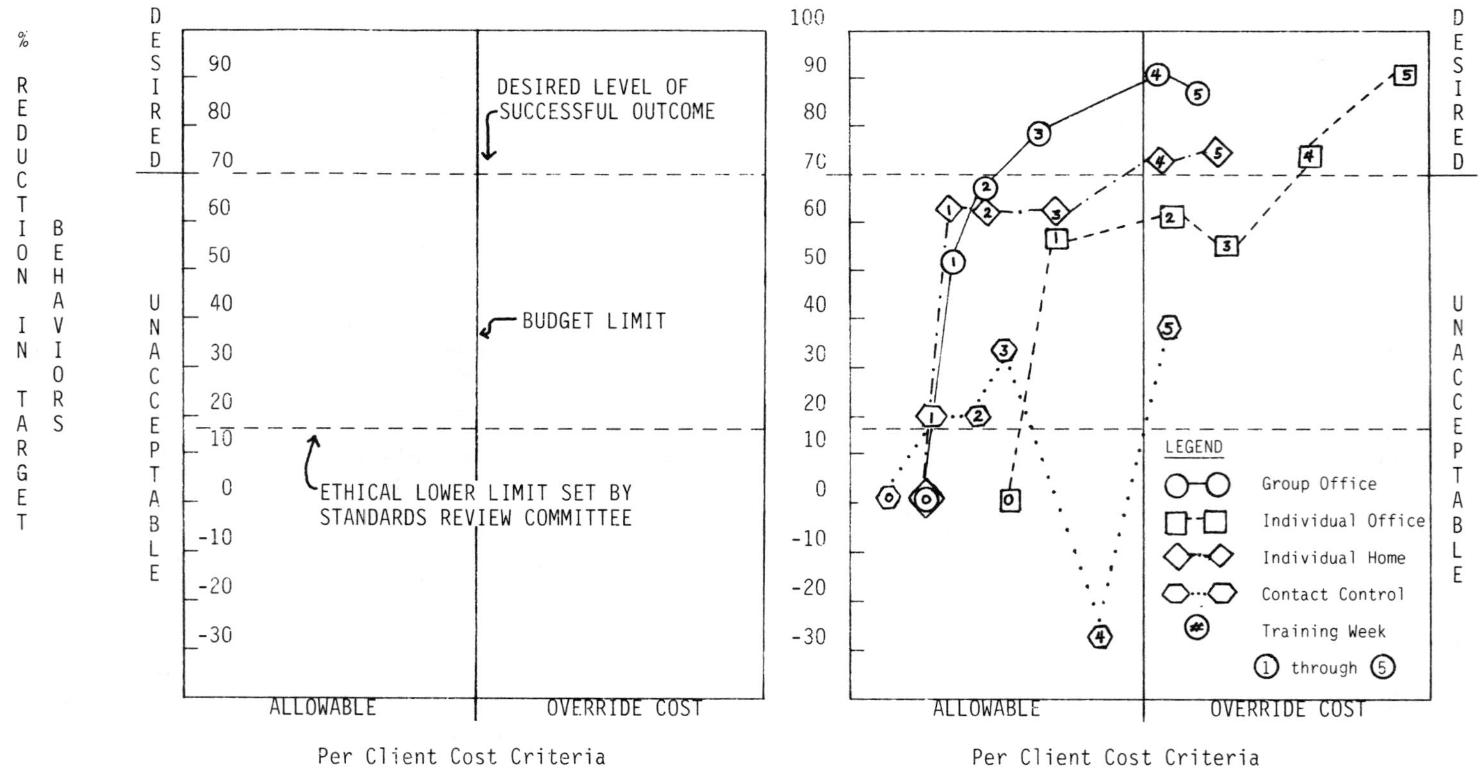

Step 1: Limits set by constraints

Step 2: Results of study

Figure 2. Graphic Description of Limits Imposed by Constraints (Left Panel) and Results of Study (Right Panel) [Adapted from Siegert and Yates (1980)]

parents reduce the frequency of problem behavior, the three differed in style and location of the counseling session:

(a) Parent group meets at clinic
(b) Parents meet with individual therapist at clinic
(c) Parents meet with therapist at parents' home
(d) Control parents meet with a counselor to discuss their problems but receive no instruction in parent-management skills.

The resources are identified in rows of Table 3, with constraints given on the right. The four alternatives are identified in the columns with the bottom row describing the outcome effectiveness. Once dollar values and desired levels of success are estimated, then the two-step graphic analysis offered in Figure 2 can be useful.

The first step is to describe the limits set by the constraints of budgets, ethical considerations, and the acceptability of different levels of outcome (left panel of Figure 2). The actual values of these limits could be set by either a mathematical procedure (e.g., linear programming) or an arbitrary standard (e.g., a professional standards committee setting a drop-out rate of 0.20 or less and an improvement rate of at least 15% reduction in problem level). The right panel describes the results of the Siegert and Yates (1980) study.

Let us inspect the enriched understanding of the results provided by the simultaneous consideration of multiple factors influencing costs and effectiveness. All three treatments were significantly better than the Contact Control condition. But by contrasting just final levels of outcome effectiveness, two procedures appeared to be approximately equivalent: Group-in-Office and Individual-in-Office. Both were approximately 15% ahead of Individual-at-Home. When considering cost efficiency within five sessions, Group-in-Office and Individual-at-Home were approximately 40% lower in per client costs. But the cost constraints suggest that only one of the procedures ought to be considered as cost effective and ethical: Group-in-Office. This conclusion is, of course, restricted to procedures for which the goals are to train parents to use behavior management techniques with their children. The results for the contact controls did suggest that simple contact and discussion of the problem may be ethically unsound. This conclusion seems warranted even though the Contact Control condition showed an average change in the reduction of problem behavior frequency which was above the ethical lower limit. Thus, the nonspecific therapeutic effects (cf. Strupp & Hadley, 1979; Strupp, Hadley, & Gomez-Schwartz, 1977) were not sufficient to be considered either cost effective or ethical. The results described in Figure 2 provide clear evidence for selecting the most cost effective and ethical approach among the alternatives considered.

CONCLUDING REMARKS

The three approaches to cost-effectiveness analysis described here are representative of many which can help us provide the most human and effective mental-health services within budgetary constraints. The issue is not whether we need to apply these procedures, but *how* to apply them. With the proper application of the procedures described in Chapters 21–24, the techniques describing *how* to do this are available to us.

— To care about another's emotional distress is humane.
— To seek the most effective means of alleviating the distress is scientifically responsible.
— To select the most effective means within our economic constraints is to be humanely responsible.

SECTION VIII

DESIGNING AND IMPLEMENTING A MANAGEMENT INFORMATION SYSTEM (MIS)

The objectives of Section VIII focus on the design and implementation of an information system to help perform managerial responsibilities, or more simply, a *M*anagement *I*nformation *S*ystem (MIS). Section VIII identifies:

— The *managerial questions* an MIS should answer as the level of responsibility shifts.
— The *shortcomings* in current MIS reports and how to correct them.
— *Practical tactics* to get an MIS started (or changed).
— The basic steps in the *system-design process.*
— The major *cost elements* of information-systems development.
— An outline for *documenting a system* through a procedures manual.

The Section is outlined to help master the essentials of MIS design and implementation:

Chapter 25: Integrating Your Information System Linkages describes how to bring together the procedures which were outlined in the preceding seven sections into an integrated system which can provide information for decisions at all levels of a mental-health program.
Chapter 26: System Design: Linking Roles and Questions in the MIS explores the role of MIS, the kinds of questions that an MIS can answer, and the kinds of questions that should be asked at varying levels of management.
Chapter 27: Implementing an Integrated System starts by suggesting some practical tactics for starting an MIS. The design process is previewed and followed by the required steps of doing a design and concludes with the costs of information systems.
Chapter 28: Assuring the Dependability of Your Fiscal Data addresses the age-old problem of accounting internal controls in mental-health organizations. The dependability of fiscal data is linked vitally to the accounting internal-control system. Many mental-health organizations have weak or inoperative accounting controls, and the fiscal data can become undependable. When fiscal data are undependable, cost analyses become unreliable. After identifying the basic elements of good accounting internal controls, detailed checklists spot major weaknesses. The lists have been designed for and used in mental-health organizations. Finally, a specific approach to organizing staff is outlined to *maximize* internal control for both small and large organizations.
Chapter 29: Documentation and a Procedures Manual outlines a general format for

writing up the MIS. Written documentation facilitates orderly system change and guards against the danger of system staff turnover. When procedures are codified, training and routine operation usually go more smoothly and the independent auditors are generally happier.

Chapter 25

Integrating Your Information System Linkages*

> Which Positions and Roles Have To Be Linked Together and in What Order?
> What Kinds of Information Need To Be Linked Together To Make a Client-Oriented Cost-outcome System Work?

To produce an ongoing client-oriented cost-outcome management system requires a crucial linkage of organizational positions through a management information system (MIS). Everyone in a mental-health organization is a manager of something. But to fulfill this managerial role requires information and clear lines of communication. Chapter 25 will reveal the critical role of the MIS in carrying out the linking process.

OUTLINE

Starting with the objective of returning the client to the community, key positions and roles are systematically interrelated. The client is linked to clinical service and case-management staff, who in turn are linked to clinical supervisory staff. Supervisory staff are then connected to consultation and education who are then linked up to the research and evaluation/MIS staff. Coming back to the client, the supportive roles of the clinical records staff and fiscal support staff are linked together. Finally, the board and top administration roles are tied in to complete the entire linking process.

The chapter is divided into 11 sections:

(1) THE BASIC CONCEPTS
(2) PREVIEW OF UNIT: LINKING KEY POSITIONS AND ROLES
(3) CLIENT RETURN TO THE COMMUNITY
(4) CLINICAL SERVICE AND CASE MANAGEMENT STAFF
(5) CLINICIAL SUPERVISORY STAFF

---

* The concept for this chapter was conceived by Barbara Buswell and the example was worked through with Fred Smith of the Pittsburgh (PA) Office of MH/MR.

(6) CONSULTATION AND EDUCATION STAFF
(7) RESEARCH AND EVALUATION/MIS STAFF
(8) CLINICAL RECORDS STAFF
(9) FISCAL SUPPORT STAFF
(10) BOARD AND TOP ADMINISTRATION
(11) SUMMARY

1. THE BASIC CONCEPTS

Chapter 25 integrates previously discussed concepts. All of the essential elements to produce a client-oriented cost-outcome system have been exposed, and now is the appropriate time to link these elements together. The MIS becomes the ''glue'' that holds all of the parts together, and the ''communications network'' that keeps all of the parts informed of what the others are doing.

Managers will see how the elusive and abstract references to ''information systems'' come into clear focus. Outside observers of the organization will be better able to pinpoint missing connections and to diagnose malfunctions. Everyone should emerge with a clear and practical understanding of the key role information systems play in producing client-oriented services.

2. PREVIEW OF THE UNIT: LINKING KEY POSITIONS AND ROLES

The objective is straightforward: Link all of the essential positions into an integrated working system. The key positions and roles start with the client, move to clinical service, case management and supervision, and then add fiscal, administrative, and Board support. Finally, Consultation and Education, and Research/Evaluation activities are added to round out the set of essential linkages.

3. CLIENT RETURN TO THE COMMUNITY

The overriding objective is the client's return to a functioning level within the community. Four critical stages are envisioned: Entry, Service Planning, Service Provision and Review, and Termination with Followup. The four progressive stages can be shown graphically with key linkages identified by 1–5 (Figure 1).

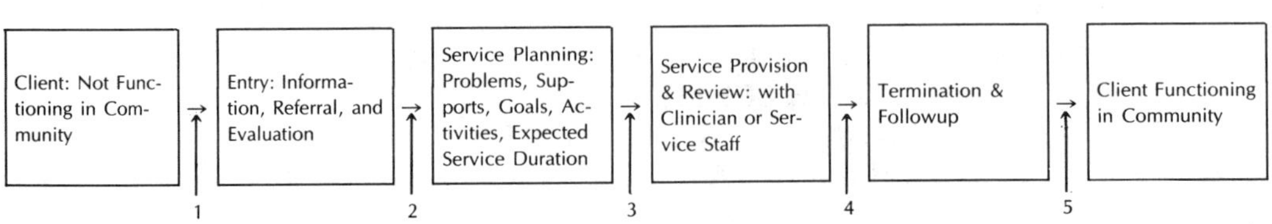

Figure 1. Linking the Four Essential Stages in Client Treatment

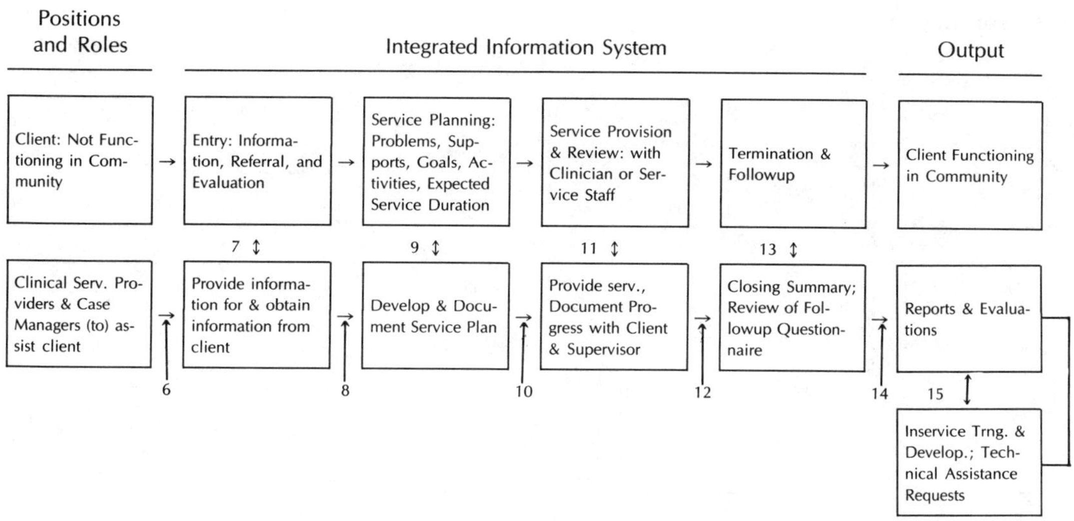

Figure 2. Linking Clinicians' and Case Managers' Roles

4. CLINICAL SERVICE AND CASE MANAGEMENT

The next essential set of positions and roles to be linked are those of the clinicians and case managers (6 in Figure 2). Linkages of the clinical processes are flagged by even numbers (e.g., 6, 8, 10), while linkages of the client to the clinical process are identified by odd numbers (e.g., 7, 9, 11). To assist the client, the client's entry requires the staff to provide as well as obtain information from the client (7). These data become the foundation for the development and documentation of a service plan (8). The process and the resulting documents become the tangible evidence of client-service planning (9). Actual service delivery is documented for review by the client and clinical supervisors (10) and (11). A closing summary review and followup questionnaire provide evidence of the client's termination and followup (12) and (13). The culmination is the creation of reports and evaluations used by clinical managers and others (14). The reports become the bases for inservice training, staff development, and technical assistance requests.

5. CLINICAL SUPERVISORY STAFF (AND EXTERNAL REVIEWERS)

Clinical activities are guided by clinical supervisors (Figure 3). Often there are external reviews from client advocates or PSROs. The positions and roles are identified by even numbers (e.g., 16, 18) and linked to clinical services by odd numbers (e.g., 17, 19). Supervisors are charged with supervising and monitoring the screening and intake standards (16), and are necessarily dependent on client data obtained by the staff (17). The supervisory process is traced into the service plans developed and documented by clinical staff (18, 19). Document reviews focus on

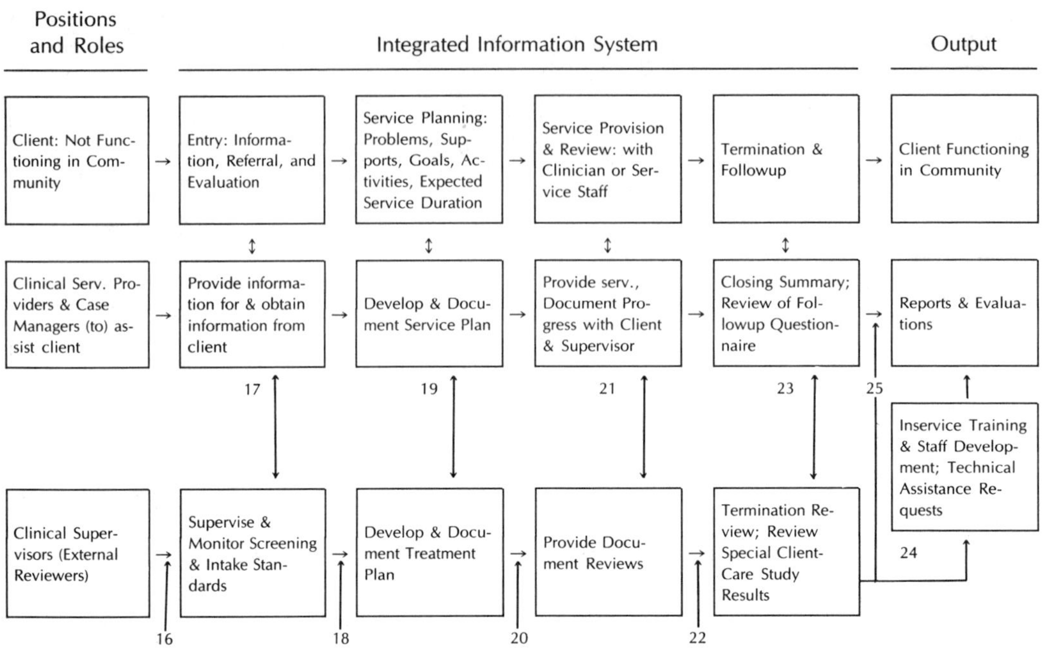

Figure 3. Linking Clinical Supervisors

- — Quality of record content
- — Concurrent progress
- — Utilization of service
- — Peer review
- — Client satisfaction
- — Special client-care studies

and link to the clinicians services, client progress and review (20) and (21). The supervisory and review process concludes with reviews of terminations and of special client-care studies (22) and (23). This latter activity also feeds requirements for inservice training, staff development, and technical assistance requests (24) and reports (25).

6. CONSULTATION AND EDUCATION

The major alternative to client service is prevention. The question is, "Is it better to treat malaria by training doctors or by spraying for mosquitos?" The former enhances direct service while the latter fosters prevention. Consultation and education (C & E) can expand the knowledge and understanding of relevant groups (e.g., teachers, judges, police) while mounting programs to help prevent mental illness. C & E staff handle community referral, agency consultation, education and liasion aimed at primary and secondary prevention (26) and (27). These efforts should be influenced by the kinds of service plans currently offered to clients (29A) as well as the results of document reviews (29B). Groups "at risk" should be identified (28, 31), and C & E programs prepared to address these identified high-risk groups (30, 33A, 33B). One direct accomplishment is a training program in coping skills for potentially vulnerable individuals (30). The revised diagram is shown in Figure 4.

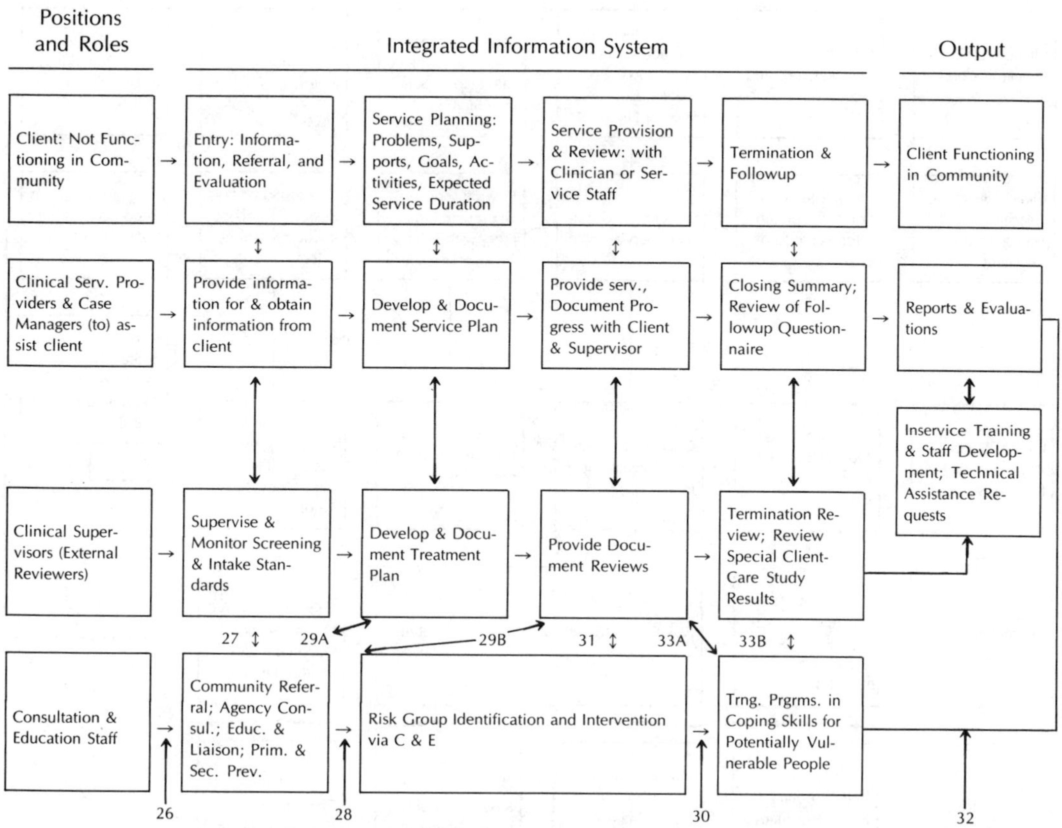

Figure 4. Linking C & E Staff

7. RESEARCH AND EVALUATION/MIS STAFF

Data retrieval and preparing reports to meet the requirements of program-oriented decision making is the role of Research and Evaluation (R & E) and MIS (Figure 5).

The various forms and reports suggested in (34) and (35) become the visible evidence and tangible products of all of the foregoing interacting positions and roles of clients, clinicians, supervisors, and C & E staff. But the model is incomplete since it has not identified the functional support provided by the clinical and fiscal records, and by the policy and procedures established by the Board and top administration. Starting again with the client, the clinical-records staff are added and followed by the administrative and policy levels.

8. CLINICAL-RECORDS STAFF

The fundamental support for clinical communication and data base for research and evaluation is lodged with the clinical records and clinical-records staff (Figure 6).

These records establish records of initial contact (38) drawn from initial client entry (39).

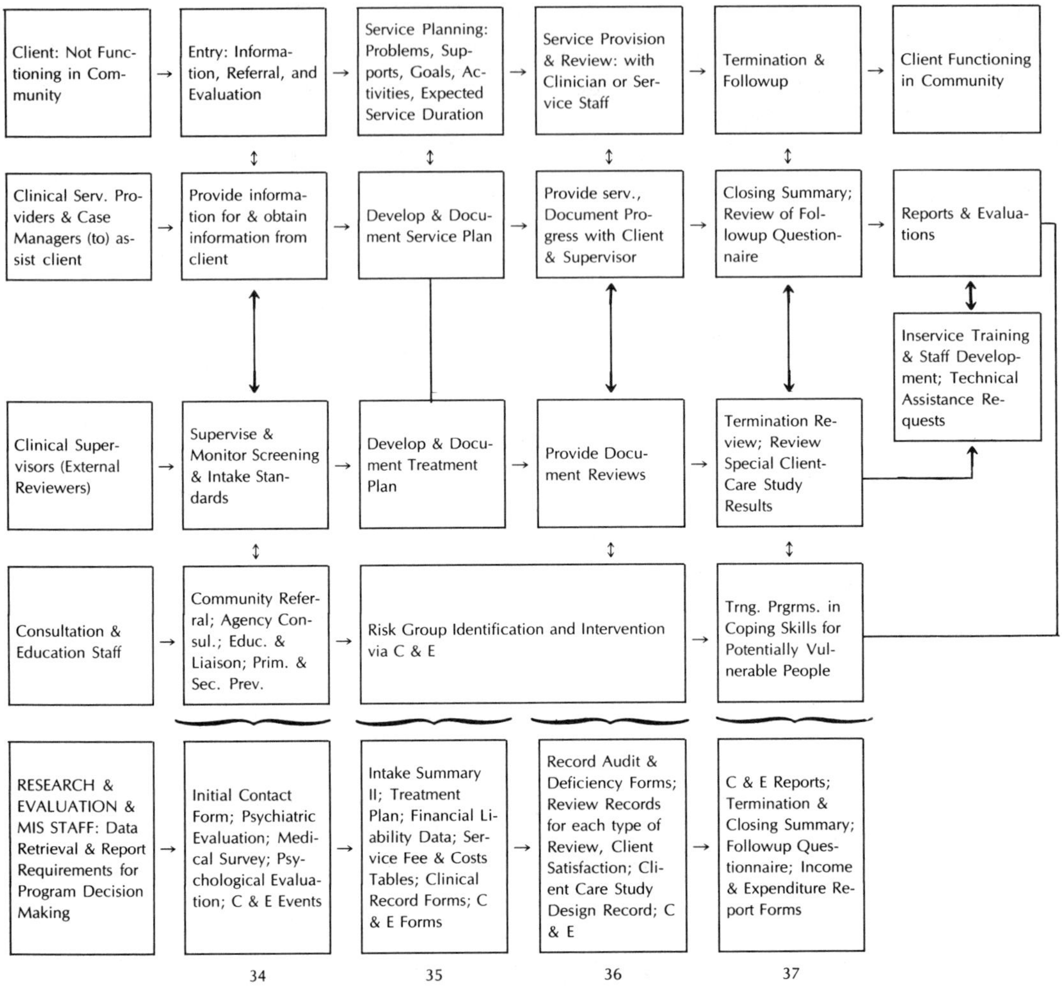

Figure 5. Linking R & E/MIS Staff

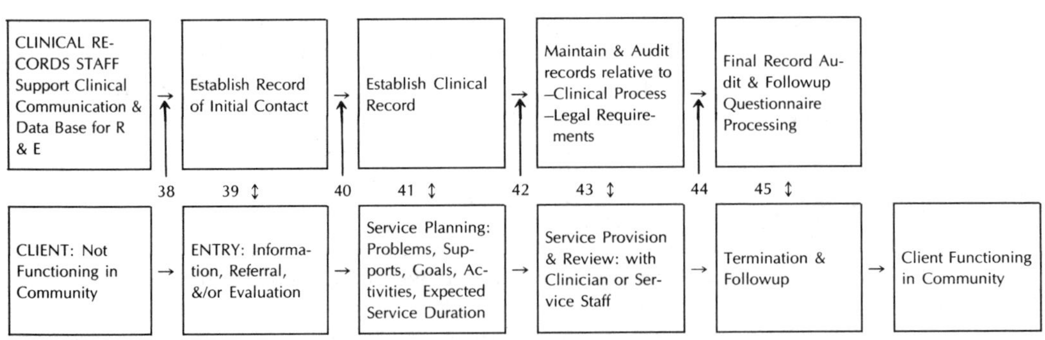

Figure 6. Linking Clinical-Records Staff

The clinical record (40) is the documentation of treatment planning (41). Evidence of services provided and satisfaction of legal requirements (42) is drawn from the provision and review of services (43). Final record audit and followup (44) link to the client termination and followup (45).

9. FISCAL SUPPORT

Fiscal staff support both clinical and administrative roles (Figure 7). Linkings (46) to (62) attempt to reveal the complex way fiscal-support staff are tied to the clinical and client positions and roles. Fiscal staff provide client information of fiscal liability (46) drawn from initial contact (47). Assessment of financial liability and payments (46) depends on service plans (49). Service activity costs, billing and collection (50) are linked to services received (51). The final account settlement (52) is tied to termination (61) and income produced from the account.

Support of administration roles starts with the budget (54) which is partially linked to fiscal liability information of clients (55). The revenue sets the limits for service costs (56) and interacts with the financial liability of first- and third-party clients (57). Service costs influence rates and payment requests (58) and are driven by service activity costs and billing (59A). However, both rates and services are interactive with service costs and financial payments from first- and third-party payments (59B). Income (60) is impacted by rates, and payment requests

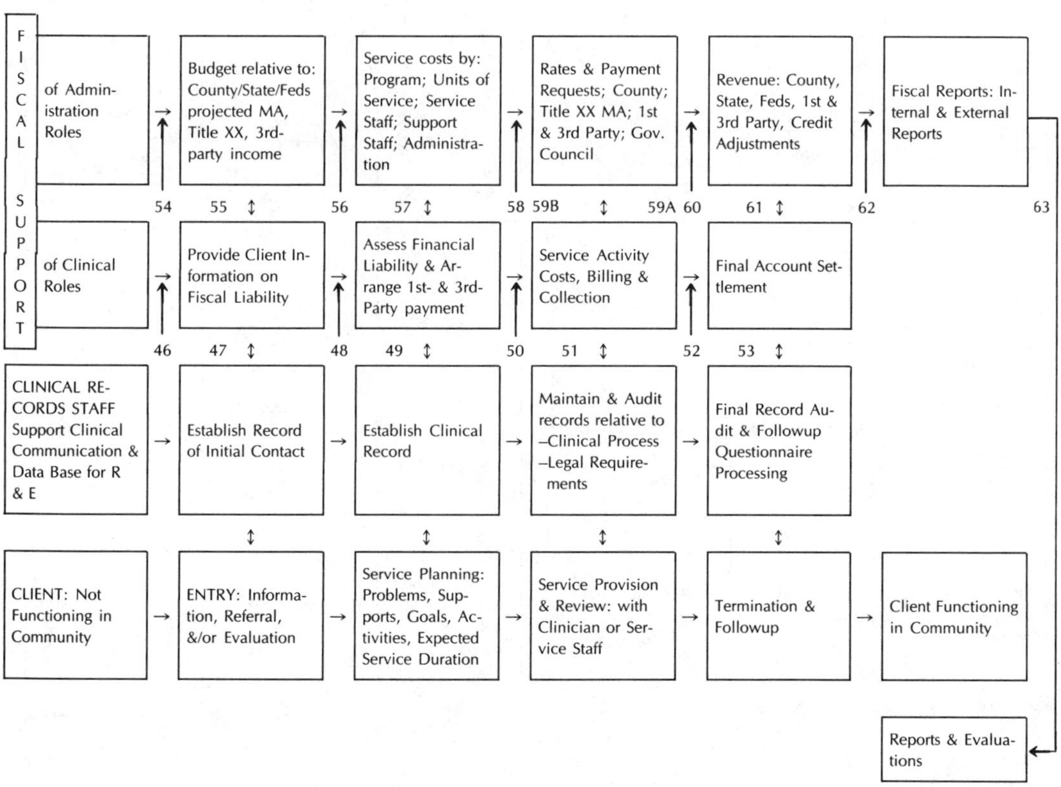

Figure 7. Linking Fiscal Support

and the final account settlement (61) converge in the fiscal reports containing both revenues and costs (62) and reports combining program evaluation and fiscal data, e.g., cost-outcome reports (63).

10. BOARD AND TOP ADMINISTRATION

The final layer is the Board and top administration (Figure 8). The Board is responsible for overall policy which is interpreted, implemented and monitored by the top administration. Procedure developed and carried out by the top administration should reflect the intent of Board policy. The Board and top administration formulate goals and objectives along with program structure (64).

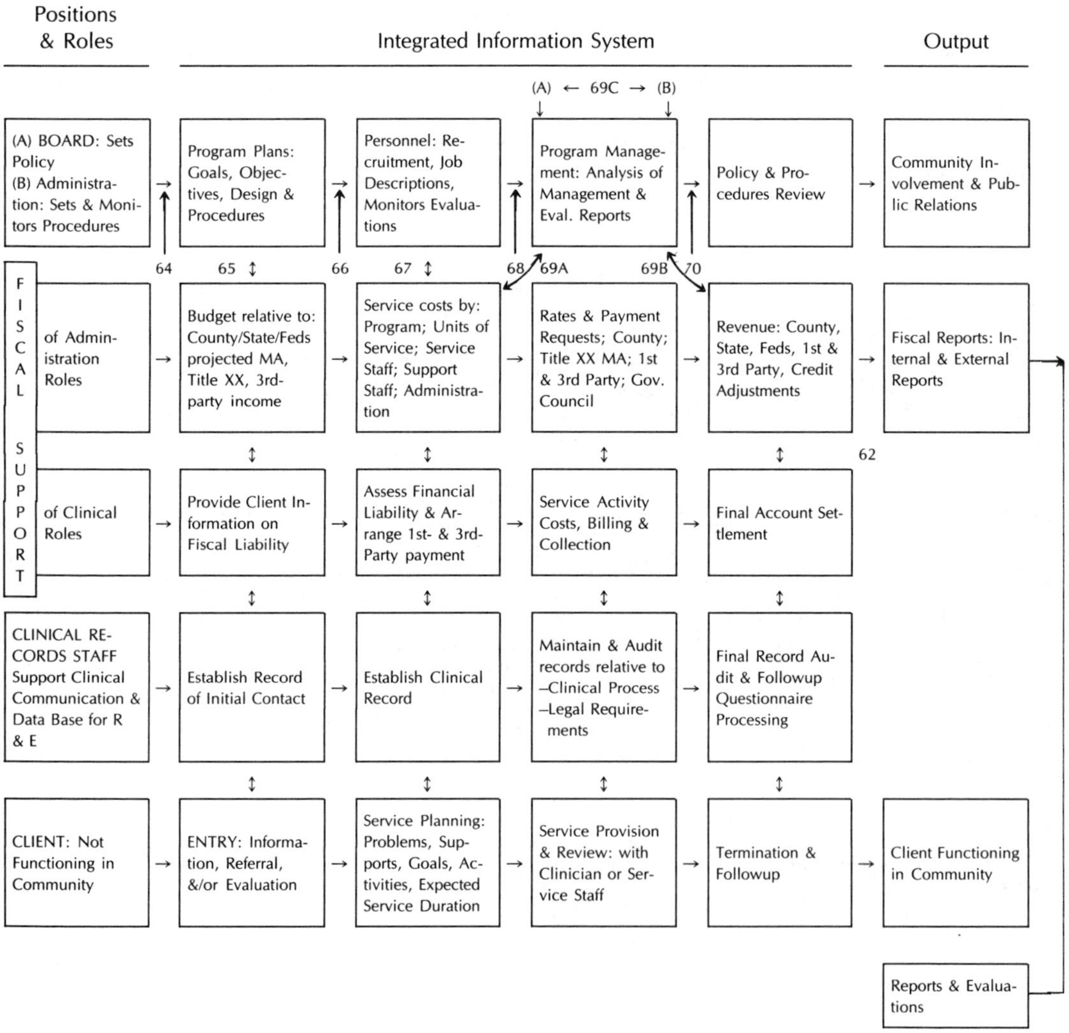

Figure 8. Linking Board and Top Administration

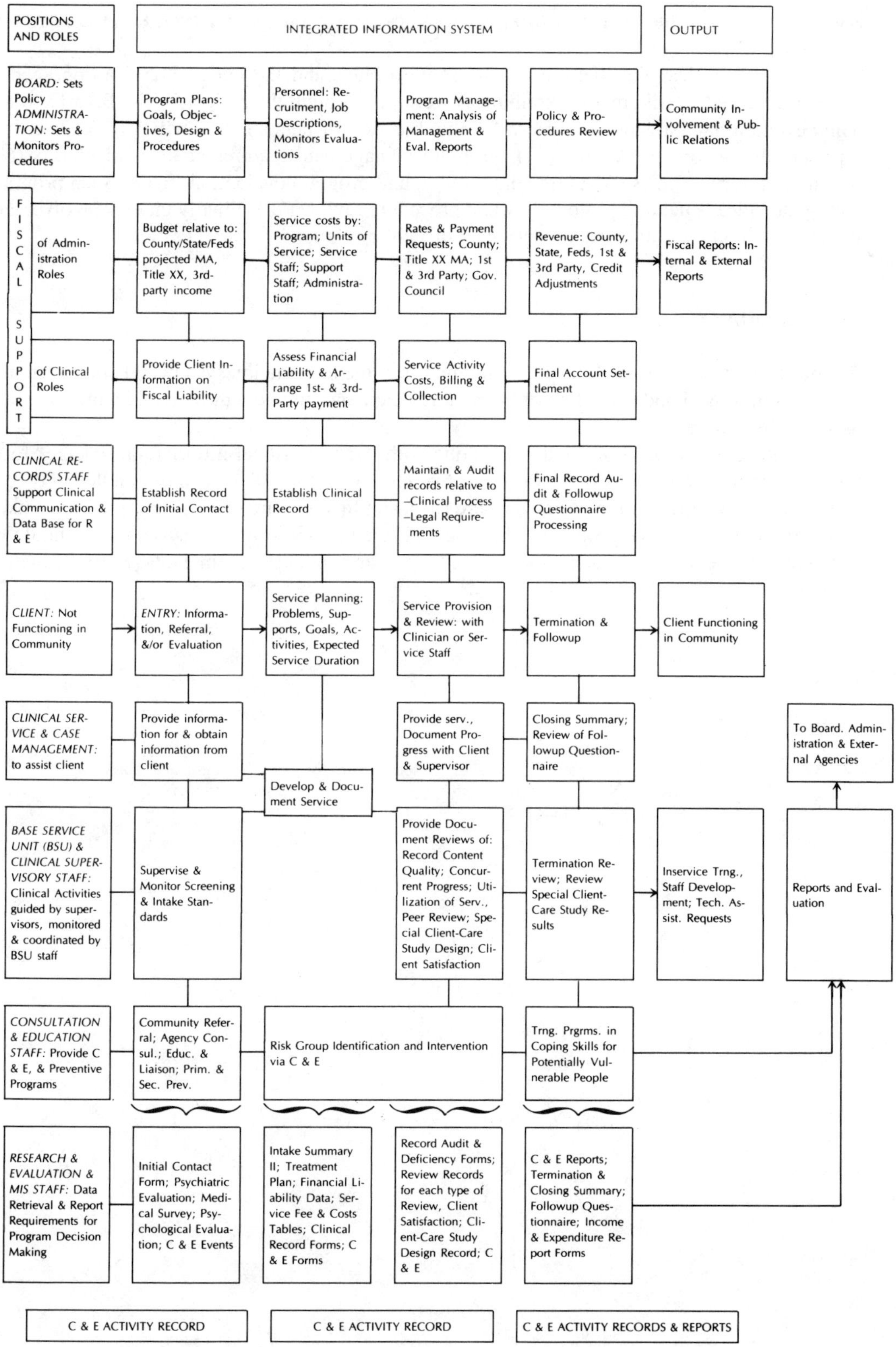

Figure 9. The Complete Integrated Information System

There is a clear link between such program plans and the budget (65). As one center director observed, ''All great program ideas work out through the budget.'' The Board and top administration have a general concern for the direction of personnel activities (66) since they represent the major service cost (67). Program management requires analysis of reports (68) prepared on service costs (69A), revenue (69B), and program evaluation (69C). Such program management leads naturally into policy and procedure review (70). Finally there is involvement in the community and the critical activities of public relations.

11. SUMMARY

By collectively viewing all of the positions and roles, the information system and outputs should lead to an improved understanding of the required elements and how they should work together, as shown in Figure 9.

Eight levels of positions and roles along with over 70 critical information linkages form the client-oriented cost-outcome management system. This complexity can be handled only by a well-coordinated information system, where roles and linkages are clearly described and linked to the program's principal products. The essential role of an information system now should be apparent. Chapters 26–28 pursue the details for the design and implementation of information systems.

Chapter 26

System Design: Linking Roles and Questions in the MIS

Since Everyone Manages Something in Mental Health Programs:
How Can the MIS Help Me?
What Are Major Management Questions I Can Answer with My MIS?
Should Team Leaders, Service Managers, Center Directors, and State Agencies Get the Same Data?

1. ROLE OF THE MIS

Developing the capacity to provide planning and performance information requires a management information system (MIS). The MIS must focus on what information is needed in decision making for the major questions faced by you as a manager.

The MIS must produce information to help you:

(1) Assess the patterns of service delivery (e.g., who receives what types and amounts of services, when, and where?)
(2) Define how current resources are being acquired and consumed (e.g., what are the major sources of revenue? What are the professional staff costs for the outpatient service?)
(3) Provide monitoring aids for various mental-health care providers and managers (e.g., were particular admissions inappropriate?)
(4) Assess outcomes of rendered services (e.g., level of functioning of client, changes in symptoms)
(5) Develop data needed for multiple reporting requirements (e.g., reporting to NIMH, funding agencies, and payment agents such as States and Social Security Administration or entities such as PSRO)
(6) Create a data base for planning (e.g., identifying changing patterns of utilization)

Good managers ask lots of questions. Our emphasis is on *comprehensive* questions. Too often, these comprehensive questions are *not* asked. In their place are detailed questions which fail to address central issues. We haven't ignored important detailed, segmented questions, since understanding *general* cost outcomes usually requires more *detailed* and more *segmented* questions.

2. QUESTIONS

Managers are likely to require select data on all clientele and on the resources acquired and devoted to providing various services (Cooper, 1973, pp. 10–11). Depending on the managerial level, managers usually require report information focused around the broad classes of information produced by the MIS.

Questions Assessing Patterns of Patient or Client Care and Services might include:

—Illustrative statistical management reports such as
- –Disposition of intakes by organizational service and entry level of functioning
- –Ethnic/racial background by sex, type of service received, and outcome
- –Clients discharged by major diagnosis and cost outcomes

Illustrative reports for resource management could include:

—Number and proportion of admissions (apparently) eligible for third-party reimbursement
—Volume of services by client problem, problem severity, type of service, and organizational unit
—Patient caseload by individual staff or staffing units, where caseload includes a description of client problem areas and level of functioning

Questions Defining How Various Types of Resources Are Acquired and Consumed require statistical and financial reports. Typical statistical reports should include:

—Distribution of staff time by discipline, service, and caseload
—Volume of services provided by staff or staffing units and caseload

The financial reports would include:

—Cost per unit of service
—Comparison of program costs and fee revenue by type of service and clients served
—Comparison of budgets and expenses by organizational components and clients served

Questions Creating Monitoring Aids for mental-health case managers for peer review and utilization review could include statistical/clinical reports such as:

—Concurrent review aids
- –Admissions not meeting admission justification profile criteria by type of admitting diagnosis or problem
- –Listing of admissions not completing treatment plans
- –Extended length of stay by service and clinical complications

—Retrospective review aids
 –Admitting diagnoses not validated by clinician
 –Admission justification not confirmed
 –Case listing of diagnoses accompanied by potentially harmful medical services

Financially oriented aid could include

—Concurrent review aids
 –Admission without determination of third-party payment source
 –Cumulative charges in excess of Medicaid or medication allowances
—Retrospective review aids
 –Cases where cost per episode differs from average cost criteria (mean ± 1 standard deviation).

When *Questions Identifying Patient Outcomes* are asked, clinical management concerns may be addressed by reports on:

—Discharge status by diagnosis, entry, and termination level of functioning
—Specific clinical complications by diagnosis and level of functioning
—Specific clinical complications by service and clinician

Financial analysis could include

—Changes in level of functioning (e.g., global outcome) and amount of resources consumed (e.g., costs) or cost outcome
—Comparisons of cost outcomes of varied services or organizational units

Usually, questions responding to *External Reporting Requirements* are completed from existing internally generated reports or by a search of an external source (e.g., census data).

Self-study Exercise: Understanding Major Management Questions

As a manager you will require some data (usually in summary form) on all clients and on the resources acquired and devoted to providing various services for those clients. Following is a series of reports answering questions about:

(A) Patterns of service delivery
(B) Acquisition and use of resources
(C) Monitoring aids
(D) Client outcomes

You are asked to:

— Classify each report in its appropriate class
— Develop a question you think the report might answer

The first report has been completed as a guide.

Report	General Class A. Patterns of Service Delivery B. Acquisition and Use of Resources C. Monitoring Aids D. Client Outcomes (please circle)	An Illustrative Management Question and Management Action: Question	Action
1. Client Load[1] by Individual Staff and Staffing Units	A. B. C. D.	Do I need to reallocate my staff to even up workload?	Reassign staff from partial care to outpatient.
2. Percentage of Staff Time Spent in Direct Service, by Client Type	A. B. C. D.		
3. Comparison of Budgeted Expenses to Actual Expenses	A. B. C. D.		
4. Number of Active Clients Not Seen in 90 Days, by Client Type	A. B. C. D.		
5. Monthly Cost-Outcome Matrix of Each Major Service	A. B. C. D.		

(Suggested solution: 2B, 3B, 4C, 5B and D)

[1]Caseload is defined by number of clients in major problem areas and by level of problem severity or functioning.

3. QUESTIONS AND REPORTS SHOULD VARY BY MANAGERIAL LEVEL

Most of the foregoing illustrative reports are focused for the manager of a mental-health service delivery organization. The type of variable and its measurement should vary depending on the *level* of the decision maker. A report on the amount of each individual's time spent in direct service may be highly significant to an outpatient team leader but dims in significance for a legislator who is more likely to focus on cost per unit of service purchased with state monies.

Selecting and focusing the measures for the level of decision making represent one of the greatest challenges in an MIS. All too often, detailed measures appropriate only for first-level supervisors are being reviewed by decision makers charged with state or regional concerns. The funding agencies have the right to all information needed to satisfy their concerns regarding the appropriate use of funds; however, detailed information on individual staff activity, for example, probably should not be reported routinely to county, state, or federal agencies. Instead, if such detailed information is needed, it is probably more appropriately obtained on an audit or

Table 1. Illustrative Reports for Varying Management Issues and Varying Levels of Decision Makers*

Major Management Issue	Service Manager	Center Director	State MH Program Office	Legislature/ Regional Office
1. Patterns of Client Care and Services	Time of day and day of week of admission	Disposition of intakes by organizational service	Clients discharged by major diagnosis and/or level of functioning	Volume of services by catchment area by case type
2. Source and Use of Resources	Volume of service and caseload by individual staff (or staffing units) Cost per unit of service	Volume of service by type of case and service and organizational unit Cost per unit of service	Total % of staff time spent in direct and indirect service by case type Cost per unit of service	Total % of staff time spent in direct and indirect service by case type Cost per unit of service
3. Monitoring Aids	Admissions not meeting admissions justification profile Listing of clients not seen in 90 days	% of admitted clients terminated without therapist approval	% of discharged ex-state-hospital patients in community service systems	% of discharged ex-state-hospital patients in community service systems
4. Planning Data (for each type of target group)	Volume of services for last three years Seasonal variations in volume of services	Volume of all services for last three years Movement of clients from more to less intensive levels of care	Level of poverty and historical utilization of services by Title XX clients	Trends in use of various services
5. Client Outcomes (by target group)	Average changes in client functioning scores for specific services	Average changes in client functioning for major target groups	Ascertain existence and function of outcome evaluation system	Ascertain existence and function of outcome evaluation system

*Sorensen, J. E., & Hanbery, G. W. *Changing the Financing, Distribution and Accountability of Mental Health Services in Arkansas.* (1978). Little Rock, AR: Division of Mental Health Services, State of Arkansas.

site-visit basis rather than via routine reporting. Centerwide summaries or trends, on the other hand, could be effectively utilized by state and federal agencies.

The development of a well planned hierarchy of reports is needed to contain unnecessary and voluminous duplications and expansive reporting activities. Table 1 attempts to illustrate potentially appropriate and relevant routine reports for five major management questions and for four varying levels of decision makers.

Self-Study Exercise: Analyzing Reports and Managerial Level

Now let's analyze the reports you currently receive, using the framework we've developed up to this point. List up to five (5) individual reports you currently receive by their title. Identify the source and frequency. Specify the management questions you ask and the action you take (or might take) using the report. (This analysis only has room for five reports. You may wish to continue this analysis for other reports on a separate form.)

Title of Report	Source	Frequency	Answers What Management Questions	Basis for What Management Actions
1.				
2.				
3.				
4.				
5.				

Are you having trouble identifying the questions? Your actions? You're not alone! In many cases, many managers find it tough to *write down* the questions a report can answer. *Specifying* the actions you do (or might) take may be even tougher. This exercise will help you see what your current reports are doing for you. For a more detailed analysis of and exercise on formulating good questions, you may wish to review Chapter 20.

Are there important questions that are *not* being answered? After reviewing the reports coming to you now, list the questions on which you would like to have complete, or more complete, answers. Suggest a title for the report. If you can, try to specify the content by identifying the labels for the rows and columns. Or, if you like, draw a graph, histogram, or chart of what the report would contain. (Again, you may wish to review Chapter 20 to assist your efforts here.)

List of Unanswered (or Poorly Answered) Questions	Suggested Titles of Reports	Suggested Contents
1.		
2.		
3.		
4.		
5.		

You have now produced information that can be *used* by an expert in system design to produce a needed management report. Until you can formulate your request in this form, the system designer will not be able to move ahead. While the designer can help you determine your information needs, you are the one who must identify your questions and the way you think they should be answered. By now, you should have a better idea of the reports you will want your information system to produce.

Chapter 27

Implementing an Integrated System

How Do I Get an MIS Started (or Changed)?
What Is Involved in the System Design Process? How Do I Do It?
How Will I Know If I Am Doing It Right?
What Are the Costs?

1. STARTING (OR REVISING) AN MIS: SOME PRACTICAL TACTICS

What are the good (and bad) tactics to follow in developing or changing an information system? Some of the approaches outlined below are drawn from actual experience. As with all tools, these tactics will have to be tuned to special situations, but some version may provide the all-important toehold (see Chapman, 1976).

Find or Create a Crisis

Organizations change when they are in a crisis situation. Decision makers can be stimulated to make changes when the pressure is on. If a funding crisis occurs, the incident may be exploited to introduce (or expand) information gathered on staff activity or cost per unit of service. Pressing problems, especially those pressures from *outside* the organization, serve as traction points to introduce changes such as a new MIS. Revisions in legislation and regulation also can serve as the impetus. Generally, few individuals or organizations will change simply because "it's good for them." So, if a natural crisis doesn't exist, lie in wait until one comes along or try to orchestrate one by seeding your environment with some explosive observations to set off a series of inquiries leading to the crisis.

Link the MIS Proposal to the Crisis Resolution. Once the crisis is understood, the solution must be clearly perceived. The proposal should be clearly linked to the resolution of the crisis and everyone should be periodically reminded about the crisis and how the plan is working toward resolution of the crisis. Periodic updates at executive and staff meetings and blurbs in the newsletter can serve this need well.

Link the MIS Proposal to the Staff's Self-concerns. The staff will consider new ideas and change if they feel the changes will benefit them. Actually have staff express their self-concerns openly, and have them describe how they see an MIS addressing these self-concerns (the products). Also have them identify what they hope the MIS will *not do* (the pitfalls). Be sure to produce a report for them, showing their statement of potential products and pitfalls.

Prepare a Realistic Plan

Often, a crisis can be identified but the proposed solutions get linked to *unrealistic* plans. A good plan will specify *realistic*

— results
— resources required
— timetable

Be sure that the staff's statement of potential products and pitfalls is clearly visible in the plan. Some slippage can be expected and should be incorporated in the timetable; nothing is more regular than irregularities. A timetable (with appropriate provision for slippage) should be met to achieve *credibility* of the proposed solution.

Secure Top-Management Commitment. Top-management commitment has to be real. Besides authorizing the resources, management must be willing to *use* the information created. When management decisions are influenced by the information produced, then organizational members will be convinced of top-management commitment. Another good tactic is to have the information-system project report to management. When the organizational chart reflects direct access to top managers, other organizational members are likely to see the project as important and having high status. Reporting through multiple layers can stifle the project by slowing its progress and degrading its importance.

Involve Staff. A design task force starts with knowledgeable MIS staff as the nucleus. Up to a dozen additional members should be added from the agency staff. The design group should be diversified since it will be the major communication link throughout the organization. Individuals with high sociometric preference should be considered for the task force, not necessarily those who hold official positions. When it comes time to sell the system, interpersonal networks can be more effective than formal lines of authority.

Regular weekly or bi-weekly scheduled meetings should be all-day commitments. Ideally, workloads are adjusted so non-MIS staff can commit their time without having to compensate for the decline in workload activity. Freeing up staff for the project also reveals another form of top-management commitment. Explicit task assignments, even in the job descriptions of the committee members, may be useful.

Document and Communicate the Decision

Thorough documentation of the decision process is essential. Documentation helps to achieve full understanding and full acceptability of the various choice points along the design path. Periodic bulletins or updates should be issued to keep the members of the organization posted. Such communication tends to ally fears and anxieties but can also trigger needed inputs from overlooked individuals who may be affected by the design.

Use Outside Consultants. Information systems involve complex technology and almost any design group will benefit from outside review. Consultants can help organize the task force, offer consultation on technical issues as they arise, and provide review of the proposed design. Often, when elements of the design are poor and need to be changed, the easiest (and safest) way to initiate the change is through an outsider.

Perform Design Reviews. For both the preliminary and detailed designs, a last step is a *review* of the design. Often anomalies surface, but only when the review process has gone through several iterations. Usually there is a need to simplify. Chapman (p. 36) captures the essence of this process in his three imperatives: "Simplify, simplify, simplify."

2. PREVIEWING THE DESIGN PROCESS

Integration of mental-health information systems begins with the design process. This stage asks questions about how the system could be designed. Although systems analysis focuses on what a system is doing or should be doing to meet user needs, system design seeks answers to how could the system best meet user requirements. System implementation focuses on the installation, development, testing, and evaluation of a detailed system design. System design involves the following:

(1) A specification of the system's goals and how they relate to the program's service goals
(2) The formulation of a conceptual model (or approach) to meet user requirements
(3) Analysis of the varying organizational constraints or requirements

- (a) Cost of acquisition
- (b) Cost of maintenance
- (c) Reliability
- (d) Life expectancy
- (e) Level of performance
- (f) Flexibility
- (g) Potential for growth
- (h) Ease of installation
- (i) Accuracy

The relative weights of constraints or requirements vary from one human-service organization to another (Weinstein, 1975). The goals, models, and constraints/requirements (especially cost, ease of installation, growth) vary widely in human-information systems.

THE SYSTEM DESIGN PROCESS[1]

The design process consists of three major phases: preliminary system design, detailed system design, and implementation of the design. Each major segment is elaborated.

---

[1] Adapted from James E. Sorensen & J. Richard Elpers (1978). Developing Information Systems for Human Service Organizations. In C. C. Attkisson, W. A. Hargreaves, & M. J. Horowitz (Eds.), *Evaluation of Human Service Programs*. NY: Academic Press.

Preliminary Design Process

The sequence of crucial events in the preliminary design is outlined as follows in ten distinct but interrelated steps:

(1) Formulation of organizational goals and objectives (see Chapters 2–7).
(2) Determination of questions (or hypotheses) to be addressed by information systems for assessing achievement of organizational goals/objectives (see Chapters 18–20, and 25).
(3) Formulation of reports that respond to the questions to be addressed by information systems (see Chapters 20–22, and 25).
(4) Determination of data elements to be used in preparing information-system reports (see Sections II, III, and V).
(5) Creation of data capture instruments to accumulate data for information-systems reports (see Chapters 10 and 11).
(6) Identification of most cost-effective approaches to error control (see Chapter 11).
(7) Estimation of volumes of data processing and storage requirements (see Chapters 10 and 11).
(8) Simplifcation of report requirements, document requirements, and error-control mechanisms (see Chapters 10 and 11).
(9) Derivation of data processing recommendations.
(10) Review of design by management and staff for decision to move to detailed design, or modify design (e.g., use a manual system by reporting requirements), or abandon the project entirely.

A common fault is to plunge into the creation of data-capture instruments (Step 5) with little regard for the crucial role of the first four steps. Inefficient and ineffective systems often result in and create frustrated and disappointed users. "Add-on" or redesigned information requirements to accommodate audit or utilization review and program evaluation are not exempt from the requirement to be developed using sound systems-design methodology. The temptation is great to pass off the preliminary design requirements as being too time consuming or too rigorous. Avoid such a temptation. Only *good* system design can produce *good* clinical and managerial information.

Detailed System Design

This phase of system design (or redesign) usually involves the following steps (Chapman, 1976, pp. 42–73):

(1) A design of improved record flow that integrates required MIS documents with existing forms. Most systems grow larger and more complex and, with the addition of new program-evaluation requirements, old forms are patched and new ones added. Data gathering becomes inefficient, accuracy drops, and staff resistance grows. An easy way to counteract opposition is to simplify through recordkeeping integration—the sequential step of charting current-record flow, integrating MIS documents with current flow, and simplifying record flow.
(2) The design of input documents or forms design. Use of demonstrated techniques on item

coding, item format, and for layout reduce the burden of recording data (written document or computer-terminal input) and enhance accuracy and completeness.

(3) The preparation of data processing specifications, including
  (a) Criteria for editing data inputs from MIS documents and internal procedures (e.g., merge edits)
  (b) Procedures for undertaking selected computations and statistical summaries (e.g., age, units of service, indices, exception listings)
  (c) Formats and guidelines for reports
  (d) Performance criteria for data processing, including programming deadlines, confidentiality, and financial arrangements

(4) The determination of firm cost estimates

(5) The design review that leads to final approval for implementing the information system

Implementation of the Design

Installing the information system requires the following (Chapman, 1976, pp. 74–85):

(1) Preparation of a detailed plan of implementation (using program evaluation and review techniques or PERT)

(2) Pretest of forms

(3) Preparation of procedure manuals and orientation and training sessions

(4) Decisions about inclusion of current caseload and historical data in the data base. (A good way to start is with the current caseload; be sure that all of the data loaded into the base have been thoroughly edited. This approach ignores most "historical data" captured under different systems, since the accuracy and completeness are nearly always seriously deficient.)

(5) Develop and test computer programs (if a computer used)

(6) Initiate collection of essential data, drawn from the existing caseload, for establishing the data base

(7) Initiate collection of current data and develop a process for distribution of reports and other MIS output products

Guidelines for Design

Though strict adherence will vary, mental-health information systems should observe the key guidelines of good system design (Burch and Strater, 1974; Davis, 1974; Murdick and Ross, 1975):

(1) Source *data* should be *collected only once* even if used several times by the system (to reduce redundancy and error)

(2) The number of *steps* in data capture should be kept at a *minimum* (to increase accuracy)

(3) *Subsystems* should produce data that are *compatible* with other subsystems; one subsystem should not have to reenter data received from another subsystem

(4) *Timing of reports* should be geared to timing and processing of supporting data; data should not be captured any sooner than required for reports.

(5) *Changes* or innovations should be *cost-effective* from an overall system perspective (e.g., cost of capturing data, correcting errors)

(6) Source *data* should be *thoroughly edited* so only valid data will be input into the information system
(7) *Audit trails* and record reproduction should be *available* upon demand
(8) *Backup and security* procedures should be maintained for all files

In summarizing a technical approach to system design and the context in which the approach can be used, Chapman (1976) observes a MIS for any organization:

(1) Can be helpful only to the extent that a climate prevails which welcomes the assistance that can be provided by a management tool.
(2) Must provide information about resource expenditures that can be compared to objectives, intuitive or structured, that can influence decisions about future resource allocations.
(3) Must determine information-collection requirements primarily in terms of the structuring of data for decisions.
(4) Must be designed by an iterative process in which the broad outlines of organizational structure, as it implies feedback needs, report requirements, data-collection needs, and methods of maintaining data integrity are determined in sequence.
(5) Must determine the details of recordkeeping integration, data-processing specification, and input-document contents and format only after a total system concept has been conceived so that implications of cost-effectiveness tradeoffs can be traced throughout the system.
(6) Must be implemented according to the carefully prepared plan that minimizes that consternation of organizational change and gets the system operational without delay and loss of credibility in the eyes of the agency staff.

Costs of Information Systems

Developing integrated systems consumes resources, and the outlays should be cost effective. Another way to state the question is: "What costs (and in what amount) will be different because of managerial and program evaluation information requirements?" Many individuals, often well-intended observers, make the mistake of thinking incremental information requirements can be added to an existing system with little or no inconvenience or expense. Others misguidedly believe the major cost of a system is the computer configuration. Costs of information systems are extensive and pervasive. A partial list follows:

(1) Costs of computer configuration
(2) Costs of renovation (e.g., facilities, air conditioning)
(3) Costs of training (e.g., including users and preparers of input)
(4) Costs of programs and program testing
(5) Costs of conversion (e.g., preparing and editing records for completeness and accuracy, setting up file library procedures, preparing and running parallel operations)
(6) Costs of operations (e.g., staff, supplies, maintenance, insurance, light and power, computer rental or amortization)
(7) Costs of professional staff and support personnel time complying with data-capture requirements
(8) Costs of error detection and correction process; costs of tracking specific cases emerging in various edit processes

(9) Costs of information-system changes or modifications elicited by changing external reporting requirements or controls

The growth of information systems costs starts with project planning and increases as the design reaches an operational state. Figure 1 is an integrated performance-cost-time (PCT) chart used for controlling the three key variables in a system development process and clearly reveals the pattern of growth of costs over time.

A useful technique for charting the path and timetable of a system design is the PERT chart (*P*rogram *E*valuation and *R*eview *T*echnique). Figure 2 provides an illustrative application for the design of a mental-health statistical-information subsystem.

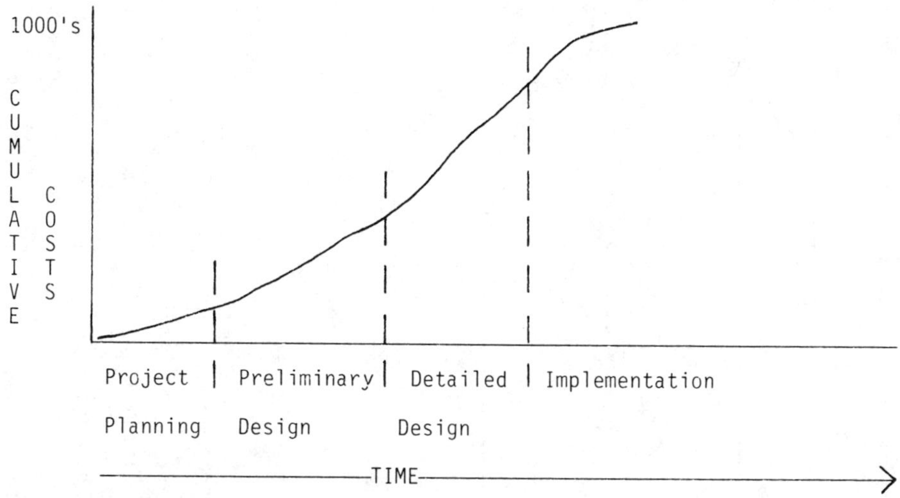

Planned Actual	Person-Hours	
Planned Actual	$ Labor	
Planned Actual	$ Materials	
Planned Actual	$ Computer Charges	
Planned Actual	Total	

Figure 1. Integrated Performance-cost-time (PCT) Chart*

* Adapted from R. G. Murdick & J. E. Ross. (1975). *Information Systems for Modern Management,* (2nd ed.). Englewood Cliffs, NJ: Prentice Hall.

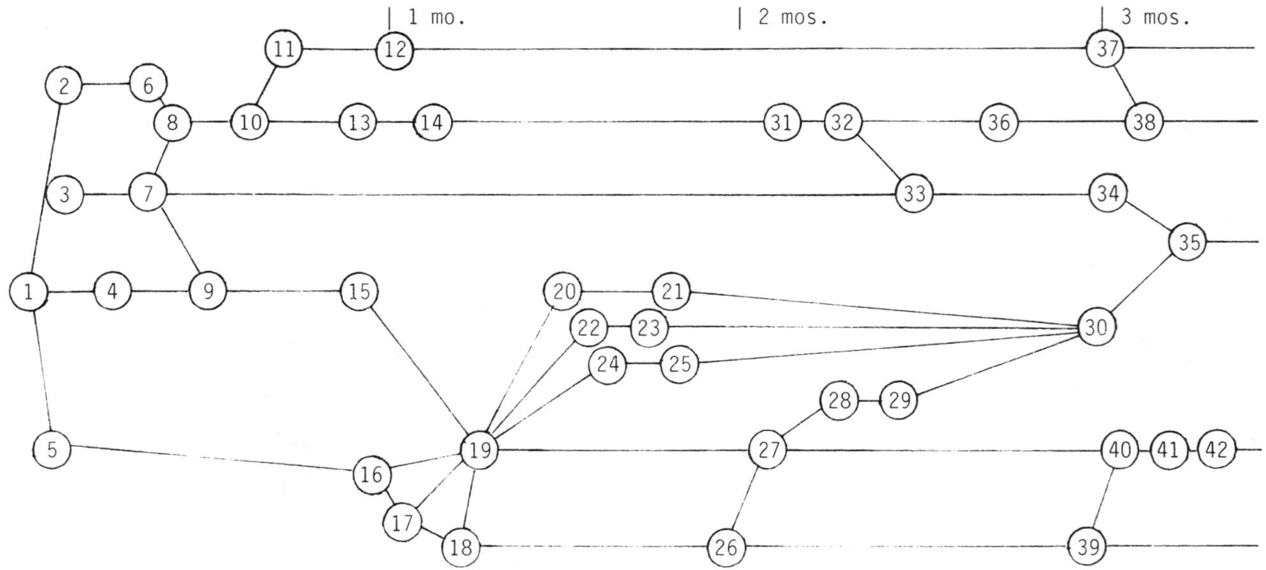

Description of Events

1. Final design approval
2. Proced Manual (PM) draft
3. Order temporary forms
4. Start test-case design
5. Sign contract for dp
6. Make copies of PM
7. Rec temporary forms
8. Start pretest of forms
9. Start forms for test cs
10. Compl pretest of forms
11. Revise form design
12. Order production forms
13. Revise procedure manual
14. Order copies of PM
15. Complete test case
16. Complete file main. pgm
17. Compl data control pgm
18. Compl programs
19. Run test case
20. Debug file main. pgm
21. Accept file main. pgm
22. Debug data control pgm
23. Accept data contr pgm
24. Debug pgm
25. Accept pgm
26. Complete Mgmt Rep pgm
27. Run Mgmt Rep pgm
28. Debug Mgmt Rep pgm
29. Accept Mgmt Rep pgm
30. Assemble accepted pgms
31 Rec copies of PM
32. Begin personnel training
33. Forms on exstg case load
34. Compl forms, exstg cs ld
35. Process existing cs ld
36. Continue personnel trng
37. Receive production forms
38. Begin collect curr data
39. Complete Stat Rep pgm
40. Run Stat Rep pgm
41. Debug Stat Rep pgm
42. Accept Stat Rep pgm

Figure 2. PERT Diagram of MIS Implementation Schedule (from Chapman, 1976)

Chapter 28

Assuring the Dependability of Cost Data*

How Can I Cut Down on Errors in My Fiscal Data?
How Do I Make Sure My Accounting System Has Good Internal Controls?
What Built-in Controls Will Make Sure Key Fiscal Data
Are Captured Completely?

Chapter 28 identifies important ways to insure the dependability of fiscal data. The time-tested techniques reviewed are used by accountants to insure good control over the collection of basic financial data. Accounting internal controls will be explored with special attention to the critical and often notably weak areas in mental-health organizations. Concrete illustrations will offer guidance in setting up good accounting systems yet recognizing the common, frequent shortage of personnel to perform the all-important accounting functions.

The chapter will cover the following points:

(1) KEY IDEAS
(2) WHAT IS ACCOUNTING INTERNAL CONTROL?
(3) CHECKING UP ON ACCOUNTING INTERNAL CONTROLS
(4) SUGGESTIONS FOR IMPLEMENTING MAXIMAL SEPARATION OF DUTIES

1. KEY IDEAS

All mental-health organizations have accounting systems of some sort. The chapter identifies *why* accounting controls are needed and *what* makes up good accounting control. Specific self-study "checklists" are provided to help evaluate accounting controls for:

— Cash and accounts receivable
— Cash and accounts payable
— Plant assets
— Budgeting

---

* Major sections of the chapter are adapted from James E. Sorensen & Glyn Hanbery. (1979). *Using Financial Management in Mental Health Organizations.* Rockville, MD: NIMH.

Finally, a matrix of people and duties is developed to suggest how effective separation of duties should be done to enhance internal controls. The matrix is sensitive to organizational size and can adjust from very small organizations to very large ones. Select up-to-date references provide access to additional and more sophisticated materials.

2. WHAT IS ACCOUNTING INTERNAL CONTROL?

An authoritative definition of accounting internal controls accepted by the accounting profession is:

> [accounting internal controls] comprise the plan of organization and all methods and procedures that are concerned mainly with, and related directly to, the safe-guarding of assets and the reliability of the financial records.

Accounting internal control procedures principally have taken the face of the more traditional control through personal supervision and observation of staff. Because of the large size and/or complex organization structures of modern entities and because of the physical separation of executives from an entity's daily operations, control by personal observation and supervision of staff becomes impracticable and ineffective. Surrogate control measures were devised to:

— Promote accurate and complete data capture, i.e., transaction control procedures
— Deter staff from misappropriation of entity resources
— Transfer risks of loss because of staff defalcation to insurance companies, i.e., bonding certain employees, recognizing that accounting internal controls are designed to deter misappropriation and not prevent it absolutely

The integrity of the centers'/clinics' accounting systems depends on:

— the adequacy of the accounting records to record and document all transactions affecting an agency's assets and equities
— the adequacy of the internal controls incorporated within an agency's accounting system to promote reliable reporting about operations and to ensure stewardship over assets

The minimal accounting internal control elements and procedures for mental-health organizations are summarized in Table 1.

Individual internal-control procedures should be adopted only in cases in which the amount of a potential injury caused by the omission of a particular internal-control procedure is reasonably expected to exceed the cost of implementing applicable internal-control procedures.

Transaction Control Procedures

Two principal accounting internal control procedures promote accurate and complete data capture:

— Qualified, well-trained personnel
— Document control, i.e., control over and accounting for all data-capture documents

Table 1. Minimal Internal Control Elements and Procedures

Internal Control Element	Objective of Internal Control Element	Internal Control Procedure
I. Transaction Control (Document control)	—To promote complete recording of transactions by requiring that data-capture documents be accounted for.	—Prenumbering documents
	—To protect against resubmission for payment of invoice already paid.	—Permanent indication of payment on paid invoices
II. Personnel Controls:		
a. Separation of Duties	—To prevent the same employee from both misappropriating assets and concealing the misappropriation.	—Assignment of following functions to different employees: –Asset custody –Accounting (recordkeeping) –Authority to acquire and dispose of assets
b. Independent check	—To provide a review by some one with no other contact with the operation under review, thus –to promote complete, accurate, and honest discharge of responsibilities –to detect errors or irregularities if made	—Reconciliations —Statements and confirmation sent to customer —Physical counts
III. Bonding employees	—To protect against loss due to misappropriation of assets by employees through insurance indemnification in event of such loss.	—Bonding employees with access to or control over liquid assets, e.g., cash
IV. Budgeting	—To establish organizational goals and objectives expressed in financial terms as a standard against which actual operations may be compared.	—Operations budgeting, i.e., budgeting expected revenues and expenses
	—To identify possible deficiencies or excesses in cash balance and plan appropriate borrowing or investments activity.	—Cash budgeting, i.e., budgeting expected cash receipts and cash disbursements.

Evaluating the degree to which personnel employed are qualified and well-trained is a difficult task matched only by the continuous challenge of acquiring and training individuals for varying positions throughout the organization.

Document control is effected by prenumbering and/or accounting for documents evidencing transactions, namely:

- Cash receipts
- Service rendered documents (or use of "control stubs" retained by receptionist/secretary and matched with completed forms)
- Checks

Also, invoices received from suppliers and other creditors should be permanently marked or stamped when paid to prevent resubmission for payment of paid invoices.

Deterrents to Employee Misappropriation of Resources

Two principal accounting internal-control procedures deter employees from misappropriating entity resources:

— Separation of duties
— Independent checks

Separation of Duties. The objective of separation of duties is to prevent one employee from both misappropriating entity assets and concealing the defalcation by altering the accounting records. This objective is accomplished, to the extent practicable, by assigning the following responsibilities and functions to *different* employees:

— Asset custody (e.g., one employee, the cashier, receives cash)
— Accounting (recordkeeping) (e.g., another employee, the accounts receivable clerk, maintains client accounts)
— Authority to acquire and dispose of assets (e.g., yet another employee may authorize write-offs of uncollectible accounts)
— Authority to set fees charged (e.g., fee is set by someone other than employee rendering service or receiving cash or a standing fee is used)

Independent Checks. An independent check is accomplished by a review of an employee's performance by another person who has no authority over or contact with the operation under review. Its objective is twofold:

— To encourage complete, accurate and honest discharge of responsibilities by employees who are aware that the independent review will be made
— To provide detection of errors or irregularities.

An example of independent checks is a bank reconciliation performed by an employee without access to cash, cash and accounts receivable accounts, and who is not involved in cash disbursements.

Bonding Certain Employees

An entity may minimize the impact of an employee's misappropriation of assets by bonding or insuring those employees with physical access to liquid (e.g., readily salable) assets. Then, if a bonded employee absconds with an entity's resources, the insurance company is obligated to indemnify the entity in accordance with the bonding agreement.

Budgeting

Accomplishment of desired goals and objectives can be better ensured by developing a plan of action, permitting subsequent comparisons of actual results with desired ones. One type of such plan is manifested by the *financial operations budget.* In this budget, expected activities are expressed in terms of financial outcomes, i.e., expected revenues and expenses of an operating period. The financial operations budget serves as a standard against which the financial results of actual operating activities can be systematically and periodically compared; timely corrective action can be taken as variances between budget and actual outcomes arise.

Another type of budget, the *cash budget,* is as much a forecast as it is a device for assisting in planning and controlling operations. This budget consists of projections of expected cash receipts and disbursements, resulting in identification of possible deficiencies and excesses in cash. Thus, plans can be developed for appropriate borrowing to cover deficiencies and for appropriate investments to properly utilize excesses.

3. CHECKING UP ON ACCOUNTING INTERNAL CONTROLS

Within CMCH's, several accounting internal-control procedures are especially critical and often notably weak. These critical areas include:

— Cash receipts
— Cash disbursements
— Related recordkeeping for accounts receivable and accounts payable
— Fixed assets
— Financial operations planning and control

Attention now focuses on:

— The objectives of accounting internal controls as applied to these traditionally weak areas
— The appropriate accounting internal-control procedures to accomplish the objectives

Cash and Related Accounts Receivable and Payable Recordkeeping

The objectives of accounting internal controls over cash and related accounts receivable and accounts payable recordkeeping are to provide reasonable assurance:

— All cash which should be received is received and recorded immediately and accurately with proper credit given to payer
— Cash disbursements are made only for authorized business purposes and are immediately and accurately recorded
— All bank accounts and cash on hand are accurately recorded and subject to appropriate safeguards
— Cash balances are maintained at adequate but not excessive levels by budgeting expected receipts and disbursements

The accounting internal-control procedures applicable to cash and related accounts receivable and accounts payable recordkeeping are contained in the questionnaire in Table 2.

Plant Assets

The objective of accounting internal controls over plant assets are:

— To provide reasonable control over plant asset expenditures
— To maintain reasonable accountability and utilization controls
— To provide information useful in computing and allocating plant asset and related expenses

The accounting internal-controls applicable to plant assets are contained in the questionnaire in Table 3.

Table 2. Accounting Internal Controls: Cash and Related Accounts Receivable and Payable Recordkeeping

Internal Control Element	Internal Control Procedure	Utilized in Center/Clinic	
		Yes	No
	CASH RECEIPTS AND RELATED ACCOUNTS RECEIVABLE RECORDKEEPING		
I. Document (Transaction) Control	—Use prenumbered cash receipts all systematically accounted for		
	—Deposit all cash receipts intact daily		
	—Deposit all branch cash receipts in a local bank subject to withdrawal only by central office		
	—Instruct the bank in writing not to cash any checks payable to the center/clinic, but to accept them for deposit only		
	—Use prenumbered service rendered documents or control stubs and systematically account for all documents		
II. Personnel Controls:			
a. Separation of duties	—Formal policies should be adopted and followed: –to assign to the following positions *exclusive* responsibility for performing certain functions, and –to prohibit these positions from performing one of the following responsibilities not assigned to it, but assigned to another position		
	—The positions with assigned and prohibited responsibilities are:		
	–Cashier: should		
	a. have exclusive responsibility to		
	1. receive cash		
	2. prepare cash receipts		
	3. prepare deposit slips and make deposits		
	b. be prohibited		
	1. access to accounting records, i.e., general ledger, journals, and subsidiary ledgers		
	2. access to bank statements and accompanying documents		
	3. involvement in reconciliation of bank account		
	4. involvement in billings or fee setting		
	5. involvement in preparation of service-rendered documents		
	6. involvement in disposition of overdue accounts		
	7. involvement in cash disbursement process		
	–Accounts Receivable Recordkeeper: should		
	a. have exclusive responsibility to		
	1. maintain accounts receivable subsidiary ledger		
	2. prepare clients' statements (i.e., billings)		
	b. be prohibited		
	1. access to cash receipts		
	2. involvement in reconciliation of bank account		
	3. involvement in determining fees charged clients		
	4. involvement in preparation of service rendered document		
	5. involvement in *deciding* disposition of overdue accounts		
	6. involvement in cash-disbursement process		
	–Credit Manager: should		
	a. have exclusive responsibility to		
	1. authorize reductions in standard fees charged individual clients		
	2. authorize write-offs of uncollectable accounts		

Table 2. (*Continued*)

Internal Control Element	Internal Control Procedure	Utilized in Center/Clinic: Yes	Utilized in Center/Clinic: No
	b. be prohibited		
	1. access to cash receipts	_____	_____
	2. access to accounts receivable subsidiary ledger	_____	_____
	3. involvement in preparation of service-rendered document	_____	_____
	–Service Deliverer or Receptionist: should		
	a. have exclusive responsibility to		
	1. prepare service-rendered document or document-service delivery, e.g., daily-activity logs, master appointment schedule, etc.	_____	_____
	b. be prohibited		
	1. access to cash receipts	_____	_____
	2. access to accounts receivable subsidiary records	_____	_____
	3. involvement in billings or fee setting	_____	_____
	4. involvement in deciding disposition of overdue accounts	_____	_____
b. Independent check	—A person who has none of the responsibilities assigned to either the Cashier or Accounts Receivable Recordkeeper should have exclusive responsibility to systematically compare		
	–cash receipts, cash deposits, and accounts receivable entries	_____	_____
	–actual fees charged for a period with accounts receivable entries (billings) for the same period	_____	_____
CASH DISBURSEMENTS AND RELATED ACCOUNTS PAYABLE RECORDKEEPING			
I. Document (Transaction) Controls	—Use prenumbered checks, all systematically accounted for (i.e., retain voided checks and cancelled checks)	_____	_____
	—Unissued (blank) checks are stored in a secure area and are accessible to only persons authorized to prepare checks	_____	_____
	—The following documents are stamped or perforated to prevent further use:		
	–voided checks	_____	_____
	–paid invoices	_____	_____
	—Check signers are not authorized to issue or sign checks payable to "cash" or "bearer"	_____	_____
	—Check signers may not sign blank checks in advance (i.e., prior to writing in payee, amount and date, and without supporting documentation)	_____	_____
	—Cash disbursements are made only on the basis of supporting documentation (i.e., authorization, invoice, receiving report)	_____	_____
	—Signature plates, if used, should be secured and accessible only to authorized persons	_____	_____
II. Personnel Control			
a. Separation of Duties	—Formal policies should be adopted and followed:		
	–to assign to the following positions *exclusive* responsibility for performing certain functions, and		
	–to prohibit these positions from performing one of the following responsibilities not assigned to it, but assigned to another position.		

(*continued*)

Table 2. (*Continued*)

Internal Control Element	Internal Control Procedure	Utilized in Center/Clinic Yes	No
	The positions with assigned and prohibited responsibilities are:		
	–Check Preparer: should		
	a. have exclusive responsibility to		
	1. maintain accounts payable subsidiary ledger	_____	_____
	2. prepare check, i.e., gather necessary supporting documentation and write on check date, payee, amount and reason	_____	_____
	b. be prohibited		
	1. from signing checks or access to signature plates	_____	_____
	2. from authorizing acquisitions of assets or services, or refunds	_____	_____
	3. from mailing signed checks or having access to or custody of unclaimed salary checks	_____	_____
	4. access to bank statements and accompanying documents	_____	_____
	5. involvement in reconciliation of bank account	_____	_____
	–Check Signer(s): should		
	a. have exclusive responsibility to		
	1. sign checks	_____	_____
	b. be prohibited		
	1. access to unissued (blank) checks	_____	_____
	2. access to accounts payable subsidiary ledger and general ledger	_____	_____
	3. from authorizing acquisitions of assets or services, or refunds	_____	_____
	4. access to bank statements and accompanying documents	_____	_____
	5. involvement in reconciliation of bank account	_____	_____
b. Independent Check	—At least two signatures should be required on all checks in excess of a specified amount	_____	_____
	CASH: GENERAL		
I. Document (Transaction) Control	—Bank statements and accompanying documents should be received directly from bank by person responsible for preparing bank reconciliation	_____	_____
	—Bank reconciliation should be performed by someone with no involvement in		
	–cash receipts	_____	_____
	–accounts receivable recordkeeping	_____	_____
	–preparation of checks	_____	_____
	–signing checks	_____	_____
II. Bonding	—*All* employees with access to cash and readily salable assets should be bonded	_____	_____
III. Budgeting	—Expected cash receipts and disbursements are projected for a reasonable period (e.g., by month for the next twelve months)	_____	_____

Table 3. Accounting Internal Controls: Plant Assets

Internal Control Element	Internal Control Procedure	Utilized in Center/Clinic Yes	No
I. Document (Transaction) Control	—Explicit policy distinguishing between capital acquisitions and expense items	___	___
	—Serially numbered plant asset acquisition documents (purchase order forms) and receiving and inspection documents with systematic accounting for all documents	___	___
	—Explicit policy requiring plant asset acquisitions be supported by:		
	–plant asset acquisition document*	___	___
	–receiving and inspection report*	___	___
	–report explaining any variance between authorized expenditure and actual costs*	___	___
	—Serially numbered, permanent I.D. tags attached to all plant assets as acquired with systematic accounting for all I.D. tag numbers	___	___
	—Serially numbered plant asset records and depreciation schedules (which may be reverse side of plant asset record), with systematic accounting for all records	___	___
	—Serially numbered requisition/utilization documents for assets for which exclusive custody and use are not assigned to specific individuals, with systematic accounting for all documents	___	___
	—Serially numbered plant asset retirement documents requiring explanation for retirement with systematic accounting for all documents	___	___
II. Personnel Controls:			
a. Separation of Duties	—Formal policies should be adopted and followed:		
	–to assign to the following positions *exclusive* responsibility for performing certain functions, and		
	–to prohibit these positions from performing one of the following responsibilities not assigned to it, but assigned to another position		
	The positions with assigned and prohibited responsibilities are:		
	–Plant Asset Account Recordkeeper: should		
	a. have exclusive responsibility to		
	1. maintain plant asset records and depreciation schedules*	___	___
	b. be prohibited		
	1. involvement in authorization of plant asset acquisition or disposition*	___	___
	–Plant Asset Custodial Personnel: should		
	a. have exclusive responsibility to		
	1. monitor utilization, through requisition/utilization documents, of plant assets for which exclusive custody and use are not assigned to specific individuals	___	___

(*continued*)

Table 3. (*Continued*)

Internal Control Element	Internal Control Procedure	Utilized in Center/Clinic Yes	No
	b. be prohibited		
	1. access to plant asset records and depreciation schedules*	_____	_____
	2. involvement in authorization of plant asset acquisition and disposition*	_____	_____
	–Plant Asset Acquisition/Disposition Manager(s): should		
	a. have exclusive responsibility to		
	1. authorize acquisitions and disposition of plant assets*	_____	_____
	b. be prohibited		
	1. access to plant-asset records and depreciation schedules	_____	_____
	2. involvement in monitoring utilization of plant assets assigned to Plant-Asset Custodial Personnel*		
	[Note: All personnel should periodically account for all plant assets within their custody.]		
b. Independent Check	—A person who has none of the responsibilities assigned to the Plant Asset Account Recordkeeper, Plant Asset Custodial Personnel, Plant Asset Acquisition/Disposition Manager(s), should have exclusive responsibility to		
	–review accounting for all serially numbered plant-asset records, i.e.		
	a. acquisition documents*		
	b. receiving and inspection documents*		
	c. I.D. tags*		
	d. plant asset and depreciation records		
	e. requisition/utilization documents		
	f. retirement documents	_____	_____
	–review accounting by all personnel for plant assets within their custody	_____	_____
	–inspect (on a sample basis) plant assets assigned to personnel and compare with accountability report submitted by such individuals		
	[Note: This procedure may be adequately performed by an independent auditor. If so, this response should be "yes."]	_____	_____
III. Budgeting	—Planning for plant asset acquisitions within the capital budget, financial operations budget or cash-flow budget*	_____	_____

*Indicates those procedures which, in our opinion, constitute minimal control procedure.

Table 4. Accounting Internal Controls: Financial Operations Planning and Control

Internal Control Element	Internal Control Procedure	Utilized in Center/Clinic Yes	No
Budgeting	—Develop comprehensive budget of expected revenues and expenses for current operating period	_____	_____
	—Periodically compare budgeted amounts with actual amounts and investigate significant variances	_____	_____

Financial Operations Planning and Control

The objectives of accounting internal controls related to financial operations planning and control are:

- To assist overall planning for and control over operations
- To provide preliminary estimates of the financial results of operations
- To aid in detection of errors or irregularities

The accounting internal control procedures applicable to financial operations planning and control are contained in the questionnaire in Table 4.

4. SUGGESTIONS FOR IMPLEMENTING MAXIMAL SEPARATION OF DUTIES

Many CMHC's have limited numbers of administrative staff and, as a consequence, abridge some of the accounting internal controls discussed previously. To address the issue of achieving adequate separation of duties with variations in staff size, Figure 1 presents suggested assignment configurations as staff size increases from four to nine individuals.

Figure 1 should be interpreted as explained. With only four persons, for example, duties should be assigned according to the content of columns one through four. With five persons available, the duties of Independent Reviewer contained in row five should be reassigned from the Credit Manager to the fifth person. Similarly, with six people, the Receptionist's duties should be reassigned from the Cashier to the sixth person.

A principal feature of this suggested duty-assignment configuration is the separation of the following responsibilities:

- Asset custody
- Recordkeeping
- Authority to approve transactions

Traditionally, CMHC's have not focused on financial information systems, so Figure 1 can provide useful guides to mental health administrators now required to develop and monitor adequate financial controls over key aspects of their operations.

		MINIMAL NUMBER FOR ADEQUATE INTERNAL CONTROL			
	Number of Personnel Available	1	2	3	4
	1–4	—Cashier –Receives Cash –Prepares Receipt –Prepares Deposit Slip and Makes Deposit	—Accounts Receivable Recordkeeping –Maintains Accounts Receivable Subsidiary Ledger –Prepares Clients' Statements	—Credit Manager –Authorizes Reductions from Standard Fees –Authorizes Write-Offs of Uncollectible Amounts	—Therapist –Prepares Services Rendered Document
ADDITIONAL PERSONNEL	9		—Check Co-Signatory –Reviews Checks and Supporting Documents –Signs Checks		
ADDITIONAL PERSONNEL	8			—Check Co-Signatory –Reviews Checks –Mails Checks	
ADDITIONAL PERSONNEL	7	—Accounts Payable Recordkeeper –Maintains Accounts Payable Subsidiary Ledger –Prepares Checks for Signing			
ADDITIONAL PERSONNEL	6	—Receptionist –Maintains Master Appointment Schedule			
ADDITIONAL PERSONNEL	5			—Independent Reviewer –Reconciles Bank Statement –Compares Daily Cash Receipts, Deposit Slips, and Accounts Receivable Subsidiary Ledger Entries –Reviews Accounting for Service Rendered Documents Issued	

Figure 1. Assignment of Responsibilities to Varying Numbers of Personnel

Chapter 29

Putting Your System Together: Developing a Procedure Manual

We close with an outline of a Procedure Manual describing how to fit the major components of a client-oriented system together as an integrated system. The outline provides a guide useful for internal staff training and guidance as well as a means of describing programs to external regulatory agencies.

The main focus up to this point has been on understanding the major features of a client-oriented system. The entire thrust has been directed toward learning concepts and constructing unique systems. Now, the central issue is how to describe your system to someone else. The goal is to help someone either to become an integral part of a service system (e.g., new staff), or to review how a service system operates (e.g., reviewers from funding, regulatory, or accreditation agencies).

TONE OF THE PROCEDURE MANUAL

The successfully constructed *Procedure Manual* communicates the system and its procedures to new staff. To be successful, new staff members need to start with a good client-oriented attitude toward their delivery of service. Thus, the general tone of the Procedure Manual should reflect an overall client orientation.

The manual has the following outline:

(1) PROGRAM GOALS AND SERVICES
(2) CLINICAL PROCESS, STANDARDS, PROCEDURES AND RECORDS
(3) FISCAL POLICIES AND PROCEDURES
(4) ADMINISTRATIVE POLICIES AND PROCEDURES
(5) PROGRAM MANAGEMENT AND PLANNING
(6) CITIZEN PARTICIPATION
(7) ADDENDUM (UPDATING MANUAL, GLOSSARY, REFERENCES)

Procedure Manual Outline	References in Text and Comments
PREFACE: WHY READ THIS MANUAL? —To learn who our agency serves —To learn how we do so —To learn what your role in this effort might be	Briefly communicate your philosophy of, and attitude toward, service. Bring the reader into your camp. Give readers an attitude with which they ought to read the manual.
1. PROGRAM GOALS AND SERVICES 1.1 Whom do we service? Target groups and needs assessment. 1.2 How do our services relate to consumers' problems? How do our services relate to other community services?	Chapter 2 provides you with the outline here.
1.3 Who helps us understand and coordinate the relationships among program goals and services? What are the supportive roles of: —The Consultation and Education staff? —The Research and Evaluation staff? —The Citizen Board and Management staff?	Use only brief summary statements here, abstracted from Chapter 25 or from Section VI, particularly Chapter 18.
2. CLINICAL PROCESS, STANDARDS, PROCEDURES AND RECORDS 2.1 How do we assist the client with our services? (An overview of the service process, case management, and continuity of care.)	Both Chapters 8 and 25 provide examples of an overview of the process.
2.2 What are the specific procedures for each of the target groups we service? The outline for each target group could be: —CLIENT ENTRY: WHO IS THE CLIENT? IS THE CLIENT AT THE RIGHT PLACE? (Admissions criteria, procedures and documents) —SERVICE PLANNING: WHAT ARE THE ISSUES? WHAT EVENTS ARE TO HAPPEN? (Problem/issues list, goal setting, service planning and case management procedures, and documents) —REVIEW: ARE EVENTS OCCURING AS PLANNED? WHAT CHANGES ARE NEEDED? (Review standards, procedures and documents) —TERMINATION AND FOLLOWUP: WERE GOALS MET? IS FOLLOWUP REQUIRED? (Termination and followup criteria, standards, procedures, and documents)	Sections II and III address these issues. As you develop these procedure sections for each target group, be sure to identify clearly how you address issues of case management, continuity of care, and cost containment. If these three issues are clearly identified, then external reviewers will be satisfied.
2.3 How do we assure that clinical data are dependable? —Staff training procedures —Review and supervisory procedures —Support provided by Research and Evaluation staff	Section IV provides the basis for this section of the manual.
2.4 How do we establish, review, and revise clinical standards? —Use of retrospective and prospective clinical care-evaluation studies?	Section II provides an outline for this. You can also use the cost-outcome and effectiveness procedures described in Section VII, Chapters 23 and 24.
3. FISCAL POLICIES AND PROCEDURES 3.1 How much do our services cost? How do we pay for providing these services? (An overview)	Section V should be useful here.

Procedure Manual Outline	References in Text and Comments
3.2 What are the roles of the client and service staff in both containing costs and obtaining maximum revenues? [Procedures and documentation for estimating client and third-party financial liability for the payment of services rendered.]	
3.3 What do external auditors look for in reviewing our fiscal affairs? —Cost finding and accounting procedures —Income and expenditure reports —Fee schedules and procedures for setting fees	
4. ADMINISTRATIVE POLICIES AND PROCEDURES	
4.1 How are we organized? —From the consumer's perspective? —From the Governing Board's perspective?	Section VI, Chapter 18's outline of: —Role responsibilities —Authority
4.2 How is a job description developed? By identifying each staff member's —Responsibility to the program's products? —Lines of coordination, accountability, and authority? —Needs for administrative support?	Chapter 18 also provides the outline for these issues.
4.3 How is a staff member supervised and evaluated? 4.4 Staff rights, privileges, and benefits. 4.5 Staff career-development and training opportunities. 4.6 How do we contract with part-time and external service providers?	Chapters 18 and 19. Except for the "Rule of Two and Five" and related discussion, these issues were not discussed in this text.
5. PROGRAM MANAGEMENT AND PLANNING	
5.1 How are the program's organizational units linked together and how does information flow through the program for communication and program management?	The discussion on "Information Systems" in Section VIII is the basis for this portion of the manual.
5.2 Who addresses what issues, and uses what data for —Routine program management (e.g., monthly reports)? —Annual program planning and budgeting?	Section VI is useful here.
5.3 How does the annual program planning and budgeting operate? Who is involved in the process? —Staff input —Administration's responsibilities —Citizen Board involvement	
5.4 How are program policies originated and reviewed? —Staff input —Administration's responsibilities —Citizen Board involvement	
5.5 What Research and Evaluation activities support the process?	Sections VI and VII, particularly Chapters 23 and 24.
6. CITIZEN PARTICIPATION 6.1 How is the community represented and how do they participate? 6.2 How is the Citizen Board structured and how does it operate?	This section should also be a synthesis of how citizen input is involved in other parts of the program's procedures.
7. ADDENDUM 7.1 How is the manual updated? 7.2 Glossary of terms 7.3 References	

REFERENCES

Arthur Andersen and Company. (1978). *A guide for studying and evaluating internal accounting control.* Chicago, IL: Arthur Andersen.

Bigelow, D. (1979, June 5). *Measurement of social functioning.* Paper presented at the National Institute of Mental Health-sponsored workshop on Client/Patient Outcome Evaluation in Mental Health Programs, Baltimore, MD.

Burch, J. G., & Strater, F. R. (1974). *Information systems: Theory and practice.* Santa Barbara, CA: Hamilton.

Campbell, D. T., & Stanley, J. C. (1963). *Experimental and quasi-experimental designs for research.* Chicago, IL: Rand McNally.

Carter, D. E., & Newman, F. L. (1976). *A client oriented system of mental health service delivery and program management: A workbook and guide.* MH Statistical Series C, No. 12. Rockville, MD: National Institute of Mental Health.

Chapman, R. L. (1976). *The design of management information systems for mental health organizations: A primer* (National Institute of Mental Health, DHEW Publication No. ADM 76-333). Washington, DC: U.S. Government Printing Office.

Ciarlo, J. A., & Reihman, J. (1977). The Denver community mental health questionnaire: Development of a multidimensional program evaluation instrument. In R. Coursey, G. Spector, S. Murell, & B. Hunt (Eds.), *Program evaluation for mental health: Methods, strategies, and participants* (pp. 131–167). New York: Grune & Stratton.

Cook, T. D., & Campbell, D. T. (1979). *Quasi-experimentation: Design and analysis issues for field settings.* Chicago, IL: Rand McNally.

Cooper, M. E. (1973). *Guidelines for a minimum statistical and accounting system for community mental health centers* (DHEW Publication No. ADM 77-14). Washington, DC: U.S. Government Printing Office.

Cox, G. B., Carmichael, S. J., & Dightman, C. R. (1979). The optimal treatment approach to needs assessment. *Evaluation and Program Planning, 2,* 269–275.

Craighead, W. E., Kazdin, A. E., & Mahoney, M. J. (1976). *Behavior modification: Principles, issues and applications.* Boston, MA: Houghton Mifflin.

Cronbach, L. J., Gleser, G. C., Nande, H., & Rajaratnam, N. (1972). *The dependability of behavioral measurements: Theory of generalizability of scores and profiles.* New York: Wiley.

Davis, G. B. (1974). *Management information systems: Conceptual foundations, structure, and development.* New York: McGraw-Hill.

Derogatis, L., Lipman, R., & Covi, L. (1973). The SCL-90: An outpatient rating scale (preliminary report). *Psychopharmacology Bulletin, 9,* 13–28.

Ellsworth, R. B. (1979). *PARS V Community Adjustment Scale.* Roanoke, VA: Institute for Program Evaluation.

Endicott, J., Spitzer, R. L., Fleiss, R. L., & Cohen, J. (1976). The global assessment scale. *Archives of General Psychiatry, 33,* 766–771.

Garfield, S. L., & Bergin, A. E. (Eds.). (1978). *Handbook of psychotherapy and behavior change: An empirical analysis* (2nd ed.). New York: Wiley.

Gottman, J. M., & Markman, H. J. (1978). Experimental designs in psychotherapy research. In S. L.

Garfield & A. E. Bergin (Eds.), *Handbook of psychotherapy and behavior change: An empirical analysis* (2nd ed.). New York: Wiley.

Hoffman, N. G., & Overall, P. B. (1978). Factor structure of the SCL-90 in a psychiatric population. *Journal of Consulting and Clinical Psychology, 46,* 1187–1191.

Jones, W. P., & Newman, F. L. (1971). Bayesian techniques for test selection. *Education and Psychological Measurement, 31,* 851–856.

Kaplan, R. M., Bush, J. W., and Berry, C. C. (1976, Winter). Health status: Types of validity and the index of well-being. *Health Services Research, 11,* 486–488.

Kiesler, D. (1978). Experimental design in psychotherapy research. In S. L. Garfield & A. E. Bergin (Eds.), *Handbook of psychotherapy and behavior change: An empirical analysis* (2nd ed.). New York: Wiley.

Larsen, D. L., Attkisson, C. C., Hargreaves, W. A., & Nguyen, T. D. (1979). Assessment of client/patient satisfaction in human service programs: Development of a general scale. *Evaluation and Program Planning, 2,* 197–207.

Luborsky, L. (1962). Clinician judgments of mental health: A proposed scale. *Archives of General Psychiatry, 7,* 407–412.

Mager, R. F., & Pipe, P. (1970). *Analyzing performance problems.* Belmont, CA: Fearon.

Mintz, J., Luborsky, L., & Christoph, P. (1979). Measuring the outcomes of psychotherapy: Findings of the Penn Psychotherapy Project. *Journal of Consulting and Clinical Psychology, 47,* 319–334.

Murdick, R. G., & Ross, J. E. (1975). *Information systems for modern management* (2nd ed.). Englewood Cliffs, NJ: Prentice-Hall.

Myers, J. L. (1979). *Fundamentals of experimental design* (3rd ed.). Boston, MA: Allyn and Bacon.

Nelson, S. M., Newman, F. L., & Hinkle, K. (1975). Purchase of service and client management: Program organization, operations and development. In R. Agranoff & A. Dykstra, Jr. (Eds.), *Mental health administration in transition.* Lansing, MI: Association of Mental Health Administrators.

Newman, F. L. (1980). Global scales: Uses and problems in program evaluation. *Evaluation and Program Planning, 3,* 257–268.

Newman, F. L., Burwell, B. A., & Underhill, W. E. (1978). Program analysis using the client oriented cost outcome system. *Evaluation and Program Planning, 1,* 19–30.

Newman, F. L., & Carter, D. E. (1975). *A strategy for studying clinical judgment and therapeutic outcome in community mental health settings.* Paper presented at the annual meeting of the Society for Psychotherapy Research, Boston, MA.

Newman, F. L., & Rinkus, A. J. (1978). Level of functioning, clinical judgment, and mental health service evaluation. *Evaluation and the Health Professions, 4,* 175–194.

Nunnally, J. C. (1975). The study of change in evaluation research: Principles concerning measurement, experimental design and analysis. In E. I. Struening & M. Guttentag (Eds.), *Handbook of evaluation research* (Vol. 1, pp. 101–138). Beverly Hills, CA: Sage.

Overall, J. E., & Groham, D. R. (1962). Brief psychiatric rating scale. *Psychological Reports, 10,* 799–812.

Riecken, H. W., & Boruch, R. F. (Eds.). (1974). *Social experimentation: A method for planning and evaluating social intervention.* New York: Academic.

Ross, D. C. (1977). Testing pattern hypotheses in multi-way contingency tables using weighted Kappa and weighted Chi Square. *Educational and Psychological Measurement, 37,* 291–307.

Ross, D. C. (in press). A test for differential response patterns in 2-treatment studies. *Educational and Psychological Measurement.*

Ross, D. C., & Klein, D. F. (1979). A comparison of analysis of covariance and the (−) technique as applied to illustrative psychopharmacological data. *Journal of Psychiatric Research, 15,* 67–75.

Schlaifer, R. (1961). *Introduction to statistics for business decisions.* New York: McGraw-Hill.

Selby, P. N. (1976). *Interpreting graphs and tables.* New York: Wiley.

Siegert, F. A., & Yates, B. T. (1980). Behavioral child-management cost-effectiveness: A comparison of individual in-office, individual in-home, and group delivery systems. *Evaluation and the Health Professions, 3,* 123–152.

Snedecor, G. W., & Cochran, W. G. (1967). *Statistical methods* (6th ed.). Ames: Iowa State University.

Sorensen, J. E., & Elpers, J. R. (1978). Developing information systems for human service organizations. In C. C. Attkisson, W. A. Hargreaves, & J. E. Sorensen (Eds.), *Evaluation of human service programs*. New York: Academic.

Sorensen, J. E., & Hanbery, G. W. (1978). *Changing the financing, distribution and accountability of mental health services in Arkansas*. Little Rock: State of Arkansas, Division of Mental Health Services.

Sorensen, J. E., & Hanbery, G. W. (1979). *Using financial management in mental health organizations*. Rockville, MD: National Institute of Mental Health.

Sorensen, J. E., & Phipps, D. W. (1975). *Cost-finding and rate-setting for community mental health centers* (DHEW Publication No. ADM 76-291). Washington, DC: U.S. Government Printing Office.

Spitzer, R. L., Endicott, J., Fleiss, J., & Cohen, J. (1970). The psychiatric status schedule: A technique for evaluating psychopathology and impairment in role functioning. *Archives of General Psychiatry, 23,* 41–55.

Steer, R. A., & Henry, M. G. (1978, December 8). *Relationship of level of functioning to indices of psychopathology*. Paper presented at Philadelphia Office of Mental Health and Mental Retardation Colloquium about Perspectives on Outcome Evaluation, Philadelphia, PA.

Strupp, H. H., & Hadley, S. W. (1979). Specific versus nonspecific factors in psychotherapy: A controlled study of outcome. *Archives of General Psychiatry, 35,* 1125–1136.

Strupp, H. H., Hadley, S. W., & Gomez-Schwartz, B. (1977). *Psychotherapy for better or worse: The problem of negative effects*. New York: Jason Aronson.

Touche Ross and Company. (1979). *Controlling assets and transactions*. New York: Touche Ross.

Waskow, I. E., & Parloff, M. B. (Eds.). (1975). *Psychotherapy change measures* (DHEW Publication No. ADM 74-120). Rockville, MD: National Institute of Mental Health.

Weinstein, A. S. (1975). Evaluation through medical records and related information systems. In E. L. Struening & M. Guttentag (Eds.), *Handbook of evaluative research* (Vol. 1). Beverly Hills, CA: Sage.

Winer, B. J. (1971). *Statistical principles in experimental design*. New York: McGraw-Hill.

Yates, B. T. (1980). *Improving effectiveness and reducing costs in mental health*. Springfield, IL: Charles Thomas.

Yates, B. T., Haven, W. G., & Thoresen, C. E. (1979). Cost-effectiveness at Learning House: How much change for how much money? In J. S. Stumphauzer (Ed.), *Progress in behavior therapy with delinquents*. Springfield, IL: Thomas.

Yates, B. T., & Newman, F. L. (1980a). Approaches to cost-effectiveness and cost-benefit analysis of psychotherapy. In G. VandenBos (Ed.), *Psychotherapy: From practice to research to policy*. Beverly Hills, CA: Sage.

Yates, B. T., & Newman, F. L. (1980b). Findings of cost-effectiveness and cost-benefit analyses of psychotherapy. In G. VandenBos (Ed.), *Psychotherapy: From practice to research to policy*. Beverly Hills, CA: Sage.

Author Index

Subject Index